Md. Torequl Islam, PhD

Methods for Laboratory Studies

Focusing Area: Natural Product Drug Discovery

nova
science publishers
www.novapublishers.com

Library of Congress Cataloging-in-Publication Data

ISBN: 979-8-89113-266-5

Published by Nova Science Publishers, Inc. † New York

Contents

Preface

Non-clinical and pre-clinical studies in drug discovery and development, especially in the area of pharmaceutical science, are one of the most popular strategies worldwide. The need for this type of research depends on the therapeutic application goal of the new drug. Non-clinical studies should follow Good Laboratory Practice (GLP) regulations while using different protocols, especially when conducting studies with experimental animals. On the other hand, early pre-clinical studies (exploratory and confirmatory) ensure the ability to make a Go/No-Go decision. In this approach, a new drug candidate should pass through a number of steps that essentially determine pharmacokinetics (e.g., absorption, distribution, metabolism, and elimination) as well as its safety profile, including toxicogenetics (e.g., toxicity, cytotoxicity, genotoxicity, and mutagenicity). Generally speaking, these exploratory investigations are exempt from GLP requirements. The purpose of these studies is to examine drug safety and gather preliminary data on how well it is tolerated across various systems in order to influence future decisions. However, other studies, such as those on repeated dosage toxicity, genotoxicity, and safety pharmacology, should be carried out in accordance with GLP criteria and are essential for the safe exposure of humans. These non-clinical and pre-clinical studies must be completed before submitting an Investigational New Drug (IND) application. Considering the non-observed adverse effect level from general toxicity studies, the package of non-clinical and pre-clinical research should therefore include all the data required for the safe transposition of pharmaceuticals from animals to people. Following IND approval, additional GLP tests are conducted during the clinical phase of development to assess the potential for carcinogenicity, genotoxicity, chronic toxicity, and reproductive and developmental toxicity. The textbook *"**Methods for Laboratory Studies**"* summarizes non-clinical and pre-clinical laboratory steps necessary for drug discovery arenas. It aims to provide easy and lucrative guidelines for undergraduate, graduate, and post-graduate students, teachers, and researchers who are working in the same or relevant fields of drug discovery.

About the Author

M. T. Islam (Md. Torequl Islam or Muhammad Torequl Islam) obtained his B. Pharm. (Hons.), M. Pharm. (Master's), and Doctorate in Biotechnology from Khulna University (Bangladesh), Southern University Bangladesh (Bangladesh), and Federal University of Piaui (Brazil), respectively. He also worked as a postdoctoral researcher at the latter institution. He has authored many hundreds of scientific articles, books (e.g., Religious books, Textbooks, eBooks), book chapters, abstracts, conferences and seminars in national and international newspapers. He has an extended research network worldwide. At present, he is working as an Associate Professor at the Department of Pharmacy, Bangabandhu Sheikh Mujibur Rahman Science and Technology University, Gopalganj (Bangladesh). He is a visiting faculty member at NGCEF (Australia). He also worked as a part-time researcher at TDTU (Vietnam) from 2018 to 2020. He has been enlisted as one of the top 2% of potential researchers in the world since 2022 by Stanford University (U.S.A.) and Elsevier.

Chapter 1

Natural Product Drug Discovery

1.1. Brief History

Humans have been using products from their natural origins and the derivatives of natural substances for many purposes, including therapeutic usages, since the beginning of the human era. However, it is very unfortunate that in the past decade, medicinal scientists have declined research into natural products due to some important burning issues, such as the lack of compatibility of the traditional substances with the natural-product chemical libraries with high-throughput screening (HTS). The history of natural products says that, among the other natural substances, medicinal plants play a pivotal role in most cultures worldwide. Research on natural products started in the 19th century (Mishra et al. 2008). It is due to the technological advances that started then. Plants have become popular with humans for their new application, which is the medical use of plants. The analgesic and sedative agent morphine was purified from opium in 1804 by Sertürner. It was an evolutionary discovery from the medicinal plant. This discovery and success stimulated others to seek “active principles” from medicinal plants. Then quinine was isolated from the cinchona bark and cocaine from coca and many other plants. Finally, the structures of cocaine, quinine, and morphine were determined in 1898, 1908, and 1923, respectively. In a laboratory, morphine was first synthesized in 1956. However, the biological activities of natural products remain the most productive hypothesis among medicinal scientists (Mayr and Fuerst, 2008).

The discovery of the antibiotic penicillin by Fleming in 1929 was a revolution in modern therapeutics. It helped to develop a number of bioassay techniques to culture and identify microbes and isolate and elucidate many antibiotics. In fact, it initiated the modern concept of microbiology and its application in modern medical and pharmaceutical science. However, the era of drug resistance in clinically important infections has limited the use of many natural antibiotics. Their discovery and development started after the Second World War. Pharma companies showed less interest in cancer therapeutic discovery and development during this era and into the 1970s. However, upon understanding the importance of cancer therapeutics, the US

National Cancer Institute took supportive action to extend an academic network for examining plant-based potential anti-cancer agents from 1960 onward. This program discovered some potential anticancer drugs, including taxol and camptothecin analogs. Unfortunately, these drugs reached the market after the early 1990s. There was a difficulty in obtaining commercial quantities of taxol, while camptothecin showed poor solubility and, consequently, a difficulty in clinical outcomes. Finally, after reaching the market, taxol became a blockbuster anticancer drug and is still known for its biological activities, including anticancer effects. To date, many derivatives of this pioneer drug have been introduced (Harvey and Cree, 2010; Mazzio et al. 2014).

1.2. Natural Products

A *natural product* refers to anything that is produced by life, including biotic materials (e.g., wood, silk), bio-based materials (e.g., bioplastics, cornstarch), bodily fluids (e.g., milk, plant exudates), and living organism derivatives (e.g., soil, coal). These are the organic compounds that are synthesized by living organisms. In the science of organic chemistry, *synthetic organic chemistry* deals with the creation of organic molecules in the laboratory, while *semi-synthetic organic chemistry* deals with the modification of existing natural products to improve or alter their activities (Newman and Cragg, 2016).

Natural product chemistry has established close interactions with many other branches, including molecular and cellular biology, medicine, biotechnology, synthetic and analytical chemistry, biochemistry, pharmacognosy, and pharmacology. Pharmacognosy-guided tools are helpful for the identification, selection, and processing of natural products for intended medicinal uses. A compound that has some form of biological activity is called an "*active principle,*" and it can act as a *lead compound* (not relevant to compounds containing the element lead (Pb)). Most often, several compounds may show some degree of biological activity. If these compounds have common chemical features, it is possible to develop one or more *pharmacophores* (molecular features that are necessary for the recognition of a ligand by a biological macromolecule at a molecular level). In this case, as a medicinal chemist, you will be able to make attempts to use *structure-activity relationships* (an approach designed to find relationships between chemical structure (structural-related properties) and biological activity (target property) of a studied compound) to improve certain features of the lead compound. *Drug design* is another important method for drug discovery. In this case, medicinal scientists study the biological and physical properties of the target. Finally, a prediction is made of the sorts of chemicals that might fit into an *active site* (Wolfender et al. 2006; Golebiowski et al. 2021).

Each natural product has a biological history. Natural products have enormous structural and chemical diversity. It has been demonstrated that about 50% of all prescribed drugs are derived from or synthesized from natural products. Animals, marine life, plants, and microorganisms are considered potential sources. However, the value of a natural product in the treatment and prevention of diseases is dependent on some criteria: (i) the rate of administration of it into a host, including its application as a template for semi-synthetic and total synthetic modification; (ii) its application to the number of diseases to be treated or prevented; and (iii) the frequency of use.

Natural products are of two types: (i) primary metabolites and (ii) secondary metabolites. A *primary metabolite* is an organic molecule having an intrinsic function essential for the survival of the organism producing it, such as nucleic acids, amino acids, sugars, and fatty acids that are required to make the major essential macromolecules of the organism: DNA, RNA, proteins, carbohydrates, and lipids, respectively (Chinou, 2008). The ultimate fates of biomolecules in living systems have been shown in Figure 1.1.

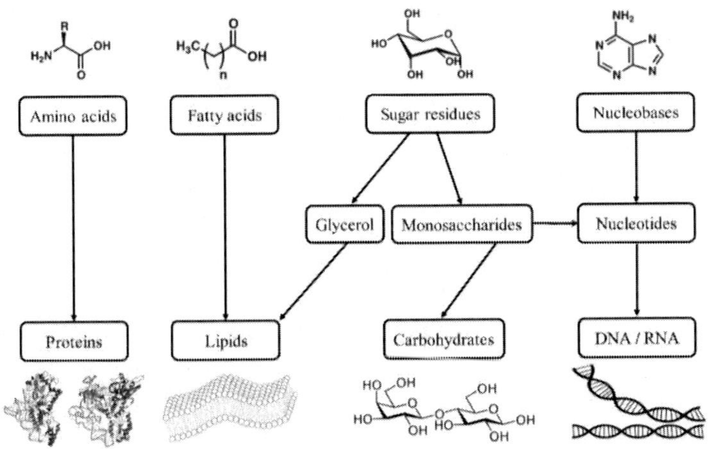

Figure 1.1. Biomolecules and their ultimate fate in living systems

A *secondary metabolite* is an organic molecule with an extrinsic function that mainly affects other organisms outside of the host. These are not mandatory for the host's survival, but these types of metabolites increase the competitiveness of the organism within its surrounding environment (Thirumurugan et al. 2018). Examples of some secondary metabolites and their building blocks have been given in Table 1.1.

Table 1.1. Building blocks of some secondary metabolites

Compound type	Building block	Example
Alkaloids	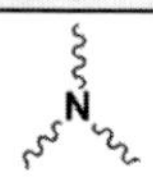 Nitrogen	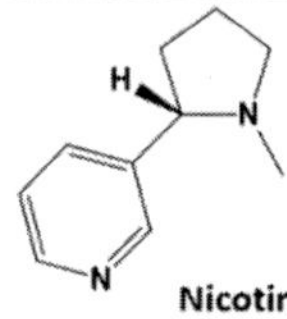 Nicotine
Phenylpropanoids	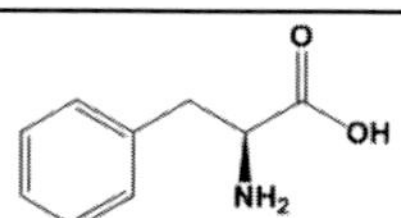 Phenylalanine	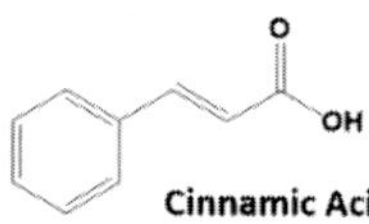 Cinnamic Acid
Polyketides	Acetate 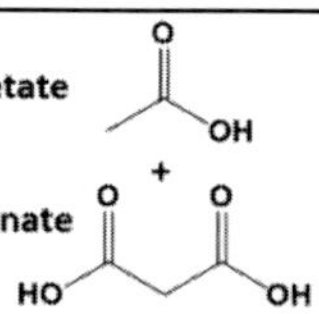 Malonate	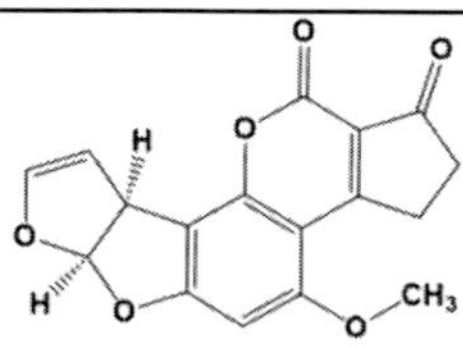 Aflatoxin B1
Terpenoids	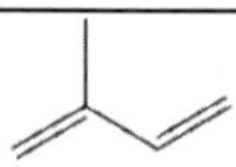 Isoprene	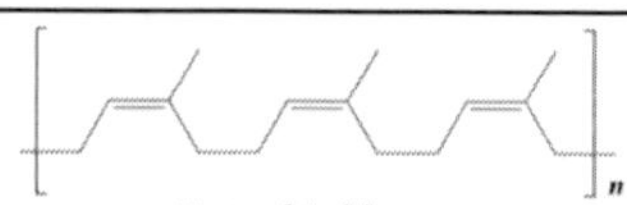 Natural Rubber

1.3. Role of Traditional Practices in Drug Discovery

Traditional medicine systems based on medicinal plants have been documented since around 2600 BCE. These systems documented the use of approximately 1,000 plant-derived substances in Mesopotamia. Traditional evidence is the basis of technical practices. The traditional basis was used to develop the concept of drugs for the treatment of diseases and disorders. The World Health Organization (WHO) estimates that approximately 75% of the world's population predominately relies on traditional medicine for their primary health care. Among them, plant-based derivatives are most prominently used, especially in fragile healthcare countries (Mukherjee et al. 2007).

Malaria remains one of the greatest health challenges worldwide. The search for better drugs for these infectious diseases is a continuous process. The *Cinchona* bark has long been used by indigenous groups in the Amazon region for the treatment of fevers and was first introduced into Europe in the early 1600s for the treatment of malaria (Gachelin et al. 2017).

Quinine was isolated from the bark of *C. officinalis* and reported in 1820 by the French pharmacists Caventou and Pelletier. Quinine was the basis for the synthesis of the commonly used antimalarial drugs chloroquine and mefloquine, which largely replaced quinine in the mid-20th century. However, the growing resistance towards these drugs has led to people searching for remedies in Traditional Chinese Medicine (TCM), such as *Artemisia annua* (Quinhaosu). At present, artemisinin analogues are used as antimalarial agents in many countries (Cheng, 2000).

Other potential drugs developed from traditional medicinal plants include: the antihypertensive agent, reserpine, isolated from *Rauwolfia serpentina* used in Ayurvedic medicine for the treatment of snakebite and other ailments; ephedrine, from *Ephedra sinica* (Ma Huang), a plant long used in TCM and the basis for the synthesis of the anti-asthma agents (beta agonists), salbutamol and salmetrol; and the muscle relaxant, tubocurarine, isolated from *Chondrodendron* and *Curarea* species used by indigenous groups in the Amazon as the basis for the arrow poison, curare; vinca alkaloids, vinblastine and vincristine, isolated from the Madagascar periwinkle, *Catharanthus roseus; taxanes from* various *Taxus* species; and so on (Pole and Sebastian, 2006).

1.4. Traditional Practice versus Technical Research

Table 1.2. Difference between traditional and technical research

Parameters	Traditional practice	Technical research
What?	Practice on the basis of traditionally passed knowledge.	Research activities are driven by a need, and are frequently used to validate traditional knowledge.
Who?	The practitioners are most often illiterate. Villagers or people from remote areas are generally familiar with natural products or religious terms.	These types of studies are conducted by highly experienced and educated people such as educationalists (e.g., teachers, researchers).
Where?	In a situation where the variables can or cannot be controlled.	In research institutes, universities, and so on.
How?	Religious or experienced viewpoints are applied to manage diseases. Major attention is given to reducing or stopping the bad impacts of diseases.	To assess a cause and effect relationship. Use less controlled procedures to understand the effects of some educational interventions. Changes can be made during the study.
Why?	To meet the needs of the general public or the poor. These are helpful to supply initial knowledge and to develop testable educational theories.	To obtain knowledge that can be applied directly to education and advanced research. To implement the observations by applying laws and regulations.

1.5. Why Pharma Companies Have Less Interest in Natural Products?

It is due to the following reasons:

1. *Time-consuming process*: It is well known that the discovery and development of medicaments from natural resources is a slow process. In general, a new drug candidate can see the light of day on the market several decades after its initial research experience. Most often, it is unable to fulfill the aim of HTS.
2. *Limited study scopes*: The number of natural products and their species is limited on this planet. On the other hand, some species, for example, certain marine species, are not easy to access. Furthermore, the differences in biodiversity and habitats, as well as the physical and chemical characteristics of each species, are quite distinct. As a result, there are currently a limited number of facilities available for the extraction and testing of all natural products that may be potential therapeutic sources. To date, 300,000–40,000 species have been recognized as higher plant species. Since the 1960s, about 19,000 species have been screened for alkaloid content. Over the last 20 years, the National Cancer Institute of the United States has collected approximately 30,000 higher plant species, including 10% of all known species.
3. *Difficulty in synthesis process*: Once a medicinal scientist gets positive signals from a lead compound derived from a natural product, he might look for mass production and further studies aiming to establish it as a new drug candidate. However, it is really difficult to synthesize a naturally occurring product-derived lead compound in a laboratory setting. It is due to the fact that, in most cases, the structures of these compounds are complex in nature and contain many similar and dissimilar functional groups. The overall process is also time-consuming and expensive. On the other hand, for commercial production, we cannot destroy the whole species, nor is it possible to cultivate the species in many different habitats.
4. *Difficulty in resupply chain*: Due to the difficulty of mass production, it is also challenging to ensure large supplies for non-clinical and pre-clinical studies of a particular natural component. Similarly, it is always challenging to collect, handle, grow, and cultivate species in a remote tropical region. Regional variations

also affect the type, quantity, and quality of the desired compounds. For example, a marine species may require expensive conditions for its growth and maintenance. Similar challenges have been reported for the growth, culture, handling, and harvesting of microbial cultures. Pharmaceutical companies need clear, predictable, controllable, and commercially available sources.

5. *Failure or challenges of combinatorial chemistry*: Although parallel synthesis techniques play an important role in the synthesis of hundreds of new compounds, combinatorial chemistry allows only a few compounds to bind to the plastic beads. As a result, the number of reactions held during the repetitive steps is limited. Therefore, only certain types of compounds are possible to use in combinatorial chemistry. Although this technique has been developed day by day, in some cases it produces very small and low-purity compounds.

1.6. Why Do We Prefer Natural Products for New Drug Discovery?

It is due to the following reasons:

1. *Bioactive secondary metabolites*: Compounds derived from natural origins are a good source of biological activity and biochemical energy. In general, each metabolite plays important roles in its host and in other biological systems. Sometimes, a certain type of metabolite may play beneficial roles in a number of systems while being harmful to others. The effects of a particular metabolite depend on its chemical nature, concentration or dose, time of exposure, ability to interact with the host's biochemistry, the pathophysiological conditions of the receiving host, and so on. It is not only an expensive but also a time-consuming process to make a bio-metabolite under laboratory conditions. It is due to the preservation of optimal metabolic energy and the endurance of genetic cost to produce a specific small molecule, which is a truly conservative process owned by the specific host(s). Moreover, bio-metabolites are diverse in their functions. This means that each molecule may interact with several biomarkers inside the hosts and play different roles in each host.

2. *Variations in chemical structures*: Nature provides multimodal and diverse biochemicals. Even for a specific target, numerous natural compounds can be found. It has been seen that compounds with diverse chemical structures are acting on the same target. Variations in the molecular skeletons of natural products are also able to change the target molecules and their mechanisms of action.
3. *Limitations of Lipinski's rule of five*: These rules aimed to strengthen the synthesis of compounds with better biophysical properties as well as better oral drug candidates. For this, the compounds must have a molecular weight under 500 Da, hydrogen bond donors <5 and acceptors <10, and a log value P<5. However, Lipinski's rule excluded natural products. Due to these reasons, certain secondary metabolites often utilize transmembrane transporters rather than passive diffusion to enter cells.
4. *Building blocks for molecular libraries*: Natural products alone or through combinatorial synthesis are capable of supplying sufficient bioactive molecules to meet the demands of modern therapeutics. It has been demonstrated over the last few decades that the combined effects of certain natural products are preferable to their individual components. Structural modifications and some other advanced strategies, such as nanotherapeutic approaches with natural products, have been well recognized for modern therapeutic purposes. Medicinal chemists are constantly on the lookout for new and alternative therapeutics, particularly from plant kingdoms and origins.

1.7. Traditional Bioactivity-Guided Isolation Phases Associated with Problems and Solutions

Bioactivity-guided isolation is a classic approach used in natural product chemistry to identify and isolate biologically active compounds from complex mixtures, such as plant extracts or microbial cultures. The process involves a series of steps aimed at isolating the active compounds responsible for the observed biological activity. Following are the traditional bioactivity-guided isolation phases:

1. *Sample preparation*: The first step involves collecting the natural source of interest, such as plants, fungi, or marine organisms. The

samples are then dried, ground, and extracted with suitable solvents to obtain crude extracts.

2. *Biological assays*: The crude extracts are tested for their biological activity against a specific target or disease model. These assays could be, for example, antimicrobial, anticancer, anti-inflammatory, antioxidant, or any other relevant activity. The goal is to identify the crude extract showing the desired bioactivity.
3. *Fractionation*: The active crude extract is subjected to fractionation, typically using chromatographic techniques such as column chromatography, thin-layer chromatography (TLC), or high-performance liquid chromatography (HPLC). This process separates the components of the crude extract into different fractions based on their physicochemical properties.
4. *Repeated bioassays*: Each fraction obtained from the fractionation step is tested again for the desired biological activity. This step helps identify the active fraction containing the bioactive compound(s).
5. *Subfractionation*: The active fraction is further fractionated, using more specific chromatographic techniques to separate the individual compounds present.
6. *Bioassay-guided isolation*: The subfractions are once again tested for bioactivity to narrow down the active compounds further.
7. *Compound identification*: The active compounds are subjected to spectroscopic and analytical techniques, such as nuclear magnetic resonance (NMR) spectroscopy, mass spectrometry (MS), and X-ray crystallography, to determine their structures.
8. *Confirmation of bioactivity*: The isolated compounds' structures are correlated with their biological activity, confirming that the active compounds responsible for the observed bioactivity have been identified.
9. *Bioactivity optimization (optional)*: If the isolated compounds show promising biological activity, medicinal chemists might further modify them through synthesis to enhance their potency, selectivity, or other desirable properties.
10. *Biological mechanism studies (optional)*: Once the active compounds are identified and optimized, researchers might delve into understanding their mechanisms of action and potential applications in medicine or other fields.

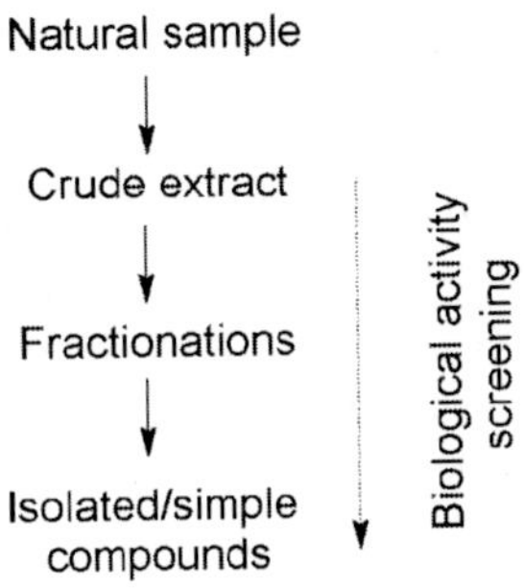

Figure 1.2. General steps of bioactivity screening of natural products

The bioactivity-guided isolation process is iterative, and several cycles may be required to purify and identify the active compounds fully. This traditional approach has been pivotal in the discovery of many natural product-derived drugs and bioactive compounds. However, with advancements in modern techniques like high-throughput screening and metabolomics, complementary or alternative approaches are often used in combination with bioactivity-guided isolation to expedite the process of natural product discovery. General steps for this purpose have been shown below (Figure 1.2).

Table 1.3 shows problems and solutions for each step of bioactivity-guided isolation process.

Table 1.3. Problems and solutions of each step

Step	Problem	Solution
Natural sample	Difficult to culture out of its indigenous environment.	New method development New models for *in situ* analysis
	Produce dissimilar natural products in different habitats	New methods for natural product synthesis Induction and stimulate for heterologous expression of biosynthetic genes
Crude extract	Presence of known natural products	New methods for dereplication
	Presence of inactive principles	Use as excipients
	Insufficient bioactive principles	New methods for extraction and pre-fractionation of extract
Isolated/simple compounds	Unknown molecular targets	New activity mechanism assay

1.8. Chemical Process for Natural Product Discovery

Natural product discovery is a multi-step chemical process aimed at isolating and identifying new and bioactive compounds from natural sources, such as plants, microbes, marine organisms, and fungi. These compounds often possess medicinal, agricultural, or industrial potential. The process generally involves the following key steps:

1. *Source selection*: Identify and collect the natural source that is likely to contain the desired bioactive compounds. This could be a plant, microorganism, marine organism, or any other organism known for its medicinal or biological properties.
2. *Extraction*: Extract the bioactive compounds from the selected natural source. This step involves grinding or crushing the material and using solvents like ethanol, methanol, or water to dissolve the compounds of interest.
3. *Fractionation*: The crude extract obtained in the previous step usually contains a mixture of various compounds. Fractionation involves separating this mixture into smaller fractions using various chromatographic techniques such as column chromatography, thin-layer chromatography (TLC), or high-performance liquid chromatography (HPLC).
4. *Bioassay-guided isolation*: Conduct bioassays to assess the biological activity of the fractions obtained in the previous step. Bioassays involve testing the fractions against specific biological targets, such as disease-causing microorganisms or cancer cell lines. The active fractions are retained for further isolation.
5. *Purification*: The active fractions obtained from the bioassays are subjected to further purification to isolate individual compounds. Various techniques, such as crystallization, precipitation, or repeated chromatography, can be employed to achieve high-purity compounds.
6. *Structural elucidation*: Identify the chemical structure of the isolated compounds using spectroscopic techniques like nuclear magnetic resonance (NMR), mass spectrometry (MS), infrared (IR) spectroscopy, and UV-Vis spectroscopy.
7. *Biological testing*: Once the structures of the compounds are known, they are subjected to comprehensive biological testing to understand their potential applications and mechanisms of action.

8. *Structure-activity relationship (SAR) studies*: By modifying the chemical structure of the isolated compounds, researchers can study the relationship between the structure and biological activity, leading to the design of more potent analogs.
9. *Scaling up and optimization*: If a compound shows promising biological activity, efforts are made to optimize its production through fermentation or synthesis.
10. *Preclinical and clinical studies*: Compounds with potential therapeutic applications undergo preclinical studies to assess their safety and efficacy in animal models. If successful, they may advance to clinical trials in humans.

The process of natural product discovery is often time-consuming and requires interdisciplinary collaboration between chemists, biologists, and pharmacologists. However, it has historically yielded valuable medicines and bioactive compounds, making it an essential area of research in drug discovery and development. General pathways have been shown below (Figure 1.3).

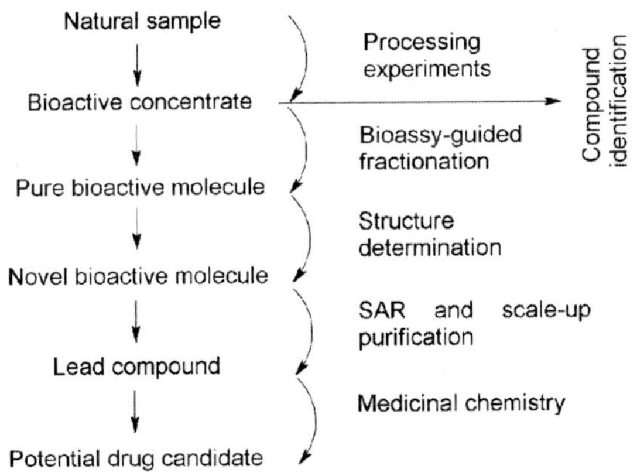

Figure 1.3. Outlines of chemical process for natural product discovery

1.9. Generic Scheme for Bioassay-Guided Fractionation

Bioassay-guided fractionation is a systematic approach used in the field of natural products chemistry and drug discovery to isolate and identify bioactive compounds from complex mixtures, such as plant extracts. This process involves a series of steps to identify the active components responsible for a specific biological activity. Here is a generic scheme for bioassay-guided fractionation of natural products:

1. *Selection of source material:* Choose a natural product source, such as plants, marine organisms, or microorganisms, based on traditional knowledge or preliminary screening results, which show promising biological activities.
2. *Preparation of extract*: Prepare the crude extract by macerating, percolating, or using other suitable methods to obtain the bioactive compounds from the source material.
3. *Biological assay:* Select a relevant and specific biological assay to evaluate the activity of the crude extract. This could be an *in vitro* assay using cultured cells or an *in vivo* assay using animal models.
4. *Partitioning/separation:* Divide the crude extract into fractions using a solvent system with increasing polarity, such as n-hexane, dichloromethane, ethyl acetate, and methanol.
5. *Biological screening:* Test the activity of each fraction using the chosen biological assay. This will help identify the most bioactive fraction(s).
6. *Repetition and convergence:* Repeat steps 4 and 5 with the most bioactive fraction(s) to further narrow down the active compounds.
7. *Column chromatography:* Apply the most active fraction to column chromatography to separate the mixture into individual compounds based on their polarity, size, and other physicochemical properties.
8. *TLC and HPLC analysis:* Analyze the fractions collected from column chromatography using Thin Layer Chromatography (TLC) and High-Performance Liquid Chromatography (HPLC) to monitor their purity and assess their composition.
9. *Structure elucidation*: Use various spectroscopic techniques like Nuclear Magnetic Resonance (NMR), Mass Spectrometry (MS), Infrared (IR), and Ultraviolet-Visible (UV-Vis) spectroscopy to determine the structure of the isolated compounds.
10. *Biological assay of pure compounds:* Test the isolated compounds individually in the biological assay to confirm their bioactivity and identify the most potent one(s).
11. *Bioactivity-guided fractionation*: If multiple bioactive compounds are identified, perform further fractionation and isolation to isolate the most active compound.

12. *Biological evaluation and validation:* Conduct additional biological evaluations to confirm the activity and potential therapeutic applications of the isolated compounds.
13. *Chemical characterization:* Confirm the chemical structure of the active compound(s) through repeated spectroscopic analyses.
14. *Structure-activity relationship (SAR) studies:* If applicable, perform SAR studies to understand the relationship between the chemical structure of the active compound and its biological activity.
15. *Mechanism of action studies:* Investigate the mechanism of action of the active compound(s) to understand how they exert their effects on the target.
16. *Lead compound identification:* Identify lead compound(s) with the desired bioactivity and potential for further development into therapeutic agents.

It is important to note that bioassay-guided fractionation is a time-consuming and resource-intensive process. However, it has been a successful strategy for the discovery of many important drugs and bioactive compounds from natural sources. General pathways have been shown below (Figure 1.4).

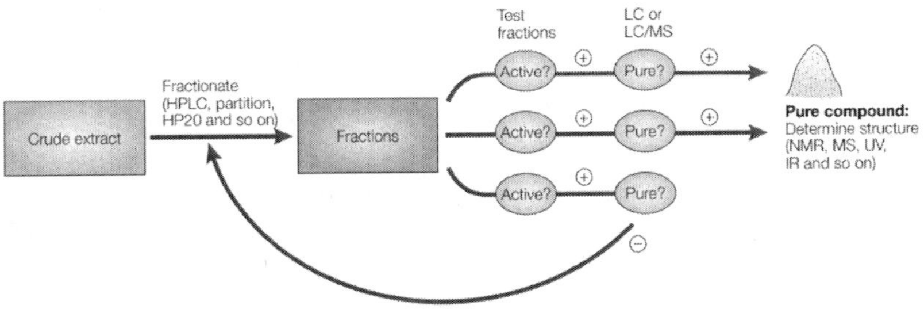

Figure 1.4. Schematic presentation of bioassay-guided fractionation

1.10. Affinity-Based Identification System for Natural Products

An affinity-based identification system for natural products is a technique used to identify and isolate specific compounds or bioactive molecules from complex mixtures of natural products. This approach relies on the use of affinity-based methods that exploit the specific interactions between the target compound and a selective binding agent. The goal is to separate and concentrate the desired natural product efficiently and selectively. The general workflow of an affinity-based identification system for natural products involves several key steps:

1. *Sample preparation:* The natural product source, which could be a plant extract, microbial culture, or other biological material, is collected and prepared for analysis.
2. *Target selection:* The specific bioactive compound or class of compounds of interest is identified for isolation and characterization. This may be based on prior knowledge of the natural product's activity or through initial screening assays.
3. *Affinity ligand design or selection:* An affinity ligand or binding agent is chosen or designed to selectively interact with the target compound. This ligand can be an antibody, a specific receptor, a molecularly imprinted polymer (MIP), or other selective binding molecules.
4. *Affinity chromatography:* The prepared natural product sample is subjected to affinity chromatography, where the chosen affinity ligand is immobilized on a solid support (e.g., a resin or a column). When the sample is passed through the column, the target compound(s) will selectively bind to the immobilized ligand, while other non-target compounds are washed away.
5. *Elution of bound target:* After the target compounds are captured on the affinity column, they can be eluted using specific conditions (e.g., changes in pH, ionic strength, or competitive binding). This step allows for the recovery of the enriched target compounds.
6. *Analytical characterization:* The eluted fraction containing the target compound(s) is analyzed using various techniques, such as mass spectrometry, nuclear magnetic resonance (NMR) spectroscopy, or other analytical methods. These techniques help in identifying the chemical structure and verifying the presence of the desired natural product(s).
7. *Biological activity testing:* Once the target compound is identified and isolated, it is subjected to biological activity testing to confirm its bioactivity and potential uses.

Affinity-based identification systems offer several advantages, including high specificity, minimal sample manipulation, and efficient isolation of target compounds from complex mixtures. They have been widely used in natural product research and drug discovery to identify new bioactive molecules with potential therapeutic applications. General pathways have been shown below (Figure 1.5).

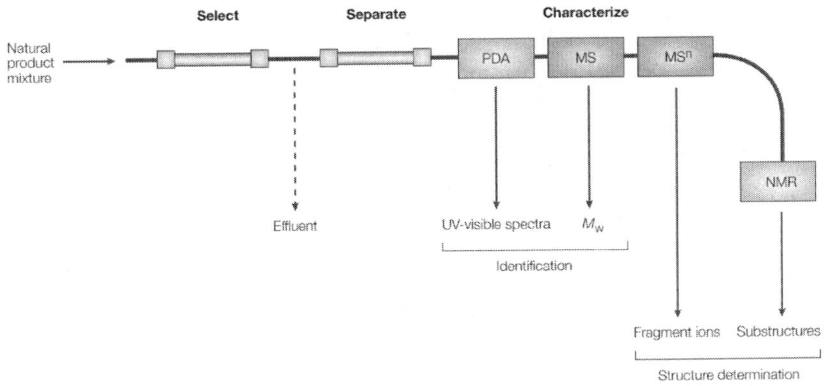

Figure 1.5. Schematic presentation of affinity-based identification system for natural products

1.11. Current Technologies for Natural-Product Lead Discovery

The discovery of drugs from natural products is a lengthy process that involves several steps, including extraction from the source, concentration from the extraction medium, fractionation and purification, and the production of a single biologically active compound. However, the overall process suffers from two common challenges: (i) Slow identification process: It is due to the slow identification of known compounds. It causes duplication of effort. However, with the application of some modern techniques, such as coupled HPLC-mass spectrometer (LC-MS) systems, this problem can be overcome. (ii) De novo structure determination of active compounds: This creates problems in coordinating the new data with the existing data. However, advances in many spectroscopic techniques (e.g., FT-IR, FT-ICER/MS), particularly in high-resolution NMR technologies, can resolve this issue. During natural product drug discovery, we can see that the lead or target compounds represent <1% by weight of the crude extract, the overall approach remains highly experimental, and the process is rate-limiting. Advances in separation technology, such as HPLC, supercritical fluid chromatography (SFC), and capillary electrophoresis (CE), have some extent rather than desirable resolving power for this problem. It is due to (***a***) the fact that you must correlate the biological signal of interest with the effector compounds and (***b***) the fact that you should then devise preparative separation methods to yield sufficient quantities of the pure material. To address these issues, a number of novel approaches have been developed to develop "on-line" bioassays that use the affinities of the desired natural ligands with the targets of interest. Hopefully, medicinal scientists are introduced to new and newer techniques and methodologies every day to get an advanced touch on natural product chemistry. For example, by using the LC-UV-SPE-NMR-MS approach, it is now possible to perform a rapid and automatic analysis of natural product extracts in which the individual components are present in 10 - 50 μg quantities.

1.12. Current Applications of Natural Products in Discovery

In the context of drug discovery and pharmaceutical research, natural products refer to chemical compounds or substances that are derived from living organisms such as plants, animals, fungi, and microorganisms. These products have evolved in nature over millions of years and often possess various biological activities. Natural products have been a valuable source of medicines and therapeutic agents throughout human history.

The discovery of natural products involves the identification, isolation, and characterization of these bioactive compounds from natural sources. This process typically includes the following steps:

1. *Collection*: Researchers collect samples from diverse natural sources, such as plants, marine organisms, soil, and microorganisms, from various geographic locations.
2. *Extraction*: The desired chemical compounds are extracted from the collected samples using suitable methods, such as solvent extraction, steam distillation, or fermentation.
3. *Isolation*: The extracted mixture is then subjected to various purification techniques, such as chromatography and crystallization, to isolate individual chemical entities with potential biological activities.
4. *Characterization*: The isolated compounds are thoroughly characterized using various analytical techniques, such as nuclear

magnetic resonance (NMR) spectroscopy, mass spectrometry, and X-ray crystallography, to determine their chemical structures.

5. *Biological screening*: The isolated natural products are then screened for their biological activities using in vitro and in vivo assays to evaluate their potential therapeutic effects, such as anti-inflammatory, antimicrobial, anticancer, or antiviral activities.
6. *Mechanism of action*: Researchers also investigate the mechanisms of action through which these natural products exert their biological effects to gain a better understanding of their pharmacological properties.

In short, natural products have been a rich source of lead compounds for drug development and have given rise to numerous pharmaceutical drugs, including antibiotics, anticancer agents, immunosuppressants, and painkillers. Additionally, they often serve as inspiration for the synthesis of novel drug candidates with improved properties and reduced side effects. However, their exploration and utilization in drug discovery require considerable effort due to factors like limited availability, complex chemical structures, and challenges in obtaining sufficient quantities from natural sources.

Current applications of natural products include:

a. *Sourcing*: Medicinal scientists are in a continuous search for new, effective, and safe therapeutic tools of natural origin. It is not restricted to the plants that grow on the land. Water covers more than 70% of the Earth. As a result, oceanic or sea areas may be one of the potential natural product resources. To date, a number of marine organisms have been identified from which many therapeutic agents have been isolated. It is because the oceans contain more than 80% of the world's plant and animal species. Therefore, marine organisms are considered a potential source of both therapeutic and cosmetic bioactive agents. In the late 1950s, Bergmann reported the first biologically active compounds of marine origin. In the 1970s, it was established that ocean derivatives are unique in genetical and biochemical aspects. To date, more than 15,000 unique natural compounds have been reported from marine sources. The classification of marine pharmacology on the basis of drug candidate sources includes (i) genetically engineered marine organisms and (ii) pharmaceuticals and nutraceuticals from marine origins.

b. *Extract libraries*: The idea of an extract library has opened a new door to drug discovery and development from natural resources. The library comprises crude extracts of plants, microbes, and animal tissues or cells. These libraries are continuously supplying screening compounds to medicinal laboratories worldwide. It is to be mentioned that many of these extracts have received FDA approval and are used for human consumption. Polyherbal preparations, super foods, and nutraceuticals are commonly known as alternative treatment approaches in the modern era. They are combined with extracts.
c. *Lead compound sourcing*: Drug discovery is a long and continuous process. Each crude extract of natural origin provides hundreds of molecules, among which many may be therapeutically active. Therefore, natural products are a great source of potential chemicals in our modern chemical library. It contains more than 100,000 compounds, and it has been shown that this library will grow over the course of the next few years. Approximately four of the ten FDA-approved drugs developed in the last four decades were derived from natural products, their derivatives, or synthetic mimetics related to natural products. More than 7,700 synthetic compounds have been identified that are similar to natural product structures.
d. *Contract research opportunities*: Drug discovery and development are complex processes. It is also expensive and time-consuming. Therefore, it is hard for a single pharmaceutical company to provide significant support to HTS discovery programs. Contact research programs might be a solution to this issue. This approach will be helpful and effective in the collection of potential natural lead substances and the conduct of screening and discovery programs to meet the basic and advanced needs of human beings. Concurrently, this approach will be able to meet the basic needs of pharmaceutical companies.
e. *Bioprospections*: To date, only a few companies or institutions have developed the unique set of skills needed to conduct bioprospecting efforts. The others are sharing products with them. This is limiting the overall success of the drug development process. Only a few companies are currently accessing and testing natural products.

Thus, the process is taking a long time and has a high price. It will not provide financial solvency for the organizations. Upon knowing this fact, a consortium approach (BioTRUST) has been founded. However, we have yet to enjoy its successes.

References

Cheng, J. T. (2000). Drug therapy in Chinese traditional medicine. *The Journal of Clinical Pharmacology*, *40*(5), 445-450.

Chinou, I. (2008). Primary and secondary metabolites and their biological activity. *Chromatographic Science Series*, *99*, 59.

Gachelin, G., Garner, P., Ferroni, E., Tröhler, U., & Chalmers, I. (2017). Evaluating Cinchona bark and quinine for treating and preventing malaria. *Journal of the Royal Society of Medicine*, *110*(1), 31-40.

Golebiowski, A., Klopfenstein, S. R., & Portlock, D. E. (2001). Lead compounds discovered from libraries. *Current Opinion in Chemical Biology*, *5*(3), 273-284.

Harvey, A. L., & Cree, I. A. (2010). High-throughput screening of natural products for cancer therapy. *Planta Medica*, *76*(11), 1080-1086.

Mayr, L. M., & Fuerst, P. (2008). The future of high-throughput screening. *SLAS Discovery*, *13*(6), 443-448.

Mazzio, E., Badisa, R., Mack, N., Deiab, S., & Soliman, K. F. A. (2014). High throughput screening of natural products for anti-mitotic effects in MDA-MB-231 human breast carcinoma cells. *Phytotherapy Research*, *28*(6), 856-867.

Mishra, K. P., Ganju, L., Sairam, M., Banerjee, P. K., & Sawhney, R. C. (2008). A review of high throughput technology for the screening of natural products. *Biomedicine & Pharmacotherapy*, *62*(2), 94-98.

Mukherjee, P. K., Rai, S., Kumar, V., Mukherjee, K., Hylands, P. J., & Hider, R. C. (2007). Plants of Indian origin in drug discovery. *Expert Opinion on Drug Discovery*, *2*(5), 633-657.

Newman, D. J., & Cragg, G. M. (2016). Natural products as sources of new drugs from 1981 to 2014. *Journal of Natural Products*, *79*(3), 629-661.

Pole, S., & Sebastian, J. (2006). *Ayurvedic medicine*. Churchill Livingstone.

Thirumurugan, D., Cholarajan, A., Raja, S. S., & Vijayakumar, R. (2018). An introductory chapter: secondary metabolites. *Secondary Metabolites-sources and Applications*, 3-21.

Wolfender, J. L., Queiroz, E. F., & Hostettmann, K. (2006). The importance of hyphenated techniques in the discovery of new lead compounds from nature. *Expert Opinion on Drug Discovery*, *1*(3), 237-260.

Chapter 2

Introduction to Non-Clinical and Pre-Clinical Studies

2.1. Non-Clinical and Pre-Clinical Studies

Non-clinical and pre-clinical studies, in general, seek to accurately model the desired biological effect(s) of a candidate molecule in laboratory animals in order to speculate on treatment outcomes in humans. Pre-clinical research is carried out before clinical testing, whereas non-clinical research refers to investigations that are not associated with, involved with, or connected with the empirical observation and treatment of living patients. This distinction must be made explicit (Pritchard et al. 2003). Therefore, both non-clinical and pre-clinical studies confirm the possibility or overall potential quality of a drug or agent entering clinical trials. This book accommodates these two types of study models cumulatively. It is because these studies share all possible beneficial and toxicological impacts associated with a drug and aim to predict its applicability (pharmacotherapy) with all possible adverse events (safety) in humans.

Currently used non-clinical and pre-clinical study models or techniques are adequately modest, as these are able to provide sufficient evidence on a drug's biological effects in laboratory microorganisms, experimental animals or their derivatives (e.g., cells, tissues, and organs), *in vitro* test systems, or even *in silico* models.

In situ (opposite: *ex situ*) is a Latin phrase meaning "on site," "in position," "on the premises," or "in place." It denotes the site where an event takes place. It can be used in many different contexts. In biological assessment, such as cell science, *in situ* stands for "intermediate between" *in vivo* and *in vitro* studies. For instance, *in situ* examination can involve analyzing a cell within an entire perfusing organ. As the donor is killed during the experiment, this would not be *in vivo*, but it would not be identical to dealing with the cell alone (a common scenario for *in vitro* experiments). *In vitro* was one of the first initiatives to qualitatively and quantitatively investigate natural events in the lab. In the end, the drawback of *in vitro* research was that it wasn't carried out in a natural setting. *In vivo* testing, which takes place inside the original creature or environment, solves this issue. *In situ* experimentation permits the regulated elements of *in vitro* research to combine with the natural ambient ingredients of *in vivo* experimentation, bridging the dichotomy of benefits that come with both approaches (Hamrell, 2010).

The inadequacies of efficacy and safety margins mean that these studies' ultimate objectives might never be fully achieved and that the clearance rate for new medication applications is still low. These studies are considered a strong foundation for the searching, identification, isolation, characterization, synthesizing, and screening of a wide variety of substances, including crude extracts of plant, microorganism, and animal origins. Many *in vitro* and *in vivo* models used for this purpose have the following merits and demerits:

2.2. *In Vitro* Versus *In Vivo* Models

An *in vitro* study refers to scientific experiments or investigations conducted outside of a living organism, typically in a controlled laboratory environment. In these studies, biological samples or cells are analyzed to observe their behavior and interactions under controlled conditions without involving a whole living organism. On the other hand, an *in vivo* study involves experiments or research conducted within a living organism. Researchers study the biological processes, effects of treatments, or interactions of substances within the context of a living system, such as animals or humans. This allows for a more realistic understanding of how various factors affect the organism as a whole. Basic differences between these two studies have been given in Table 2.1.

If their products have yet to be tested on humans, numerous pharma and biotech businesses describe themselves as being in the pre-clinical stage of research. Certain service providers, however, refer to their animal lab capacities as non-clinical in order to include research carried out after an IND submission, such as reproductive or chronic toxicity research. Because of how similar and overlapping the two research categories are, the terms are frequently used interchangeably, and either one could be used to refer to studies that enable INDs.

Table 2.1. Difference between *in vitro* and *in vivo* methods

Parameters	***In vitro* method**	***In vivo* model**
Economy and preparation	Animal cells or cell lines having a long lifespan are used for this purpose. These models are effective, easy to find, and reasonably priced. Generally, it requires no ethical concerns.	Experimental animals or human volunteers are used for this purpose. It requires ethical concerns and is expensive in nature.
Time	Relatively rapid.	It usually requires more time to reach the conclusion.
Findings	Outcomes need to be confirmed on live volunteers by applying one or more *in vivo* methods.	More specific and detailed.
Testing regulations	More relaxed.	Strict.
Implementation	Generate new therapies and research methodologies.	Generate new therapies and study plans.

2.3. Non-Clinical Study Types

1. Pharmacodynamics (PD)

- *Primary:* These *in vitro* and/or *in vivo* experiments ascertain how the treatment affects the body's response (efficacy).
- *Secondary:* These kinds of investigations ascertain how the intervention affects various bodily functions (i.e., other than the target).
- *Safety:* These kinds of investigations pinpoint adverse impacts on crucial physiological processes at therapeutic dose levels and above. These examinations assess the functions of the circulatory, pulmonary, and central nervous system (CNS).

2. Pharmacokinetics (PK)

- *ADME:* It is the study of A (absorption), D (distribution), M (metabolism), and E (excretion) in your test sample.
- *Toxicokinetics:* It examines how much of an intervention is within the body and where and when unfavorable consequences occur.

3. Toxicology

To evaluate the toxic impacts of your test sample:

- *Single-dose study:* Identify the toxic effects on target organ(s), determine the maximum tolerable dosage, determine the non-observed adverse reaction level, and set doses for the next toxicity study or first-in-human administration. These experiments are first carried out on rodents (such as mice or rats), then on larger species of animals (e.g., dogs).
- *Repeated-dose studies:* These studies aim to evaluate the chronic toxicity of your test sample. The typical time frames are as follows: I Sub-chronic: 7, 14, and 28 days, and 3 months; (ii) Chronic: 6, 9, and 12 months.
- *Genotoxic effect study:* These investigations look for possible interactions between your test sample and DNA or chromosomes that could cause gene mutations or other chromosomal harm.

- *Carcinogenicity:* The two-year rat bioassay and the 26-week transgenic mouse are two examples of this.
- *Studies on development and reproductive toxicology:* (i) Fertility (usually rat); (ii) teratology (the comparison of two formulations of the same medication in the same dosage form with a similar bioavailability; typically rat and rabbit); and (iii) peri- and post-natal toxicity (typically rat).
- *Initial human dosage calculation (clinical study):* Protection of subjects taking part in first-in-human studies depends on estimation of the initial dosage in people (Phase I trial). Although all pertinent non-clinical data should be taken into account, the no-observed-adverse-effect level (NOAEL) provides the most crucial details. Non-clinical data may be used to estimate doses for exploratory clinical research in people; the regulatory guidelines include criteria for establishing the beginning dose.

2.4. Strength of Non-Clinical Study

Non-clinical research is primarily used to identify target organ safety, which can then be used to either halt product development or monitor potential human toxicity. Nevertheless, the following non-clinical events have the potential to halt the discovery of a novel drug:

1. Identification of target organ safety; for instance, if a substance is hepatotoxic (toxic to the liver) in animals, continued research may be reexamined, albeit the predictive validity of animal experiments may be contested.
2. Investigation of weak PK characteristics, such as when a substance accumulates, causes toxicity, or doesn't reach its target. This also underlines the need for early ADME investigations, which are carried out to maximize the selection of promising product candidates.

2.5. Special Type Non-Clinical Studies

Higher animal biologics, including humans, can be used as therapeutic leads. Compared to tiny molecules, these are more complicated (e.g., large molecules, tissues, cells, and proteins). Despite sharing the same fundamentals, the non-clinical development plan for biologics must be modified on a case-by-case basis. In contrast to those for small molecules, which have been well established, the conventional planning process for biologic drugs is also starting to emerge as a result of lessons learned from past experiences and fresh regulatory guidance.

In short, non-clinical studies are carried out throughout all stages of drug discovery and development. It aims to investigate the safety level and pharmacokinetic and toxicokinetic properties of a drug candidate. Adequate precautions taken can identify the main 'knock-out' criteria of a drug candidate. Thus, it can maximize the goals of your study.

References

Hamrell, M. R. (2010). Non-clinical Assessment of New Drug Products. *Drug Development*, *5*.

Pritchard, J. F., Jurima-Romet, M., Reimer, M. L., Mortimer, E., Rolfe, B., & Cayen, M. N. (2003). Making better drugs: decision gates in non-clinical drug development. *Nature reviews Drug discovery*, *2*(7), 542-553.

Chapter 3

Collection and Extraction of Materials

3.1. Collection and Management of Plant Sample

Whole plants or their parts collected for the pre-clinical studies are mainly based on ethnobotanical information obtained from the local people, including the traditional practitioners and users (Jachak and Saklani, 2007). However, medicinal scientists can grossly collect medicinal plants or plant parts to investigate their possible biological outcomes. Literature evidence suggests that a significant amount of research is done on phytochemical and pharmacological investigations into medicinal plants in many countries around the world, including Bangladesh, India, and China. Universities, research organizations, and pharmaceutical companies mainly take care of this type of research worldwide. Nowadays, plants of marine origin have gained much attention in the drug discovery and development arena.

The investigators are concerned about the existing literature reports, promising parts or extracts, and folk evidence on the target medicinal plants to be investigated. Sources of crude drugs of plant origin include:

1. Organized drugs

- *Overground parts:* Herbs, leaves, flowers, fruits, seeds, barks, and woods
- *Underground parts:* Roots, rhizomes, bulbs, and corms

2. Unorganized drugs: Juices, lattices, extracts, alkaloids, glycosides, tannins, resins, volatile and fixed oils, fats, waxes, mucilage, and gums

While collecting a medicinal plant or its parts to be investigated, you should be concerned with the following seven facts:

- *Identification*: Proper identification prior to mass collection of a crude sample (e.g., plants or microorganisms) is essential in drug discovery and development. Identify your sample with the help of a taxonomist, then go for an extensive literature survey on the identified sample. This will help you see its current status and make a decision about your study design.

- *Time of collection*: Many plant species grow and produce optimum metabolites (primary and secondary) in certain seasons of the year. Thus, collection time directly affects the phytochemical and biological activities of a plant or its parts. Before collection, a study of the sample's morphology and physiology is a must for your research study.
- *Collection method/technique*: This is important for the rapid, economic, appropriate, and optimum collection of a sample under investigation.
- *Required parts*: It is highly appreciated to collect only your required parts (a sample) from the whole mass. Save time and resources while saving lives on Earth.
- *Adulteration*: Most often, samples of natural origin contain other (similar or dissimilar) substances. Take additional care to collect an adulteration-free sample.
- *Drying and processing*: Grossly, drying is done for the purpose of storing crude samples. Drying reduces the moisture content of your sample. Drying is also necessary to facilitate the course grinding of your sample, especially for plant samples. After drying, extraction is carried out with a suitable solvent or solvent combination. Shade drying may preserve all types of essential components in your sample. However, sun drying is evident in the loss of some components, such as light-sensitive compounds and volatile components. The leaves of aromatic plants are often dried prior to extraction. Moreover, the drying or fermentation processes of some plants may produce new compounds that are not present in their fresh contents, for example, vanilla.
- *Storage conditions*: Storage facilities (e.g., place, container, temperature, humidity) also affect crude drugs. After extraction, all crude extracts should be preserved in amber-colored containers (glass or plastic) at 4 ^{O}C or in a dark and cool place.

Besides these, be concerned about other factors, including temperature, humidity, climate conditions, and the growing environment, that also affect crude drugs' quality and quantity.

3.2. Extraction of Plant Materials

The initial stage in separating the intended natural products from raw ingredients is extraction. In chemistry, the technique for separating a material from a matrix is known as separation. It mainly aims to extract certain components present in plants. Components present in pant materials are dissolved in appropriate solvent(s) and thus separated after actions such as filtration, elution, or other means. It is a type of solid/liquid separation process in which the solid object (e.g., powdered plant materials) is made available in contact with a suitable fluid (solvent), and the components present in the solid phase are then solubilized and contained within the solvent. Thus, the type of solvent used to extract your plant material will be largely dependent upon the type or nature of components present in your plant material (Salim et al. 2008). Commonly used solvents for the extraction of crude drugs are shown in Table 3.1.

Equipment: Tools, instruments, or devices used for a specific task or purpose.

Apparatus: A set of equipment designed for a particular function or experimental setup.

Machine: A mechanical device with moving parts designed to perform tasks or work.

Method: A systematic approach or procedure used to achieve a specific goal or solve a problem.

Methodology: The overall framework or set of principles guiding a particular research or work process.

Strategy: A carefully planned and coordinated series of actions to achieve long-term goals or objectives.

Alcohols are frequently used in the extraction of natural products. It is because alcohols allow the extraction of both water-soluble and oil-soluble components. Moreover, alcohols are bactericidal solvents. Thus, these can also preserve your extract for long-term use. Research evidence suggests that methanol is the most efficient extraction solvent. You will get the highest yield value (33.2%) if you use this solvent. The maximum amounts of phenolics (13.36 mg GAE/g DW), flavonoids (1.92 mg QE/g DW), alkaloids (1.40 mg AE/g DW), and terpenoids (1.25% w/w) are obtained via methanol extraction. [**N.B.** - GAE: Gallic acid equivalent; QE: Quercetin equivalent; AE: Atropine equivalent; DW: Distilled water]

Table 3.1. Polarity of some commonly used extraction solvents

Solvent	Polarity
n-Hexane	0.009
Petroleum ether	0.117
Diethyl ether	0.117
Ethyl acetate	0.228
Chloroform	0.259
Dichloromethane	0.309
Acetone	0.355
n-Butanol	0.586
Ethanol	0.654
Methanol	0.762
Water	1.000

Ethanol, on the other hand, can be used to extract plants with great efficiency and safety. It will take a lot of oil out of the plant before it evaporates entirely. As a result, your plant produces the most output that may be used in both nutritional and commercial products. However, you should keep in mind that to extract, you need the concentration and evaporation of the solvent to be at their optimum values. For example, at 70%, the high value of ethanol doesn't evaporate too much.

Percentage **yield** = (Extraction wt (gm) ÷ Powdered material wt (gm)) ×100

A list of inorganic and organic solvents used in active compound extraction is shown in Table 3.2.

Table 3.2. Inorganic and organic solvents used in active compound extraction

Water	Ethanol	Methanol	Chloroform
Anthocyanin Saponins Tannins Terpenoids	Alkaloids Flavonoids Polyphenol Tannins Terpenoids	Anthocyanin Polyphenol Saponins Tannins Terpenoids	Flavonoids Terpenoids
Dichloromethanol	**Ether**	**Acetone**	
Terpenoids	Alkaloids Terpenoids	Flavonoids	

Table 3.3. Widely used extraction methods for natural products (Zhang et al. 2008)

Technique	Solvent	Temperature	Pressure	Time	Solvent volume	Polarity of extraction products
Maceration	Water, aqueous and non-aqueous solvents	Ambient	Normal (atmospheric)	Long	Large	Solvent-dependent
Percolation	Water, aqueous and non-aqueous solvents	Ambient, occasionally under heat	Normal (atmospheric)	Long	Large	Solvent-dependent
Maceration	Water, aqueous and non-aqueous solvents	Ambient	Normal (atmospheric)	Long	Large	Solvent-dependent
Decoction	Water	Under heat	Normal (atmospheric)	Moderate	None	Polar compounds
Refluxing	Aqueous and non-aqueous solvents	Under heat	Normal (atmospheric)	Moderate	Moderate	Solvent-dependent
Soxhleting	Aqueous and non-aqueous solvents	Under heat	Normal (atmospheric)	Long	Moderate	Solvent-dependent
Pressurized liquid	Water, aqueous and non-aqueous solvents	Under heat	High	Short	Small	Solvent-dependent
Supercritical fluid	Usually S-CO2, occasionally with modifier	Ambient	High	Short	None or small	Non- to moderately polar compounds
Untrasound assisted	Water, aqueous and non-aqueous solvents	Ambient or under heat	Atmospheric	Short	Moderate	Solvent-dependent
Microwave assisted	Water, aqueous and non-aqueous solvents	Ambient	Atmospheric	Short	None to moderate	Solvent-dependent
Pulsed-electric field	Water, aqueous and non-aqueous solvents	Ambient or under heat	Atmospheric	Short	Moderate	Solvent-dependent
Enzyme assisted	Water, aqueous and non-aqueous solvents	Ambient or heated after enzyme treatment	Atmospheric	Short	Moderate	Solvent-dependent
Hydro-distillation and steam distillation	Water	Under heat	Atmospheric	Short	None	Non-polar (e.g., essential oil)

Small-scale crude extraction methods like maceration and percolation are typically ineffective, sluggish, and time-consuming. To extract materials at a laboratory size more quickly and efficiently, these procedures are typically adjusted. Large-scale industrial batch processes require further changes to the extraction process. In general, for laboratory studies, we perform cold maceration and hot Soxhlet apparatus techniques for the extraction of plant materials. See Chapter Four: Islam (2021). Table 3.3 presents widely used extraction methods for natural products.

3.3. Fractionation of Crude Extract

In general, fractionation aims to isolate more than two components in a mixture in a single run. Different types of separation techniques are used for this purpose. The basic differences between extraction and fractionation include that your plant material (e.g., powder) will be in contact with a suitable solvent that will be able to dissolve or contain components from the plant material having similar polarities. On the other hand, fractionation includes a step-by-step extraction of components using either of the extracting solvents.

Compounds having similar physico-chemical properties in a crude extract are separated by this process. Fractionation can be done in various ways. However, each technique has one or more unique features. The type and quality of the extract and the solubility, size, shape, electrical charge, etc. properties of the chemical groups influence the fractionation process. Precipitation, solvent-solvent extraction, distillation, dialysis, chromatographic processes, and electrophoresis are common techniques used for crude fractioning or extract clean-up. The selection of a typical fractionation technique largely depends on the following: properties of the extracted compounds; immediate fate of the separated fractions; cost and accessibility of the necessary tools and materials; and safety for the overall process, people, and chemical compounds.

3.3.1. Precipitation

When a substance's solubility is exceeded by its concentration within the solution, precipitation happens. A chemical can be precipitated through a variety of techniques, each of which involves changing a solubility-influencing component. Precipitation can be used to either remove the desired chemicals or to remove the undesirable material while keeping the desired substances in solution. Examples of some precipitating techniques along with the precipitating groups are shown in Table 3.4.

Table 3.4. Examples of some precipitating techniques along with the precipitating groups

Precipitation/complexation reagent	**Type of precipitated phytochemical (groups)**	**Revising conditions**
Lead subacetate ($Pb_3(OH)_4(O_2CCH_3)_2$) solution (10%)	Flavonoids, chlorophyll, polyphenols	Aqueous alkali
Powdered hide	Polyphenols, tannins	
Gelatin solution (5%)		
Polyvinylpolypyrrolidone (PVPP)		
Ca(OH)2 (paste form)	Polyphenols, tannins, alkaloids	Excess dilute acid
Picric acid ($(O_2N)_3C_6H_2OH$)	Alkaloids	Non-polar solvent precipitates with aqueous alkali Dichloromethane for extract alkaloids
Dragendorff's reagent (potassium iodobismuthate, BiI7K4) or Mayer's reagent (potassium iodomercuarte, K2[HgI4]) or Ammonium reineckate	Alkaloids	Dissolve precipitation in acetone : methanol : water (6:2:1) and pass through anion-exchange column

3.3.2. Solvent-Solvent Extraction

- *Immiscible solvent technique*: Two layers are created by adding a liquid to an extract that has already been dissolved in a different liquid that does not mix with the first (Figure 3.1). Any mixture component will be soluble in one of the two layers (often referred to as phases), and over a period, the two layers' concentrations will balance out at this point. In a stoppered separating flask, mixing the two phases fairly vigorously reduces the time needed to reach equilibrium.
- *Cracking emulsion technique*: To separate the emulsion from the other stages, pour it into a spotless separating funnel. You can then try the following therapies:

Step 1. With your fingers or a blunt, robust rod, lightly tap the edges of the separating funnel while slowly rotating it in a vertical orientation.

Step 2. A small amount of methanol or ethanol is added, and the mixture is treated as in Step 1. Alcohol makes it easier for the two phases to separate by lowering the interfacial tension between them.

Step 3. Filtration using filter paper with silicone treatment that is available commercially but at a lower pressure. The water component cannot flow through, but the non-polar phase can.

Step 4. Filtration under decreased pressure can be done if there are any tiny particles present. The construction and use of a kieselguhr bed are typically used for filtering since the particles are frequently so minute that they would quickly obstruct the holes in standard filter paper.

- *Multiple extraction technique*: By repeatedly extracting the initial phase in question from the opposing phase, it is possible to further fractionate a chemical into only one phase. Instead of using one large amount of the whole volume, it is preferable to use multiple subsequent relatively small volume elutions. For example, a chemical, A, with a partition coefficient of K (chloroform:water) of 4:1, is present in a 100 mL aqueous extract. Either one 100-mL aliquot or four subsequent 25-mL aliquots of chloroform are used to extract the substance.

Partition coefficient $\kappa = [A]_{\text{Chloroform}} \div [A]_{\text{Water}} = 4$
Extraction with 4×25 mL aliquots
After equilibrium $[A]_{\text{Chloroform}} = x/25$
$[A]_{\text{Water}} = (100 - x)/100$
From κ above $x/25 = 4\ [(100 - x)/100]$
$100x = 4 \times 25(100 - x)$
$100x = 10000 - 100x$
$200x = 10000$
$x = 25$

i.e., from the water phase into the chloroform, 50% of A is eliminated. Therefore, 93.75% of the original is eliminated after four extractions, which is equal to 50% of the original plus 50% of 50% (25%) plus 50% of 25% (12.5%) plus 50% of 12.5% (6.25%).

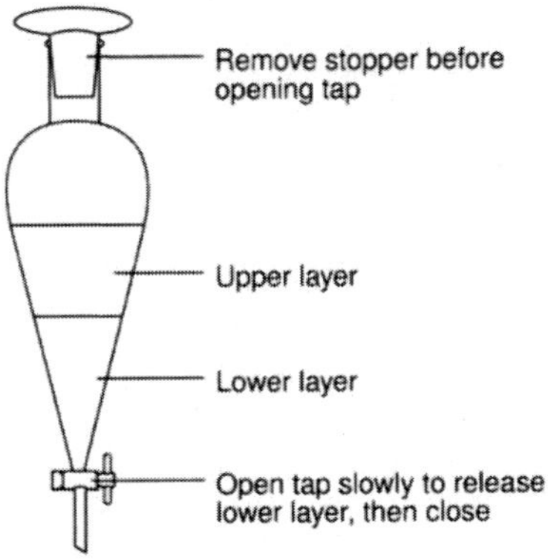

Figure 3.1. Separating funnel for solvent-solvent extraction.

3.3.2.1. Using one 100 mL aliquot for the extraction

[A] in chloroform = 4 [A] in water due to both being 100 mL = 80.0% removed into the non-polar solvent chloroform, i.e., the extraction is less efficient than using 4 × 25 mL aliquots of this solvent. Immiscible liquids with a variety of polarities can be used in consecutive liquid extraction processes. Thus, hexane, dichloromethane, ethyl acetate (or dichloromethane: ethanol 3:1), and butanol can be used in succession to extract aqueous extracts. This series' extraction solvents have progressively higher levels of polarity. In contrast, a solvent series exhibiting reducing polarity, such as water, water: ethanol 3:1/water: ethanol 2:1/water: ethanol 1:1, may be used to extract a petrol or dichloromethane extract. It is typical to combine related phases and extract one phase many times from the other. Follow the following scheme (Figure 3.2):

- *Salting out technique*: By "salting out," it is possible to improve the extraction of medium-polar chemicals from aqueous extracts by relatively immiscible solvents like butanol or methyl ethyl ketone. When a sizable quantity of an extremely soluble inorganic salt is added to the solution, the solubility of many non-ionic compounds in water is significantly reduced. If there isn't any other solvent available, the non-ionic substance may precipitate out, but if there is, it will often dissolve into another moderately polar solvent. Because it is inexpensive and generally available. Sodium chloride is frequently used for this purpose, but ammonium sulphate and other substances are also frequently utilized. Polar solvents like acetonitrile and methanol become insoluble when 1 g/mL sodium chloride is added to water, making them suitable for solvent-solvent extraction.

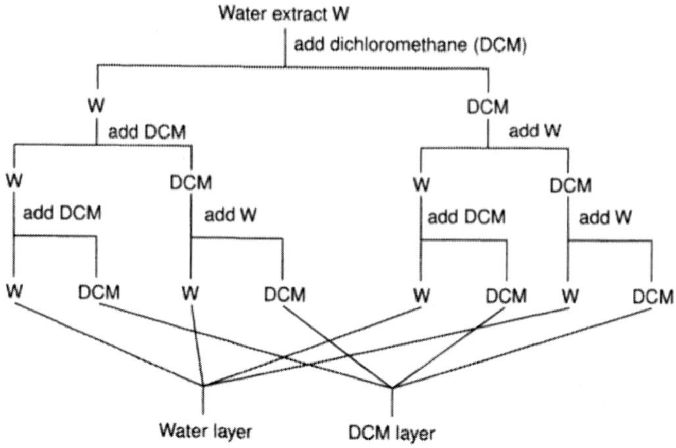

Figure 3.2. Scheme of a typical multi extraction strategy

- *pH change technique*: Acidic and basic portions can be created and recovered from extracts by taking advantage of the generally non-polar pH-dependent differences in water miscibility of acidic and basic substances. Basic substances can be separated as follows (Figure 3.3):

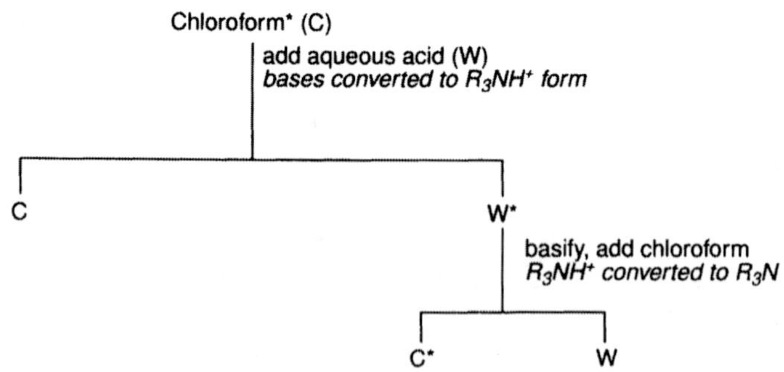

Figure 3.3. Scheme of pH change strategy

- *Solvent removal technique*: Organic extracts usually contain a small amount of another solvent, such as water. Therefore, you can take the necessary steps to remove it from your extract by adding anhydrous sodium sulphate. Upon salt addition, it can be seen to seem more crystalline when properly mixed by agitation or swirling, and the organic solvent frequently appears to be much more translucent. Since only one molecule of anhydrous sodium sulphate consumes 10 water molecules during the crystallization process, the upshot of this process is that water is added while the organic solvent is left "dry." A significant quantity of sodium sulphate is added gradually at first until no additional crystalline material appears to be forming. The solid residue is filtered off, and the remaining water is removed by using absorbent cotton (cotton wool), in which the cellulose in the cotton fibers absorbs a lot of water, or filter paper impregnated with silicone, which prevents water from passing through.

3.3.3. Distillation

Fractional distillation can help separate a mixture of volatile substances. Because this method is very useful for extracting volatile (also known as "essential") oils, it has very limited use in extract fractionation but is widely used in the petrochemical industry. The temperature differential created with a condensing column placed at the upper level of a boiling liquid is what supports fractional distillation. The most volatile substances condense far away from the boiling chamber, whereas the least volatile ones do so. The liquid condensate drawn from each of the withdrawal sites will have a different composition, as demonstrated in the following (Figure 3.4).

3.3.4. Dialysis

The basic idea behind this technique is compound separation on the basis of molecular size. Molecules having less than 1000 Da molecular mass can pass through a semipermeable membrane made of a thin polymeric substance. Larger molecules cannot, or only with great difficulty, pass through. In the prescnce of pressure or an osmotic differential, almost all of the small molecules in a mixture move through the membrane while the larger molecules are left behind. Therefore, the efficiency of this technique depends on the quality or composition of the porous materials, the pore size of the semipermeable membrane, the size and physicochemical nature of the materials to be separated, and so on.

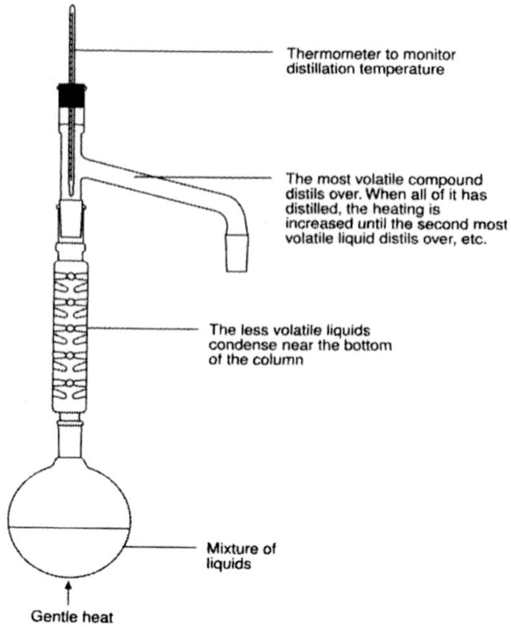

Figure 3.4. A typical distillation setup

The technique of desalting, which is frequently used in the purification of proteins and polysaccharides, involves dialysis. The big molecule-containing aqueous extract is contained by a membrane and submerged in water. An osmotic gradient causes water molecules to move one way through the membrane while low-molecular-mass compounds like salts, carbohydrates, and other things move in the opposite direction. As a result, the small molecular mass components of the big molecules kept within the membrane are removed, but the fluid becomes more diluted. If tiny molecules are the main interest, the same procedure can also be employed to eliminate compounds with large molecular masses. The aqueous phase of the membrane outside must be frequently refreshed to enable complete removal of tiny molecules, as transport throughout the membrane won't happen until the concentration on either side is equal.

3.3.5. Electrophoresis

The process of electrophoresis is used to separate a mixture of materials that are capable of carrying electrical charges. In this case, the charged species move at different rates in the presence of an electrical field depending on the size, shape, and overall electrical charge they have. For small samples of mixtures of charged molecules, especially proteins, peptides, and amino acids, electrophoresis is frequently used as an analytical method rather than a fractionation approach. It can be utilized in a manner analogous to preparative layer chromatography to separate the constituent parts of relatively simple mixtures. Analytical electrophoresis has seen a huge upsurge in attention recently due to the discovery of the technique known as capillary zone electrophoresis (CZE). Since this method may be modified to study both charged and uncharged compounds, it offers an edge over prior ones. This approach has not yet been used in preceding applications.

3.3.6. Cautions

It is crucial that volatile solvents and warm or hot aqueous media not be combined. The stopper will be blown off, and the contents of the separating funnel will be sprayed out as a result of the significant increase in vapour pressure caused by this. If an exothermic reaction occurs, such as the mixing of acids and bases or the diluting of strong acids, this could also happen with cold fluids.

Some organic phases easily combine with aqueous phases to produce emulsions, especially if there are any tiny particles or precipitate-formed particles. These emulsions are most likely to be created by the chlorinated solvents dichloromethane and chloroform. The simplest way to prevent the creation of emulsions is to either avoid using these solvents altogether or, if you must, mix the two phases extremely slowly. Emulsions frequently generate an opaque third layer at the intersection of the two clear phases when they are created. According to the adage "like dissolves like," the solubility of an uncharged material in any phase at a certain temperature depends on how similar it is to the liquid phase in terms of polarity. In this scenario, "opposites attract" because charged molecules have a strong attraction to liquids with lots of ions with the opposite charge. For example, acidic compounds will dissolve more readily in a basic than in a neutral or acidic aqueous phase. The ratio of a substance's concentrations in the two distinct phases is known as the partition coefficient, or K. Because different substances have different partition coefficients, a substance's partition coefficient in relation to the more polar phase is much larger for a moderately polar molecule than it is for a non-polar compound. Therefore, when an extract is exposed to two immiscible liquids, distinct solutes will distribute themselves in different ways. If a substance's partition coefficient is higher than 100, the majority of it will be concentrated in just one phase.

For chromatographic description see Chapter Four: Islam (2021).

3.4. Chemical Investigations in Plants

This is an important step in identifying the biologically important candidate compounds in plants, which could ultimately result in the discovery and development of new drugs. The identification of chemical groups in plant extracts leads to compound isolation, identification, and characterization in phytochemistry. Evaluation of biological effects in various test models is the ultimate objective of this purpose. Not only does this help to identify the components of plant extracts and which one dominates compared to the others, but in addition, it aids in the hunt for bioactive compounds that could be used to create valuable medications. Thus, it is crucial to find new sources of substances like alkaloids, flavonoids, phenolic compounds, saponins, steroids, tannins, and terpenoids that are both therapeutically and commercially significant. Additionally, you can investigate the presence of different metals, vitamins, and ionic content in your plant sample.

3.5. Qualitative Identification of Secondary Metabolites

Thousands of phytochemicals have been discovered in vegetables, fruits, beans, whole grains, nuts, and seeds. These chemicals are synthesized in each and every part of the plant. Such phyto-components collaborate with nutrients and fibers to create an integrated element of the body's defense mechanism against numerous illnesses and stressors. Phytochemicals are classified into two types based on their roles in plant metabolism: primary and secondary metabolites. Carbohydrates, amino acids, proteins, and so on are examples of primary (main) metabolites, whereas secondary components include alkaloids, phenolic compounds, flavonoids, tannins, glycosides, terpenoids, saponins, etc. Table 3.5 presents a list of chemical group tests for natural products.

Table 3.5. Test for chemical groups in natural products (Islam, 2021)

Test for alkaloids
Mayer's test: 1 mL extract + 2 mL freshly prepared Mayer's reagent (add side-by-side to test tube) → Dull white or creamy precipitates indicate alkaloids.
Dragendorff's test: 1-2 mL Dragendorff's reagent + 1 mL extract → Yellow or orange red precipitates indicate alkaloids.
Hager's test: 2-3 drops Hager's reagent (saturated aqueous solution of picric acid) + 1 mL extract → Yellow precipitates indicate alkaloids.
Wagner's test: 1 mL extract + 2 mL Wagner's reagent (add side-by-side of the test tube) → Reddish brown precipitates indicate alkaloids.
Tannic acid test: 2-3 drops tannic acid (10%) + 1 mL extract → Buff colour indicates alkaloids.
Ammonia Reineckate test: Extract solution + slightly acidified (with HCl saturated solution of ammonia reineckate) → Pink flocculent precipitate indicates alkaloids.
Vitali-Morin test: Extract treated with fuming nitric acid (HNO_3) → Evaporate to dryness + Add methanolic potassium hydroxide (KOH) solution → Violet colour indicates tropane alkaloids.
Silver nitrate test: Silver nitrate (AgNO3) solution + extract solution → Yellowish white precipitate (insoluble in HNO_3, but soluble in dilute ammonia (NH3)) → Hyoscine derivatives.
UV test: Ergot (indole alkaloid) under UV light → Red-colour fluorescence.
Dissolve your extract in CHCl3 and sodium carbonate (Na_2CO_3) → Separate CHCl3 layer + p-dimethylaminobenzaldehyde (0.1 g), H_2SO_4 (35%, v/v, 100 mL) + 5% ferric chloride ($FeCl_3$) (1.5 mL) → Deep blue colour confirms ergot.
Strychnine test: Extract + ammonium vanadate and H2SO4 → Purple color indicates strychnine.
Potassium dichromate test: Extract + potassium dichromate ($K_2Cr_2O_7$) + conc. H_2SO_4 → Violet colour gives strychnine.
Brucine test: Extract + conc. HNO_3 → Yellow to orange color indicates brucine.
Pilocarpine test: Extract + dil. H_2SO_4 + hydrogen peroxide (H2O2) solution + benzene and potassium chromate (K_2CrO4) solution → Shake → Bluish-violet colour (organic layer) and yellow colour (aqueous layer).
Thalleioquin test: Extract + one drop dil. H_2SO_4 + 1 mL distilled water + bromine water drop wise → Permanent yellow colour + 1 mL dil. NH3 solution → Emerald green colour indicates quinine alkaloids.
Sulphuric acid – UV test: Extract + H_2SO_4 → under ultraviolet (UV) light → Blue fluorescence indicates methoxy group of quinine and quinidine alkaloids.
Emitine test: Extract (0.5 g) + HCl (20 mL) + water (5 mL) → Filter + (2 mL) potassium chloride (KCl) (0.01 M) → Yellow colour develops (on standing for 1 h) → Gradually changes to red indicates emitine.
Aqueous extract + $FeCl_3$ solution + HCl → Deep reddish purple colour indicates meconic acid.
Extract + conc. H_2SO_4 + formaldehyde (HCO) → Dark violet colour indicates morphine.
Extract + HCl + potassium chlorate ($KClO_3$) crystals → Heat to dryness + dil. NH3 → Purple colour (caffeine) and murexide colour (purine alkaloids).
Extract + tannic acid (C76H52O46) solution → White precipitate indicates caffeine.
Amino alkaloid test: Extract (10 mg) in water (1 mL) + dil. HCl (0.2 mL) + copper sulphate ($CuSO_4$) (0.1 mL) + sodium hydroxide (NaOH) solution (2 mL) → Liquid turns violet + ether (2 mL) → Shake vigorously → Ethereal layer (purple) and aqueous layer (blue).
Colchicine test: Extract + H_2SO_4 (70%) or conc. HCl → Yellow colour indicates colchicine alkaloids.

Table 3.5. (Continued)

Test for glycosides
Keller-killiani test (test for deoxy sugars): 0.5 gm extract + 5 mL distilled water + 2 mL glacial acetic acid + one drop FeCl3 solution + 1 mL conc. H_2SO_4 → Brown ring at the interface (deoxysugar characteristic of cardenolides) or violet ring below the brown ring and greenish ring in the acetic acid layer (just above the brown ring and gradually spread throughout this layer).
Modified Borntragers test: 2-3 mL dil. HCl + 1 mL extract + a few drops $FeCl_3$ solution → Boil, cool and filter the extract with benzene + treat chloroform layer with 1 mL NH3 → Red colour in the ammoniacal layer indicates anthraquinone glycosides.
Borntragers test: 2-3 mL dil. H_2SO_4 + 1 mL extract → Boil, cool and filter with 3 mL $CHCl_3$ → Separate chloroform layer + 1 mL NH3 (10%) solution → Pink colour (glycosides) and red colour in the ammoniacal layer (anthraquinone glycosides).
Legal test: 50 mg extract + pyridine + sodium nitroprusside ($C_5FeN_6Na_2O$) solution + 10% NaOH → Pink color indicates glycosides.
Baljet test: 1 mL extract + 1 mL sodium picrate ($C_6H_2N_3NaO_7$) solution → Yellow to orange colour indicates aglycones or glycosides (cardiac glycosides).
Mineral acid test: Extract + strong mineral acid → Lemon yellow to dirty greenish brown colour indicates glycosides.
Boil 1 g extract with 10 mL water for 1 minute and strain → 1-2 drops of this solution + 2 mL NaOH solution → No rose colour indicates glycosides.
Haemolysis test: 1 drop blood + 2-3 drops aq. Extract → RBC's rupture indicates saponin glycosides.
Foam test: 1 gm extract → 10–20 mL distilled water → Shake few minutes → Foam formation persists for 1-2 min indicates saponin glycosides.
Libermann burchard test: Alcoholic extract → Evaporate to dryness and extract with $CHCl_3$ → 1-2 drops acetic anhydride ($C_4H_6O_3$) + conc. H_2SO_4 (side wall manner) → Violet to blue colour ring at the junction of two liquids indicates steroid glycosides.
Salkowaski test: Alcoholic extract → Evaporate to dryness and extract with $CHCl_3$ + conc. H_2SO_4 (sidewall-wise of the test tube) → Yellow colour ring at the junction of two liquids → Turns red after 2 min indicates steroid glycosides.
Zimmermann test: Meta dinitrobenzene solution + Alcoholic solution of your extract (containing alkali) → Heat → Violet colour indicates keto steroid glycosides.
Antimony trichloride test: Alcoholic extract → Evaporate to dryness and extract with $CHCl_3$ + Saturated solution of antimony trichloride (SbCl3) to $CHCl_3$ containing 20% C4H_6O_3 → Heat → Pink colour indicates steroids and triterpenoid glycosides.
Trichloro acetic acid test: Extract + saturated solution of trichloro acetic acid ($C_2HCl_3O_2$) → Coloured precipitates indicate triterpenoid glycosides.
Tetranitro methane test: Extract + tetranitro methane → Yellow colour indicates unsaturated steroids and triterpenoids glycosides.
Borntrager's test: 1 gm extract + 5–10 mL dil. HCl → Boil in a water bath for 10 min → Filter and cool → Extract with carbon tetrachloride (CCl4)/benzene + equal amount of NH3 solution → Shake → Pink or red colour in the ammoniacal layer indicates anthraquinone glycosides.
Modified borntrager's test: 1 gm extract + 5 mL dil. HCl + 5 mL $FeCl_3$ (5% w/v) → Boil 10 min, cool and filter → Extract with CCl4/benzene + an equal volume of NH3 solution → Pink to red colour indicates anthraquinone moiety (C-type anthraquinone glycosides).

Alcoholic extract + an equal volume of water + 0.5 mL strong lead acetate ($Pb(C_2H_3O_2)_2$) solution → Shake and filter → Extract with an equal volume of CHCl3 → CHCl3 extract evaporate to dryness → Dissolve the residue in 3 mL of glacial acetic acid + a few drops of $FeCl_3$ solution → Transfer the solution to a test tube containing 2 mL conc. H_2SO_4 → Reddish brown layer (turns bluish green after standing) indicates digitoxose (cardiac glycosides).
Alcoholic extract + an equal volume of water + 0.5 mL of strong ($Pb(C_2H_3O_2)_2$) solution → Shake and filter → Extract with an equal volume of $CHCl_3$ → CHC_{13} extract evaporate to dryness → Dissolve the residue in 2 mL pyridine (C_5H_5N) + 2 mL $C_5FeN_6Na_2O$ + NaOH solution → Pink colour indicates glycosides or aglycon moiety (cardiac glycosides).
3,5-dinitro benzoic acid test: Alcoholic solution + a few drops of NaOH + 2% solution of 3,5-dinitro benzoic acid ($C_7H_4O_6N_2$) → Pink colour indicates cardiac glycosides.
$FeCl_3$ test: Concentrated alcoholic extract + a few drops alcoholic $FeCl_3$ solution → Deep green colour + conc. HNO_3 → Yellow indicates coumarin glycosides.
Fluorescence test: Alcoholic extract + 1 N NaOH solution (one mL each). → The Blue-green fluorescence indicates coumarin glycosides.
Sodium picrate test: Powdered extract + moisten with water + few drops conc. H2SO4 → Impregnate filter paper with sodium picrate ($C_6H_2N_3NaO_7$) solution + $NaCO_3$ solution → Brick red colour indicates volatile hydrogen cyanide (HCN) in the presence of cynophoric glycosides.
Ammonia test: Dip filter paper + alcoholic solution of extract + expose to NH3 vapor → Yellow spots on filter paper indicates flavonoid glycosides.
Shinoda test: Alcoholic extract + magnesium (Mg) turning → dil. HCl → Red colour indicates flavonoids.
Alcoholic extract + zinc (Zn) turning + dil. HCl → Deep red to magenta colour indicates dihydro flavonoid glycosides.
Vanillin HCl test: Vanillin HCl + alcoholic solution → Pink colour indicates flavonoid glycosides.
Borax test: 10 mL extract solution + 0.5 gm borax ($Na_2[B_4O_5(OH)_4]\cdot 8H_2O$) → heat → Green colour fluorescence indicates aloe-emodin anthranol.
Modified anthraquinone test: 0.1 gm extract + 5 mL FeCl3 (5%) solution + 5 mL dil. HCl → Heat in a water bath for 5–6 min and cool + benzene or $CHCl_3$ → Shake → Separate organic solvent layer → equal volume dil. NH3 → Pinkish red colour indicates anthraquinone.
Bromine test: 5 mL extract solution + equal volume bromine solution → Bulky yellow precipitate indicates tetrabromaloin.
Flavone glycoside test: Extract + 80% H_2SO_4 → Orange yellow colour indicates chalcone glycoside isoliquiritin.
Dip a strip of white filter paper in 10% aqueous solution of picric acid ($C_6H_3N_3O_7$) → Drain and dip in 10% $NaCO_3$ solution → Drain again + Water → Trap the $C_6H_2N_3NaO_7$ paper on the neck of the flask with cork → Brick red colour indicates volatile HCN (cyanogenic glycosides).
Extract + 3% aqueous solution of mercurous nitrate ($Hg_2(NO_3)_2$) → Reduction to metallic mercury (Hg) indicates cyanogenic glycosides.
Test for phenols/lignins
Ferric chloride test: 2 mL extract + few drops of 5% $FeCl_3$ solution → Blue green colour indicates phenolic compounds.
Lead acetates test: 50 mg extract + distilled water + 3 mL 10% lead acetate ($Pb(C_2H_3O_2)_2$) solution → Bulky white precipitates indicate phenolic compounds.
Gelatin test: 50 mg extract + 5 mL distilled water + 2 mL 1% solution of gelatin containing 10% sodium chloride (NaCl) → White precipitates indicate phenolic compounds.
Potassium dichromate test: Extract + $K_2Cr_2O_7$ solution → Precipitation confirms tannins and phenolics.

Table 3.5. (Continued)

Alkaline reagent test: Extract + NaOH solution → Yellow to red precipitates indicate phenolic compounds.
Phloroglucinol-HCl test: Alcoholic extract + few drops of phloroglucinol ($C_6H_6O_3$) + conc. HCl → Red color indicates lignins.
Test for flavonoids
Alkaline reagent test: Extract + few drops NaOH solution → Intense yellow color + dil HCl → Colorless solution indicates falvonoids.
Shinoda (Magnesium hydrochloride reduction) test: 0.2 g (4 mL) extract + 2 mL 50% methanol (CH3OH) → Heat + a chip of Mg metal + few drops conc. HCl → Red or orange colour indicates flavonoids (occasionally, green to blue color also appears after a few minutes).
Ethyl acetate- Ammonia test: Powdered sample + 10 mL ethyl acetate → Heat in a water bath for 3 min → Filter → 4 mL of filtrate + 1 mL dil. NH3 → Shake → Yellow colour indicates flavonoids.
Pew's test: 5 mL aqueous extract + 0.1 g Zn + 8 mL conc. H_2SO_4 → Red colour indicates flavonols.
Test for tannins
Ferric chloride test: 0.5 g extract + 10 mL distilled water → Boil and filter + few drops of 0.1% FeCl3 → Brownish green or blue-black colour → Blue color (gallic tannins) and green black (catecholic tannins).
Lead acetate test: Extract + 1 mL $Pb(C_2H_3O_2)_2$ solution → White precipitate indicates tannins.
Potassium dichromate test: Extract + $K_2Cr_2O_7$ solution → Precipitate confirms tannins and phenolics.
Phenazone test: 5 mL aqueous extract solution + 0.5 g sodium acid phosphate (NaH2PO4) → Heat, cool and filter + 2% phenazone ($C_{11}H_{12}N_2O$) solution → Bulky coloured precipitates indicate all tannins.
Gelatin test: 1% gelatine solution + little 10% NaCl solution → 1% extract solution → Precipitation of gelatin indicates tannins.
Test for catechin (Matchstick test): Dip a matchstick in the dilute extract → Dry, moisten with conc. HCl, and warm it near a flame → Wood pink or red colour indicates catechin.
Extract + vanillin (C_8H8O_3) + HCl → pink or red colour indicates catechin.
Lime water ($Ca(OH)_2$) + aqueous crude extract → Brown colour, which turns to red precipitate on standing indicates tannins.
Dil. Extract solution + ferric ammonium sulphate ($NH_4Fe(SO_4)_2$) → Green colour + NaOH → Purple colour indicates tannins.
Extract + ferrous sulphate (FeSO4) → Green color. Extract + alkali (e.g., KOH) → Violet colour.
Extract + minerals → Precipitation indicates tannins.
Chlorogenic acid test: Dil. extract solution + aq. NH3 → Exposed to air → Green colour indicates chlorogenic acid.
Vanillin-hydrochloric acid test: Extract + vanillin: alcohol: dil. HCl in the ratio of 1:10:10 → Pink or red colour indicates tannins.
Test for saponins
Frothing test: 0.5 g extract + 5 ml distilled water → Shake vigorously → Stable and persistent froth + 3 drops of olive oil → Re-shake vigorously → Emulsion formation.
Sodium bicarbonate test: Few mg extract + few drops sodium bicarbonate ($NaHCO_3$) → Shake well → Honey comb like frothing indicates saponins.

Test for terpenoids
Salkowski's test: 0.5 g extract + 2 mL $CHCl_3$ + 3 mL conc. H2SO4 → Reddish brown ring between the interfaces indicates terpenoids.
Liebermann - Burchard's test: 4 mg extract + 0.5 mL $C_4H_6O_3$ + 0.5 mL $CHCl_3$ + conc. H_2SO_4 → Red violet (terpenoids) and green bluish (steroids).
Hesse's reaction: Extract + $CHCl_3$ (4 mL) + equal quantity conc. H_2SO_4 → Pink colour ring → Shake diffuse in both layers indicates sterols.
Test for steroids/triterpenoids
Libermann- Buchard test: Extract + few drops $C_4H_6O_3$ → Boil and cool + conc. H_2SO_4 → Brown ring at the junction of two layers → Upper layer turns green (steroids) and deep red colour (triterpenoids).
Salkowski test: Extract + $CHCl_3$ + few drops conc. H_2SO_4 → Shake well and allow → wait for a few minutes → Red color in the lower layer (steroids) and yellow colour in the lower layer (triterpenoids).
Acetic anhydride-H_2SO_4 test: Extract + 2 mL $C_4H_6O_3$ + 2 mL conc. H_2SO_4 → Violet to blue or green indicates steroids.
Libermann sterol test: Extract + glacial acetic acid + one drop conc. H_2SO_4 → Rose, red, violet, blue and green colours indicate steroids.
Test for sugar/carbohydrates (Dissolve 100 mg of extract in 5 mL of distilled water and filter through Whatman No.1 filter paper. Subject the filtrate to the following tests.)
Molish's test: 2 mL filtrate + 2 drops alcoholic 1-naphthol (20% in ethyl alcohol) solution → Shake properly + 1 mL conc. H_2SO_4 → Allow to stand → Reddish violet ring indicates carbohydrates.
Fehling's test: 1 mL extract (filtrate) + 1 mL each of Fehling solutions A and B → Boil in a water bath → Brick red precipitate indicates sugars.
Barfoed's test: 1 mL extract (filtrate) + 1 mL Barfoed's reagent → Heat in a boiling water bath for 2 minutes → Red precipitate indicates sugars.
Benedict's test: 0.5 mL extract (filtrate) + 0.5 mL Benedict's reagent → Heat in a boiling water bath for 2 minutes → Characteristic colour precipitates indicate sugars. (Reddish brown precipitates → Reducing sugars. Filtrate + strong H_2SO_4 → Camnelization carbohydrates).
Iodine test: 1 mL extract + 3 drops iodine solution → Blue colour indicates starch.
Osazone test: Extract + phenylhydrazine hydrochloride + sodium acetate + acetic acid → Heat → Yellow crystals indicates carbohydrates.
Selivanoff's test (resorcinol test for ketones): A resorcinol crystal + extract + equal volume conc. HCl → Warm in a water bath → Rose colour indicates ketones like fructose, honey or hydrolysed inulin.
Test of pentose sugar: Extract + equal volume HCl (containing a little phloroglucinol) → Heat → Red colour indicates pentoses.
Keller-Kiliani test: Extract + acetic acid + trace amount $FeCl_3$ + conc. H_2SO_4 → Reddish-brown colour at the junction of two liquids indicates deoxysugar (in cardiac glycosides) → Gradually becomes blue.
Furfural test: Extract + a drop of syrupy phosphoric acid (H_3PO_4) → Heat. Filter paper moistened with a drop of 10% solution of aniline in 10% acetic acid → Place over the mouth of this tube → Heat (30-60 sec) the bottom of the test tube → Pink or red colour appears on the reagent paper indicates carbohydrates.
Hemicellulose test: Extract + iodine and H_2SO_4 → Blue colour indicates hemicellulose.

Table 3.5. (Continued)

Test for amino acids/proteins (Dissolve 100 mg of extract in 10 mL of distilled water and filter through whatman No.1 filter paper. Submit the filtrate to tests for proteins and amino acids.)
Millon's test: 2 mL extract filtrate + few drops Millon's reagent (approx. 2 mL) → White precipitate indicates proteins.
Biuret test: Aliquot (2 mL) filtrate (extract) + 1 drop (2%) $CuSO_4$ solution + 1 mL ethanol (95%) + excess KOH pellets → Pink colour in the ethanolic layer indicates proteins. (Dipeptide does not give this test).
Ninhydrin test: 2 drops ninhydrin solution (10 mg of ninhydrin in 200 mL of acetone) + 2 mL aqueous filtrate (extract) → Purple color indicates amino acids.
Gelatine test: Extract + gelatin (1 g) + soda lime → Heat produces a smell of NH3. Extract + $C_6H_3N_3O_7$ + gelatin → Yellow precipitate. Extract + gelatin (0.5 g) in water (10 mL) + tannic acid (10%) → White buff-colour precipitates.
Xanthoproteic test: 1 mL extract + 1 mL conc. nitric acid (HNO_3) → White precipitate → Boil and cool + 20% NaOH or NH3 → Orange colour indicates aromatic amino acid.
Test for fats and fixed oils
Spot test: Extract → Between two filter papers → Press → Oil stains indicate fixed oils.
Saponification test: 1 mL extract + few drops (0.5 N) alcoholic KOH + 1 drop phenolphthalein ($C_{20}H_{14}O_4$) → Heat in a water bath for 2 hrs → Neutralize with soap indicates fixed oils.
Bandouin's test: Extract (2 mL) → Shake with conc. HCl (1 mL) containing 1% sucrose → Pink color indicates sesamol.
Villavecchia test: Extract (2 mL) → Shake with conc. HCl (1 mL) containing 1% furfural → Pink color indicates sesamolin or free sesamol.
Test for volatile oils
A thin section of the sample + alcoholic solution of Sudan III → Pink color indicates volatile oils.
A thin section of the sample + tincture of alkane → Red colour indicates volatile oils.
Test for resins
Extract + water → Trituration → Milky emulsion indicates resins.
Extract (approx. 0.5 g) + HCl (5 mL) → Boil for a while → Filter and take filtrate + NH3 → Blue fluorescence indicates resins.
Extract + FeCl3 in alcoholic solution → Green colour indicates resins.
Extract on TLC → Spray phosphomolybdic acid (H_3PMo12O40) → Nerolidol.
Extract (0.1 g) + acetic acid (10 mL) + 1 drop conc. H_2SO_4 → Purple colour changes to violet colour indicates resins.
Alcoholic extract + conc. solution copper acetate ($Cu(CH_3COO)_2$) → Brown precipitate or green colour without precipitate indicates podophyllum resin.
Test for other groups
Extract (5 g) + 10% aqueous potassium permanganate ($KMnO_4$) solution → Heat → Bitter almond-like odour indicates cinnamic acid (carboxylic acid).
Alcoholic extract solution + $FeCl_3$ solution → Green colour indicates phenolic compound coniferyl benzoate.
Extract (1 drop) solution + $CHCl_3$ (1 mL) + H_2SO_4 (1 drop) → Violet colour changing to purple or brown indicates vitamin A.
Extract (1 mL) + $CHCl_3$ (10 mL) + few drops of saturated solution of antimony trichloride in $CHCl_3$ → Blue colour indicates vitamin A.

0.5 g extract + $CHCl_3$ + 1 mL acetic anhydride + 2 drops H_2SO_4 → Deep green colour indicates cholesterol.	
Extract + diphenyl carbazone → Purple colour indicates barbiturates.	
Extract + bromothymol blue Extract + Light-green colour indicates lipids.	
Extract + 2, 4 – di-nitro phenyl hydrazine → Yellow-red colour indicates aldehydes and ketones.	

3.6. Example of Isolation and Identification of Compounds in a Crude Extract

The dried and powdered flowers of plant X are extracted for 48 hours at room temperature using a mixture of 7:3 methanol and water. After filtration and reduced-pressure evaporation of the organic solvent (methanol), the appropriate aqueous extract is produced. The equivalent extracts are produced by progressively extracting the resulting aqueous extract with dichloromethane, ethyl acetate, and n-butanol. Figure 3.5 shows a typical fractionation scheme.

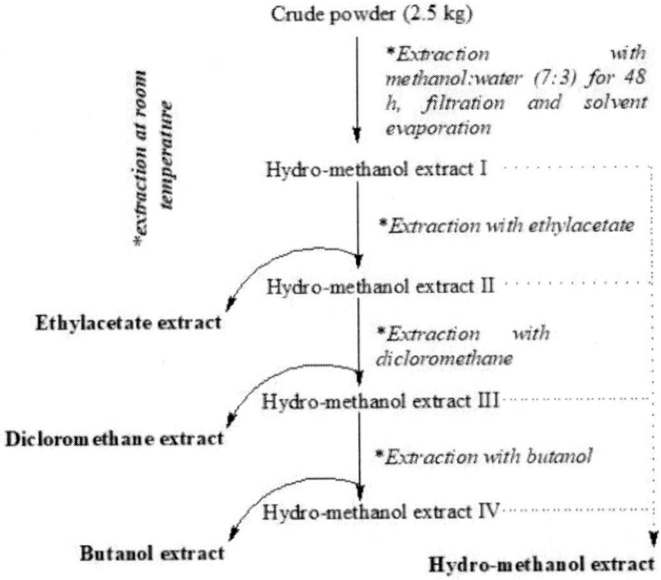

Figure 3.5. A typical fractionation scheme

Only ethyl acetate (25 g) is further processed using silica gel column chromatography, which elutes with dichloromethane/methanol gradients from each crude extract. There are six major fractions (250 mL × 6). By employing column chromatography over silica gel with dichloromethane/ methanol (9:1) as the eluent, fraction 5 (19 g) is purified to provide isosalipurposide 1 (18 g) and quercetin 2 (50 mg).

Use the methanol/HCl concentrated system at reflux for two hours to perform hydrolysis. The result is the compound Y. A Bio-Rad spectrophotometer with a resolution of 4 cm^{-1} and a wavelength range of 400 to 4 000 cm^{-1} is then used to create FT-IR spectra.

On a Bruker AC-300, deuterated CD3OD ^{1}H-NMR and ^{13}C-NMR spectra are obtained at 300 and 75 MHz, respectively. The values (mg/L) for all chemical changes are presented. For a thorough assignment of the proton and carbon signals in the NMR spectra, double resonance, COSY, and HMBC studies are conducted. Whenever possible, mass spectra are collected using an automass multi-thermo-finingam ES-MS spectrometer. On SDS silica gel 60 F254 (70-200 m), column chromatography is carried out with a dichloromethane and methanol mixture as the eluent (Ghribia et al. 2014).

3.7. Drugs from Animal Origins

The bloodletting technique used by leeches (*Hirudo medicinalis*) is an ancient treatment strategy. Later, it was discovered that leeches' saliva contains lepirudin, which is known to prevent blood coagulation in animals. Following the example of another anticoagulant compound, *hirudin* was developed. It also acts as a thrombin inhibitor. In Mayan culture, ants were crushed and used as toothaches. Moreover, ant bites were used for joint pain. Nowadays, a number of animal-origin biochemicals are used as pharmacotherapeutic agents, such as *heparin, insulin*, and *pituitary hormones.* These examples are some stimulants for the discovery and development of new drug candidates from animal origins.

Insulin, discovered in 1920, is widely used in diabetes (Type 2: IDDM). Porcine or bovine pancreas are used to prepare commercially available insulin. On the other hand, *heparin* was extracted from the dog's liver. Now it is used to treat a number of coronary and cardiovascular diseases. In contrast, *protamine sulfate* was isolated from salmon sperm following production by genetic engineering (recombinant DNA technology). In the 1970s, *captopril* was isolated from a Brazilian snake (*Bothrops jararaca*), which was the first ACE inhibitor. Similarly, *eptifibatide* was isolated from a dwarf rattlesnake (*Sistrurus miliarius barbouri*). It is a platelet glycoprotein receptor IIb/IIIa inhibitor and is used in thrombosis. Another important animal-based drug is thyroid (porcine thyroid glands), which is one of the best-known drugs for hypothyroidism. Besides these, we have many important excipients that are frequently used in pharmaceutical manufacturing, such as *gelatin* (porcine or bovine origin), which is used for the production of capsules. Table 3.6 presents a list of animal-origin drugs.

Table 3.6. Animal drug pipeline from natural sources

Drug	Therapeutic use
Porcine drugs	
Enoxaparin	Anticoagulant, Antithrombotic
Pancrelipase	Digestive supplements and cholelitholytics
Pancrelipase	Digestive supplements and cholelitholytics
Poractant alfa	Respiratory agent
Dalteparin	Anticoagulant
Normal immunoglobulin (Human)	Immunoglobulin
Heparin sodium	Anticoagulant
Heparin sodium	Anticoagulant
Heparin sodium	Anticoagulant
Rabies immune globulin (human)	Rabies immune globulin (human)
Measles, mumps and rubella virus vaccine live	Vaccine
Susoctocog alfa	Haemostatic agent
Danaparoid	Haemostatic agent
Amylase, Lipase, Pancrelipase, Protease	Digestive supplement
Human prothrombin complex	Haemostatic agent
Measles, Mumps, Rubella and Varicella Virus Vaccine Live	Vaccine
Human rotavirus live attenuated vaccine	Vaccine
Rotavirus vaccine live oral pentavalent	Vaccine
Live varicella vaccine.	Vaccine
Zoster virus vaccine live	Vaccine
Bovine drugs	
Aprotinin (synthetic), factor XIII, fibrinogen, thrombin and calcium chloride dihydrate	Surgical antiseptics and applications
Lactobacillus acidophilus, Bovine colostrum	Digestive supplements
Lactobacillus acidophilus, Bovine colostrum	Digestive supplements
Gelatin succinylated	Plasma volume expander
Polygeline	Plasma volume expander
Inactivated Japanese encephalitis vaccine	Vaccine
Methylprednisolone sodium succinate	Adrenal steroid hormones
Measles, mumps and rubella virus vaccine live	Vaccine
Eptacog alfa(activated)	Haemostatic agents
Beractant	Pulmonary surfactant
Thyrotropin alfa	Diagnostic Agents

Table 3.6. (Continued)

Drug	Therapeutic use
Aprotinin - Factor XIII - Fibrinogen, Calcium chloride dihydrate - Thrombin	Haemostatic agent
Bovine colostrum	Anti-diarrhoeal
Varicella zoster vaccine, live	Vaccines
Hepatitis A vaccine; Salmonella typhi vaccine	Vaccines
Drugs from Chinese hamster ovary	
Tocilizumab	Immunomodifiers
Brentuximab vedotin	Antineoplastic
Octocog alfa	Haemostatic agent
Rurioctocog alfa pegol	Haemostatic agent
Fremanezumab	Antimigraine preparations
Laronidase	Enzyme replacement therapy
Darbepoietin	Haemopoietic agent
Bevacizumab	Antineoplastic
Interferon beta-1a	Immunomodifier
Avelumab	Antineoplastic
Follitropin alfa (rch)	Pituitary hormone
Nonacog alfa	Haemostatic agent
Inotuzumab ozogamicin (rch)	Antineoplastic
Blinatumomab (rch)	Antineoplastic
Etanercept.	Antirheumatoid agents
Cerliponase alfa	Endocrine and metabolic agents
Mycophenolate mofetil	Immunomodifiers
Imiglucerase	Enzyme replacement therapy
Secukinumab (rch)	Immunomodifier
Daratumumab	Antineoplastic
Dupilumab (rch)	Immunomodifier
Corifollitropin alfa	Pituitary hormones
Galcanezumab	Antimigraine
Etanercept	Immunomodifier
Vedolizumab	Immunomodifier
Epoietin-alfa	Haemopoietic agent
Aflibercept	Ophthalmic medication
Agalsidase beta	Enzyme replacement therapy
Benralizumab	Immunomodifier
Follitropin alfa	Pituitary hormone
Lenograstim	Supportive therapy
Emicizumab	Haemostatic agent
Trastuzumab	Antineoplastic agent
Normal immunoglobulin (human) with vorhyaluronidase alfa	Immunoglobulin
Tildrakizumab (rch)	Immunomodifier
Trastuzumab emtansine.	Antineoplastic agent

Drug	Therapeutic use
Trastuzumab	Antineoplastic agent
Pembrolizumab (rch)	Antineoplastic agent
Octocog alfa	Haemostatic agent
Alemtuzumab (rch)	Immunomodifier
Lutropin alfa	Pituitary hormone
Alemtuzumab	Antineoplastic agent
Rituximab	Antineoplastic agent
Tenecteplase	Fibrinolytic agent
Methoxy polyethylene glycol- epoetin beta	Haemopoietic agent
Mycophenolate	Immunomodifiers
Alglucosidase alfa	Endocrine and metabolic agents
Galsulfase (rch)	Endocrine and metabolic agent
Epoietin beta	Haemopoietic agent
Epoetin lambda	Haemopoietic agent
Eptacog alfa	Haemostatic agent
Mepolizumab	Respiratory agent
Susoctocog alfa	Haemostatic agent
Trastuzumab.	Antineoplastic agent
Trastuzumab	Antineoplastic agent
Nivolumab	Antineoplastic agent
Abatacept	Immunomodifier
Choriogonadotropin alfa	Pituitary hormone
Follitropin alfa (rch)/lutropin alfa (rch)	Pituitary hormone
Pertuzumab	Antineoplastic agent
Alirocumab (rch)	Hypolipidaemic agent
Denosumab	Affects calcium and bone metabolism
Dornase alfa	Respiratory agent
Follitropin beta	Pituitary hormone
Interferon beta-1a	Immunomodifier
Recombinate antihaemophilic factor	Haemostatic agent
Follitropin delta	Pituitary hormone
Evolocumab	Hypolipidaemic agent
Recombinant Coagulation Factor IX (rFIX), Nonacog gamma (rch)	Haemostatic agent
Asfotase alfa rch	Endocrine and metabolic agent
Siltuximab (rmc)	Antineoplastic agent
Thyrotrophin alfa	Diagnostic agent
Trastuzumab	Antineoplastic agents
Panitumumab	Antineoplastic agents
Elosulfase alfa (rch)	Endocrine and metabolic agent
Denosumab	Antineoplastic agent
Omalizumab	Respiratory agent
Moroctocog alfa	Haemostatic agent
Ipilimumab	Antineoplastic agent
Bezlotoxumab	Antibiotics and anti- infective
Murine drugs	
Octocog alfa	Haemostatic agent
Rurioctocog alfa pegol	Haemostatic agent

Table 3.6. (Continued)

Drug	Therapeutic use
Ofatumumab	Antineoplastic agent
Bevacizumab	Antineoplastic agent
Protein C	Anticoagulant, antithrombotic
Ramucirumab	Antineoplastic agent
Elotuzumab	Antineoplastic agent
Cetuximab	Antineoplastic agent
Obinutuzumab	Antineoplastic agent
Trastuzumab	Antineoplastic agent
Infliximab	Immunomodifier
Trastuzumab	Antineoplastic agent
Octocog alfa	Haemostatic agent
Tisagenlecleucel	Antineoplastic agent
Alemtuzumab	Immunomodifier
Ranibizumab	Ophthalmic medication
Alemtuzumab	Immunomodifier
Rituximab	Antineoplastic agent
Eptacog alfa	Haemostatic agent
Trastuzumab	Antineoplastic agent
Trastuzumab	Antineoplastic agent
Idarucizumab	Detoxifying agent, antidote
Octocog alfa	Haemostatic agent
Infliximab	Immunomodifier
Infliximab	Immunomodifier
Rituximab	Antineoplastic agent
Somatropin	Pituitary hormone
Golimumab	Antirheumatoid agent
Basiliximab	Immunomodifier
Eculizumab	Immunomodifier
Siltuximab	Antineoplastic agent
Palivizumab	Immunomodifier
Trastuzumab	Antineoplastic agent
Natalizumab	Immunomodifier
Omalizumab	Respiratory agent
Axicabtagene ciloleucel	Antineoplastic agent
Equine	
Equine Antithymocyte globulin	Immunomodifier
Black snake antivenom	Antivenom
Brown snake antivenom	Antivenom
Death adder antivenom	Antivenom
Conjugated estrogens/bazedoxifene.	Gonadal hormone
Brown snake antivenom, Death adder antivenom, King brown snake antivenom, Taipan antivenom, Tiger snake antivenom	Antivenom
Oestrogens, Conjugated	Gonadal hormone
Red back spider antivenom	Antivenom

Drug	Therapeutic use
Sea snake antivenom	Antivenom
Stonefish antivenom	Antivenom
Human fibrinogen and human thrombin	Surgical Preparation
Taipan antivenom	Antivenom
Tiger snake antivenom	Antivenom
Drugs from egg/chicken	
Quadrivalent influenza vaccine	Vaccine
Influenza virus vaccine	Vaccine
Clevidipine	Antihypertensive agent
Olive oil and soya oil	Parenteral vitamins, minerals and nutrition
Propofol	Anaesthetics
Influenza virus vaccine	Vaccine
Influenza virus vaccine	Vaccine
Quadrivalent influenza vaccine	Vaccine
Quadrivalent Influenza Vaccine	Vaccine
Trivalent influenza vaccine	Vaccine
Propofol	Anaesthetics
Influenza virus vaccine	Vaccine
Soya oil	Parenteral vitamins, minerals and nutrition
Sebelipase alfa	Endocrine and metabolic agent
Measles, mumps and rubella virus vaccine l	Vaccine
Measles, mumps and rubella virus vaccine	Vaccine
Measles, mumps, rubella and varicella vaccine	Vaccine
Propofol	Anaesthetics
Coxiella burnetii vaccine	Vaccine
Rabies vaccine	Vaccine
Risperidone	Antipsychotic agent
Yellow Fever Vaccine	Vaccine
Influenza virus vaccine	Vaccine
Verteporfin	Ophthalmic medication
Drugs from other animals	
House dust mite extract	Antiallergy preparation
Box Jellyfish Antivenom	Antivenom
Chondroitin	Complementary osteoarthritis
Digoxin binding antibody Digoxin-specific antibody fragment	Antidote
Inactivated influenza vaccine	Vaccine
SARS-CoV-2 or its derivatives	Vaccine
Funnel web spider antivenom (rabbit)	Antivenom
Glucosamine	Complementary osteoarthritis
Phleum pratense.	Antiallergy preparation
Insulin	Insulin preparation
Adalimumab	Immunomodifier
Eptacog alfa	Haemostatic agent
Eicosapentaenoic acid (EPA) ethyl ester, docosahexaenoic acid (DHA) ethyl ester.	Cardiovascular agent
Antithymocyte globulin (rabbit)	Immunomodifier

Table 3.6. (Continued)

Drug	Therapeutic use
Bovine-Indirect	
Pertussis vaccine, Diphtheria toxoid, Tetanus toxoid, Poliomyelitis vaccine	Vaccine
Acellular pertussis, diphtheria, tetanus and poliovirus type 1, 2 and 3	Vaccines
Hepatitis A vaccine	Vaccine
Diphtheria toxoid, Tetanus toxoid, Pertussis vaccine	Vaccine
Diphtheria toxoid, Tetanus toxoid, Pertussis vaccine, Poliomyelitis vaccine	Vaccine
Hepatitis B vaccine	Vaccine
Hepatitis A vaccine	Vaccine
Hepatitis A vaccine	Vaccine
Diphtheria, tetanus, pertussis, hepatitis B, poliomyelitis and Haemophilus influenzae type b conjugate vaccine	Vaccine
Haemophilus B conjugate vaccine	Vaccine
Diphtheria, tetanus, acellular pertussis (DTPa) vaccine	Vaccine
Diphtheria, tetanus, acellular pertussis (DTPa) and inactivated poliovirus vaccine	Vaccine
Generic name	Therapeutic class
Poliovirus (inactivated)	Vaccine
Rabies vaccine	Vaccine
Measles, mumps and rubella virus vaccine live	Vaccine
Meningococcal group C polysaccharide conjugate vaccine	Vaccines
Pneumococcal purified capsular polysaccharides	Vaccine
Measles, mumps & rubella vaccine	Vaccines
Varicella zoster vaccine, Rubella vaccine, Mumps vaccine, Measles vaccine	Vaccines
Measles, Mumps, Rubella and Varicella (Oka/Merck) Virus Vaccine Live	Vaccines
Pertussis vaccine acellular, diphtheria and tetanus toxoids (adsorbed), inactivated poliovirus types 1, 2 and 3	Vaccines
Rabies vaccine	Vaccines
Human Rotavirus (live attenuated oral vaccine)	Vaccines
Generic name	Therapeutic class
Rotavirus vaccine	Vaccines
Somatropin (rmc), recombinant human growth hormone	Pituitary hormones
Yellow Fever Vaccine	Vaccines

Drug	Therapeutic use
Pertussis vaccine- acellular, combined with diphtheria and tetanus toxoids	Vaccines
Combined hepatitis A and hepatitis B vaccine	Vaccines
Salmonella typhi Vi polysaccharide vaccine	Vaccines
Live varicella vaccine	Vaccines
Varicella zoster vaccine, live	Vaccines
Influenza virus vaccine	Vaccine
Diphtheria toxoid	Vaccine

Table 3.7. Marine medicine pipeline from natural sources

Clinical status	Compound name	Marine organism	Chemical class	Disease area
Approved	Cytarabine, ara-C	Sponge	Nucleoside	Cancer, leukemia
	Brentuximab vedotin (SGN-35)	Mollusk/cyanobacterium	ADC (MMAE)	Cancer, lymphoma
	Vidarabine, ara-A	Sponge	Nucleoside	Anti-viral
	Omega-3-acid ethyl esters	Fish	Omega-3 fatty acid	Hypertriglyceridemia
	Ziconotide	Cone snail	Peptide	Pain
	Eribulin mesylate (E7389)	Sponge	Macrolide	Breast cancer
	Trabectedin (ET-743)	Tunicate	Alkaloid	Cancer
Phase III	Plitidepsin	Tunicate	Depsipeptide	Cancer
	Tetrodotoxin	Pufferfish	Guanidinium alkaloid	Chronic pain
	Soblidotin (TZT 1027)	Bacterium	Peptide	Cancer
Phase II	DMXBA (GTS-21)	Worm	Alkaloid	Cognition, Alzheimers disaese, schizophrenia
	Plinabulin (NPI-2358)	Fungus	Diketopiperazine	Cancer
	Glembatumumab vedotin	Mollusk/cyanobacterium	ADC (MMAE)	Breast cancer, melanoma
	Elisidepsin	Mollusc	Depsipeptide	Cancer
	PM1004	Nudibranch	Alkaloid	Cancer
	Tasidotin, synthadotin (ILX-651)	Bacterium	Peptide	Cancer
	Pseudopterosins	Soft coral	Diterpene glycoside	Wound healing
Phase I	Bryostatin 1	Bryozoa	Polyketide	Cancer
	Pinatuzumab vedotin (DCDT-2980S) and (DCDS-4501A)	Mollusk/cyanobacterium	ADC (MMAE)	Non-Hodgkin lymphoma, chronic lymphocytic leukemia
	Hemiasterlin (E7974)	Sponge	Tripeptide	Cancer
	HuMax®-TF-ADC	Mollusk/cyanobacterium	ADC (MMAE)	Cancer for ovary, endometrium, cervix, prostate
	Marizomib (salinosporamide A)	Bacterium	Beta-lactone-gamma lactam	Cancer
Preclinical	Chrysophaentin A	Alga *Halobacillus salinus*	Shikimate	Bacterial infections
	Phenethylamine	Bacterium lyngbyoic acid	Shikimate	Bacterial infections
	Geodisterol sulfates	Sponge	Peptide	Fungal infections
	Pseudoalteromonas sp. metabolites	Bacteria	Polyketide	Bacterial infections
	Peziza vesiculosa β-carboline	Bryozoa	Alkaloid	Fungal infections
	Bromophycolides	Alga	Terpene	Malaria
	Plakortin	Sponge	Polyketide	Malaria
	Homogentisic acid	Sponge	Shikimate	Malaria
	Cladonia cervicornis diterpene	Alga	Terpene	Protozoal infections
	Hymenidin	Sponge	Alkaloid	Tuberculosis
	Ggyrosanols	Soft coral	Terpene	Viral infections
	Dysidine	Sponge	Terpene	Diabetes
	Arenamides A and B	Bacteria	Peptide	Inflammation
	Capnellene	Soft coral	Terpene	Inflammation
	Floridosides	Alga	Glycolipid	Inflammation
	Grassystatins A-C	Bacteria	Peptide	Immunity
	Callyspongidiol	Sponge	Polyketide	Immunity
	Calyculin A	Sponge	PKS/NRPS	Nervous system
	Pulicatin A	Bacteria	Alkaloid	Nervous system
	Dysideamine	Sponge	Terpene	Nervous system

ADC: Antibody drug conjugate, MMAE: Monomethylauristatin E, PKS: Polyketide synthases, NRPS: Nonribosomal peptide synthases, DMXBA: 3-(2,4 dimethoxy) benzylidene-anabaseine

3.8. Drugs from Marine Sources

Seawater makes up a large portion of the earth's surface. Thus, most of the plants, microbes, and animals have marine origins. The present medical era is much more concentrated on marine drugs. Marine Pharmacognosy is a special branch of the main course in Pharmacognosy. It deals with naturally occurring, medicinally useful bioactive chemicals that are produced by marine creatures. These marine organisms have been used to produce numerous anti-viral, anti-parasitic, anti-viral, and anti-cancer medications. One of the most significant cytostatics for the treatment of several types of leukemia has been obtained from a marine sponge in conjunction with sources from different terrestrial animals. The *Caribbean sponge* was used to produce *cytotarabine,* which is derived from the name of the original component that was obtained, *cytosine arabinoside* (*Cryptotheca crypta*). *Halichondrin B*, which is again derived from a marine sponge but this time from the species *Halichondria okadai*, has cytostatic properties. Table 3.7 presents a list of marine-origin drugs.

3.9. Extractions from Microorganisms

Not only plants but also microorganisms, including bacteria, fungi, etc., are the sources of naturally derived drug candidates. The era of this noble field began with the discovery of Penicillin. Now we have hundreds of diverse antibiotics. The main six groups include penicillins, cephalosporins, tetracyclines, aminoglycosides, macrolides, and fluoroquinolones. So far, hundreds of thousands of microbial secondary metabolites have been discovered, serving as the foundation for numerous clinically significant pharmacological therapies. Thus, besides antibiotics, medicinal scientists have developed a number of anti-microbial, anti-cancer, and anti-parasitic drugs from microorganism origins. It is to be noted that 42% of the pharmaceutical medications with the highest sales in 1997 were made from microbial metabolites. As a result of contemporary understanding of microbe genetics, drug development has undergone multiple revolutions. To date, many successful vaccines have been developed from viruses. Moreover, many other human ailments can be treated with microbe-derived drugs.

3.9.1. Bacterial Material Extraction: Isolation and Identification of Antibiotic Drug Candidates

The extraction of bacterial materials and subsequent isolation and identification of active compounds from the extract can be outlined as below:

Step 1. Collect, identify, and characterize the bacterial colony or species. Mass grow or perform a mass collection for extraction purposes. To get a pure culture, perform a serial dilution and subsequent incubation at a specified temperature for a specified period.

Step 2. Filtrate to get cell mass, add a solvent at 1:1, and agitate overnight.

Step 3. Separate by using a separating funnel. Collect the bioactive components from the upper layer.

Step 4. Concentrate the extract through a vacuum rotatory evaporator at a low temperature.

Step 5. Isolate and identify drug candidates from the extract by applying different chromatographic and spectroscopic techniques. Then perform different biological tests to prove the compound's potential as a drug candidate.

3.9.2. Fungal Material Extraction: Isolation and Identification of Drug Candidate from Fungi

The extraction of fungal materials and subsequent isolation and identification of active compounds from the extract can be outlined as below (Maljurić et al. 2018):

Step 1. Collect, identify, and characterize the fungi. For mass growing or performing a mass collection for extraction purposes.

Step 2. Chop the fungal material and add a suitable solvent (e.g., ethanol) to it.

Step 3. Incubate the fungi-solvent mixture at room temperature for 24 hours.

Step 4. After this period, filter the extract through Whatman filter paper No. 1.

Step 5. Evaporate the solvent, keeping the extract overnight at an ambient temperature.

Step 6. Reconstitute the dried extract with a suitable solvent combination (e.g., acetonitrile: water ---- 50:50, v/v) and filter through a 0.22 μm nylon filter (if necessary). Then they perform different biological tests.

Step 7. Isolate and identify drug candidates from the extract by applying different chromatographic and spectroscopic techniques. Then perform different biological tests to prove the compound's potential as a drug candidate.

N.B. – Isolation processes for some potential lead compounds are described in Chapter 3.

3.10. Advances in Compound Identification and Structural Characterization

This section deals with the isolation, identification, and purification of natural compounds from crude extracts. For this, the separation of lead compounds is done by applying a number of chromatographic techniques, which mainly act through the following mechanisms: adsorption, partition, molecular exclusion, and affinity. Examples include some important chromatographic techniques: PC, TLC, HPTLC, HPLC, CC, FCC, GC, DCCC or DCC, IEC, etc. Identification is done by applying various spectroscopic approaches, including UV, UV-Vis, IR, NMR, MS, and FTIR. Medicinal scientists also use combinations such as GC-MS and LC-MS for this purpose (Islam, 2021).

After these processes, the compounds are subjected to biological activity evaluations and the lab synthesis of their derivatives. All isolated compounds or their derivatives also go through a round of toxicological studies prior to entering clinical trials. The modern era introduces targeted approaches to drug discovery.

Some approaches developed recently are quickly expanding with promising successes, such as molecular diversity, compound library design, protein 3D structures, NMR-based screening, 3D-QSAR in current drug design, physicochemical principles, computer-aided drug design utilizing various tools, drug toxicity prediction, and metabolism prediction (Islam, 2021). Figure 3.6 presents an overall pathway of drug discovery and development from natural origins.

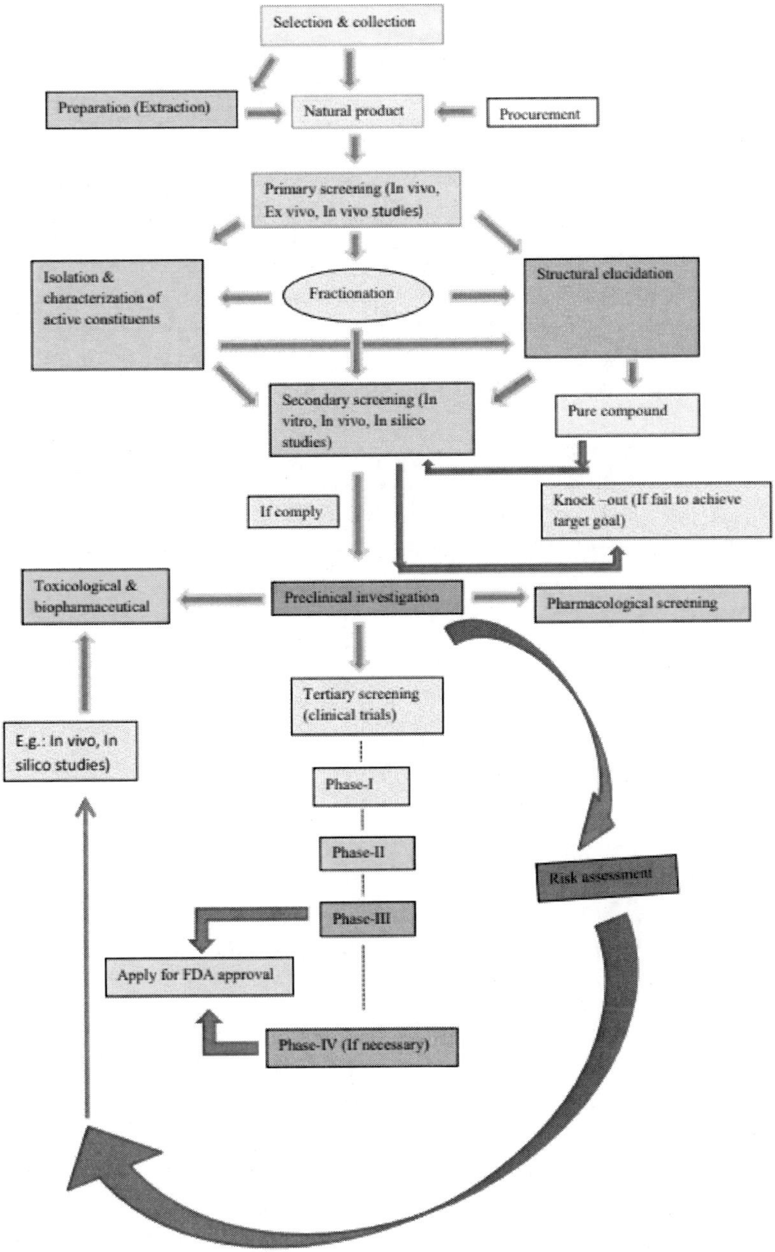

Figure 3.6. An overall pathway of drug discovery and development from natural origins

References

Ghribia, L., Ghouilaa, H., Omrib, A., Besbesb, M., & Janneta, H. B. (2014). Antioxidant and anti–acetylcholinesterase activities of extracts and secondary metabolites from *Acacia cyanophylla. Asian Pacific Journal of Tropical Biomedicine*, *4*, S417-S423.

Harhorne, J. B. (1991). Phytochemical Methods, 2nd Ed., Chapman & Hall, London. Ikan, R. (1991) Natural Products - A Laboratory Guide, 2nd edn, Academic Press, London.

Islam, M. T. (2021). PHARMACOGNOSY in natural product drug discovery. Mahi Publications, *Ahmedabad-380007,* India 2021 (ISBN: 978-93-90651-94-8).

Jachak, S. M., & Saklani, A. (2007). Challenges and opportunities in drug discovery from plants. *Current science*, 1251-1257.

Maljurić, N., Golubović, J., Ravnikar, M., Žigon, D., Štrukelj, B., & Otašević, B. (2018). Isolation and determination of fomentariol: Novel potential antidiabetic drug from fungal material. *Journal of Analytical Methods in Chemistry, 2018.*

Salim, A. A., Chin, Y. W., & Kinghorn, A. D. (2008). Drug discovery from plants. *Bioactive molecules and medicinal plants*, 1-24.

Zhang, Q. W., Lin, L. G., & Ye, W. C. (2018). Techniques for extraction and isolation of natural products: A comprehensive review. *Chinese Medicine*, *13*, 1-26.

Chapter 4

Isolation of Lead Compounds

4.1. Herbal Remedies

According to the World Health Organization (WHO), "Traditional medicine" refers to "the knowledge, skills, and practices based on the theories, beliefs, and experiences indigenous to different cultures and used in the maintenance of health and in the prevention, diagnosis, improvement, or treatment of physical and mental illness." Among the different systems of traditional medicinal care, a plant-based strategy has been recognized as a leading approach. Medicinal plant-based treatment strategies are emphasized not only for disease management but also for user health maintenance. It is because herbs and plants are rich in a variety of compounds that are essential to maintaining good health and fighting against ailments (De Smet, 2002).

Traditional Chinese Medicine (TCM) has a history of more than 3000 years. The book, *The Devine Farmer's Classic of Herbalism,* was compiled about 2000 years ago in China. TCM uses holistic approaches (the patient and the patient's symptoms, expressed in terms of the balance of Yin and Yang) in the diagnosis and management of diseases and disorders in humans and other animals with the help of herbs and their derivatives. Yin refers to the earth, cold, and femininity, whereas Yang refers to the sky, heat, and masculinity (Wachtel-Galor and Benzie, 2011). Thus, these two words' interaction comprises the action of the five vital elements: metal, wood, water, fire, and earth.

The development of chemically synthesized drugs and their mass production have significantly grown over the past 100 years. It could be due to the large number of research studies conducted in this eminent field. It should be noted that a significant proportion of the population in developing countries still relies on traditional medicine for the management of various diseases and disorders. For example, in Africa, India, China, Hong Kong, and the USA, up to 90, 70, 40, and >15% of the population depend on traditional medicine for their health care needs, respectively (Cheng, 1984; Ernst, 2005).

In general, most people use traditional medicine because it is readily available and affordable, has patient compatibility, is less toxic or even non-toxic than chemical (synthetic) drugs, and allows satisfactory personalized health care as well as greater public access and health information regarding a particular treatment. These are mainly used for health promotion and the treatment of chronic diseases. Most often, it takes time to cure a disease, but the mode of treatment is long-lasting. However, most people use traditional medicine when their conventional treatments do not work. Traditional remedies are considered natural, safe, and non-toxic therapeutics. The prescribers do not recommend these drugs with prescription drugs, over-the-counter medications, or other herbs. It is due to a lack of adequate quality control information on herbal remedies.

Currently, herbal drugs are used in the treatment of many chronic and acute diseases, including cardiovascular disease, prostate problems, depression, inflammation, and immunological problems. Traditionally, in China and Africa, traditional herbal medicines are used for severe acute respiratory syndrome (SARS) and HIV infection in humans (Chaachouay and Zidane, 2021). It should be noted that herbal remedies are commonly used in European countries. They have processed the herbs, plants, and their derivatives in different ways and forms. For this, they use the whole herb; teas, syrups, essential oils, ointments, salves, rubs, capsules, and tablets that contain a ground or powdered form of a raw herb or its dried extract. Plant and herb extracts vary in the solvent used for extraction, temperature, and extraction time and include alcoholic extracts (tinctures), vinegars (acetic acid extracts), hot water extracts (tisanes), long-term boiled extracts, usually roots or bark (decoctions), and cold infusions of plants (macerates). Hopefully, many countries and drug approval systems, including European countries and USA-based drug administration systems, are developing and applying rules and regulations on standardization, commercialization, and uses of herbal drugs on a regular basis. There is mounting evidence that herbal medicine factories are springing up all over the world.

Q. What is an herb?

Ans. The word "***herb***" (Latin *"herba"* and an old French word *"herbe")* refers to any part of a plant, such as roots, stigmas, bark, stems, fruit, seeds, flowers, flowering tops, etc. It also means a non-woody plant. In earlier reports and still now in the classification of plants, the word "herb" was meant for non-woody plants.

4.2. Plant-Origin Bioactive Ingredients

Plants (including those from the land and the aqueous environment) cover a large portion of the earth's surface. Using plants and their derivatives has been around since the beginning of human civilization. Even at present, there is a growing interest in medicinal plants and their derivatives in various fields, including botany, pharmacy, biotechnology, food, and agriculture. In the pharmaceutical context, plants are one of the major sources of promising and new bioactive compounds. To date, many drug candidates have been introduced from the same plant. Moreover, a significant number of the world's general population still relies on plant extracts and formulations in complementary and alternative therapies. The history of their use of these formulations is somewhat prehistoric. The polyherbal and functional food approaches recently introduced have gained the attention of people of every class. These are commonly introduced as nutraceutical strategies (Balunas and Kinghorn, 2005; Wan et al. 2015).

It should be noted that plants provide approximately 25% of modern prescription drugs (both modified and unmodified). However, medicinal scientists' report that we have yet to investigate 95% of plant species for this purpose. Current discovery approaches are more concentrated on synthetic medicine chemistry for clinical uses from plants and other natural sources. In the context of drug discovery and development, finding new lead compounds and advancements in phytochemistry, especially in the diversity of this pathway, makes this pathway more challenging and interesting. At present, advancements in bioassay screening modalities, identification and isolation techniques, and structural elucidation have shortened and accelerated the whole drug discovery process in medicinal chemistry. Alongside this, there is an increasing interest in standard development and practices in the safety, quality, and efficacy management of herbal drugs and formulations. This chapter will discuss the isolation steps of important plant metabolite constituents.

4.2.1. Atropine

Atropine, an optically inactive laevorotatory isomer of hyoscyamine, is a tropane alkaloid. It is found in many members of the Solanaceae family, including *Atropa belladonna*, *Datura stramonium*, and *Hyoscyamus niger*.

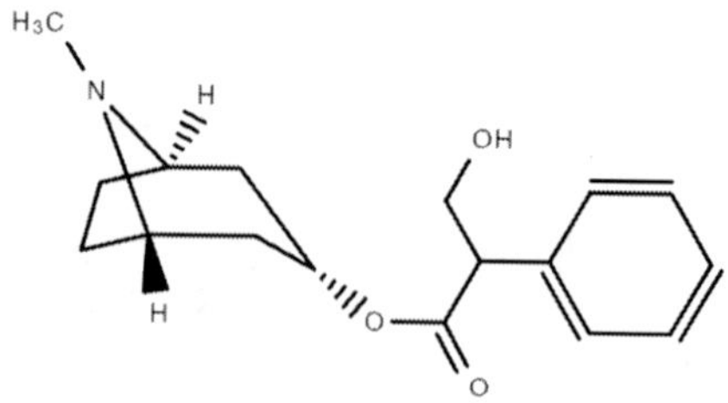

Atropine

Isolation steps:

You can isolate atropine by following the below-mentioned steps:

Step 1. Collect the target plant and make a powder of the drug materials.

Step 2. Moisten the crude materials with an aqueous solution of sodium carbonate and extract with ether or benzene. Extract the alkaloidal free bases with water acidified with acetic acid.

Step 3. Shake the acid solution with ether. This will help to remove color-related matters. Sodium carbonate will precipitate the alkaloids, filter them off, wash them off, and dry them.

Step 4. Dissolve the dried materials in ether or acetone, dehydrate with anhydrous sodium sulfate, and filter. This will yield crystals of hyoscyamine and atropine upon concentration and cooling.

Step 5. Separate the crystals, dissolve them in alcohol, and add the sodium hydroxide solution. This will recimize hyoscyamine completely to atropine. Confirm it by checking optical activity.

Step 6. Purify crude atropine by crystallization from acetone. The presence of a colorless crystalline powder indicates atropine sulfate. It is soluble in water and alcohol but insoluble in ether and chloroform.

4.2.2. Andrographolide

Andrographolide is a diterpenoid lactone that is bitter. *Andrographis paniculata* (family: Acanthaceae) is the source of it.

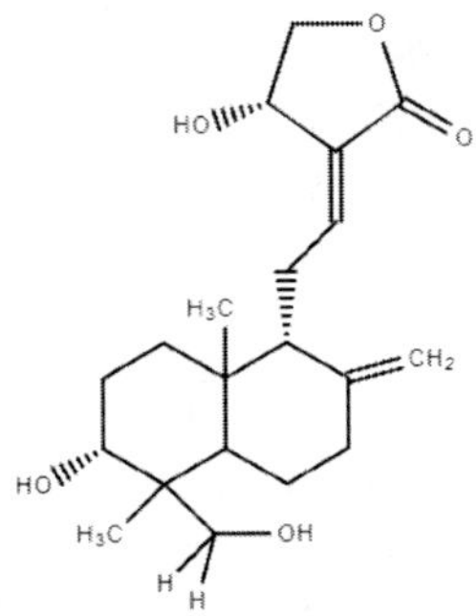

Andrographolide

Isolation steps:

You can isolate andrographolide by following the below-mentioned steps:

Step 1. Collect dried herbs, clean and remove foreign materials, and crush them into a coarse powder.

Step 2. Extract the powdered materials with a methanol:ethylene dichloride (1:1) mixture.

Step 3. Concentrate the extract and subject it to treatment with activated charcoal.

Step 4. Filter and get a pastey mass. Dissolve the mass in hot methanol.

Step 5. Again, treat it with charcoal (or pass it through a mix of charcoal and Hyflo bed).

Step 6. Reduce the volume to half of the resultant clear, light yellow-colored solution, subject to crystallization; filter the crystals after 24 h; and wash with chilled methanol.

Step 7. Dry the crystalline product in a vacuum dryer at a temperature of not more than 50 °C. You may get 1.25 - 1.75% of andrographolide by this process.

4.2.3. Bacosides

Bacosides (triterpenic saponins) are isolated from various parts of *Bacopa monnieri* (family: Scrophulariaceae). Bacosides A and B are the most common and important bacosides of this plant.

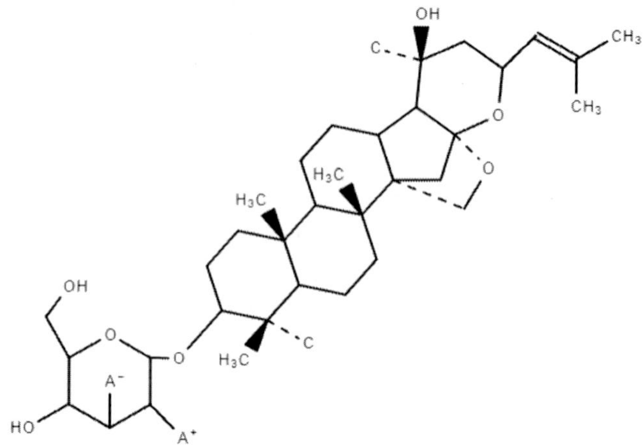

Compounds	R	R1
Bacoside A1	-H	-arabinosyl
Bacoside A3	-arabinosyl	-β-D-glucosyl

Isolation steps:

You can isolate bacosides by following the below-mentioned steps:

Step 1. Collect the fresh parts of the herb, dry them, and crush them into a coarse powder.

Step 2. Extract with ethyl alcohol and concentrate to dryness.

Step 3. Dissolve in 60% alcohol and separate the benzene and alcohol-soluble parts using a separating funnel.

Step 4. Further divide the alcohol-soluble part (the slimy mass) into ether and petroleum ether parts.

Step 5. Concentrate the alcohol-ether-petroleum ether mixture. Macerate the residue with acetone and filter it. Partition the acetone-insoluble powder between butanol and water.

Step 6. During the concentration of the butanol solution, separate the precipitate that settles down and code it as A1.

Step 7. Again, concentrate the filtrate and precipitate with acetone and ether and code it as A2. You will get mother liquor (brownish powder). Code it as A3. Bacoside A dominates fractions A1, A2, and A3.

Step 8. Store the acetone-soluble fraction in a cool place for a few days. As the solid settles, filter it and wash it with acetone. It mainly consists of bacoside B.

4.2.4. Caffeine

Caffeine (1,3,7-trimethylxanthin), a purine-base alkaloid, is present in many plant species, including coffee, tea, cocoa, and guarana. It was discovered in coffee by Robiquet in 1821 and in tea leaves by Oudry in 1827. Its major sources are tea leaves (1 - 4%) and coffee seeds (1 - 2%).

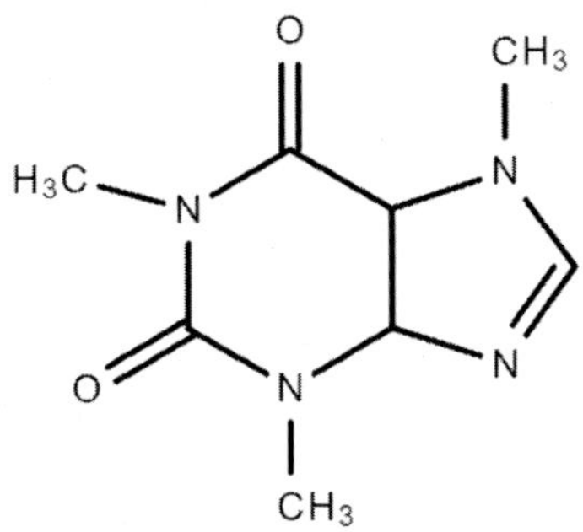

Caffeine

Isolation steps:

You can isolate caffeine by following the below-mentioned steps:

Method 1: Extract the teat leaf into a coarse powder with boiling water and filter. Treat the extract with lead acetate. This will precipitate tannins and filter them. Precipitate and separate out the excess lead acetate with dilute sulfuric acid; filter and boil the solution with charcoal. This will remove the coloring materials (if any). Filter again to remove charcoal. The solution is then evaporated by the extract using chloroform. It consists of caffeine as white matter and re-crystallizes with alcohol.

Method 2: Extract tea leaves finely (or coarsely) powdered with hot ethanol (in a Soxhlet extractor). Add magnesium oxide and mix well with 10% H_2SO_4. Then extract with chloroform and re-crystallize.

Method 3: Leach coffee beans in distilled water for 30 minutes at 75 °C.

Method 4: You can also use supercritical fluid extraction for caffeine extraction. In this case, in a pressure vessel, moist coffee provides caffeine. Then it passes through a second pressurized vessel containing an adsorbing medium such as activated carbon, resin, or water, which retains caffeine. Separate the adsorbed caffeine by adding chloroform.

4.2.5. Camphor

Camphor (a bicyclic monoterpene ketone, an optically inactive mixture) is isolated from *Cinnamomum camphora* (family: Lauraceae). It is also synthesized from pinene.

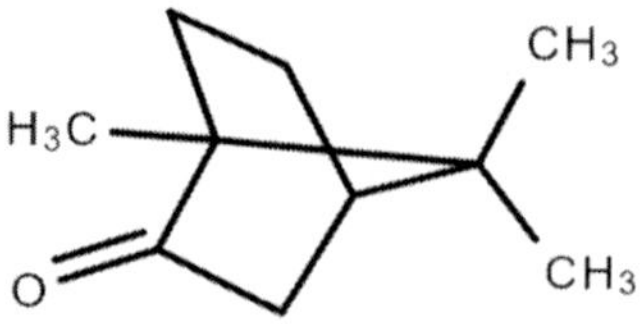

Camphor

Isolation steps:

You can isolate camphor by following the below-mentioned steps:

Step 1. Collect camphor oil through the steam distillation process. It contains about 50% camphor.

Step 2. Separate camphor by cooling and centrifugation.

Step 3. Perform fractionation. It will give two types of oils: (i) white camphor oil-first distillation fraction with a cineol-like odour, containing 35% of cineol; and (ii) brown camphor oil-fraction with a higher boiling point, containing 80% of safrol.

4.2.6. Capsaicin

Capsaicin (8-methylN-vanillyl non-6-enamide; pungent compound) is present in *Capsicum annum var. minimum* and *C. fruitescens* (family: Solanaceae). It is mainly present in the dissepiment of fruits.

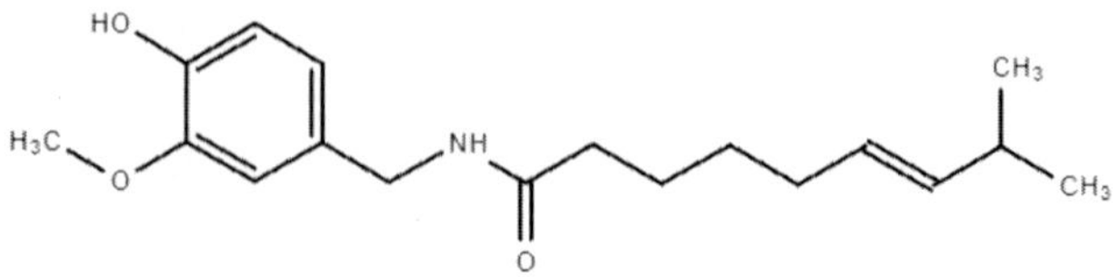

Capsaicin

Isolation steps:

You can isolate capsaicin by following the below-mentioned steps:

Step 1. Collect dried, ripe fruits of capsicum, coarsely powder them, and extract them with hot acetone or alcohol (90%). Then concentrate the extract and let it dry.

Step 2. Further extract the dried residue with cold alcohol (90%). Evaporate to dryness. This oleoresin contains approximately 8% capsaicin.

4.2.7. Colchicine

Colchicine (a tropolone group alkaloid) is isolated from many species of Colchicum, including *Colchicum autumnale* (family: Liliaceae).

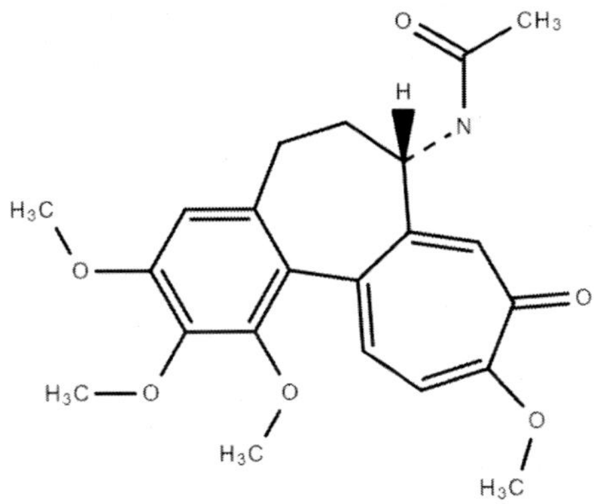

Colchicine

Isolation steps:

You can isolate colchicine by following the below-mentioned steps:

Step 1. Extract the materials with ethanol, concentrate, and dry to get a syrupy residue.

Step 2. Add the water. This will precipitate insoluble fats and resins. Filter the extract and extract it with chloroform or digest it with lead carbonate.

Step 3. Re-filter, evaporate the materials, and re-extract with chloroform. This will give it a crystalline complex.

Step 4. Completely evaporate the solvent, chloroform. This yields an amorphous colchicine, which can be crystallized from ethyl acetate as pale yellow needles.

4.2.8. Curcumin

Curcumins or curcuminoids (diaryl heptanoids) are isolated from *Curcuma longa* (family: Zingiberaceae).

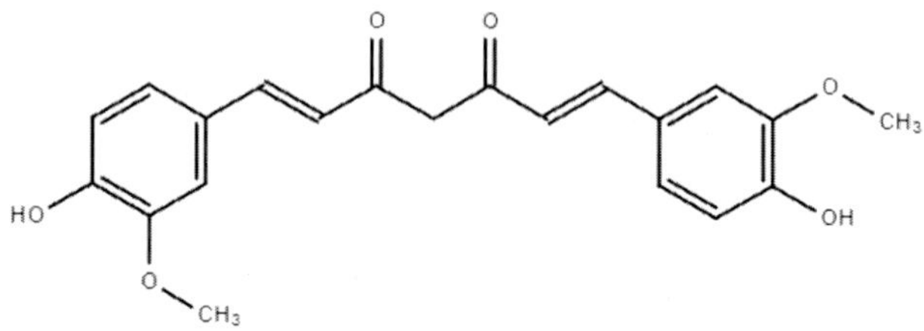

Curcumin

Isolation steps:

You can isolate curcumin by following the below-mentioned steps:

Step 1. Extract the turmeric powder with hot alcohol such as ethanol (in a Soxhlet extractor).

Step 2. Concentrate it under reduced pressure and allow it to dry. You can extract the turmeric powder with hexane, followed by acetone, and concentrate to get curcumin.

Step 3. Throw the ethanol extract into superior-grade kerosene. This will separate a solid mass. Strip off the mass with petroleum ether and re-crystallize with ethanol (orange-red needles).

4.2.9. Digoxin

Digoxin (Lanoxin), a widely used cardiac glycoside, is isolated from the *Digitalis lanata* leaf (family: Scrophulariaceae). It yields digoxigenin as an aglycone and three moles of digitoxose upon acid hydrolysis.

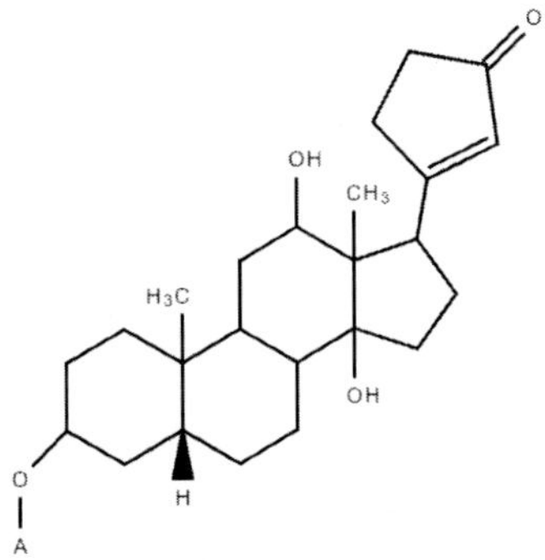

Digoxin

Isolation steps:

You can isolate digoxin by following the below-mentioned steps:

Step 1. To extract lanatosides, grind fresh leaves with neutral salt. This will inactivate the enzymes. Extract the pulp with ethyl acetate.

Step 2. Defat the leaves with benzene prior to extraction. It will yield a glycoside. Concentrate the ethyl acetate extract, dry it, and subject it to chromatographic purification. It will give you lanatoside A (46%), lanatoside B (17%), and lanatoside C (37%).

Step 3. Crystallize the fraction of alcohol. Subsequent hydrolysis of lanatoside C gives digoxin.

4.2.10. Diosgenin

Diosgenin is isolated from the tubers (dried) of many species of Dioscorea, including *Dioscorea deltoidea* Wallich (family: Dioscoreaceae).

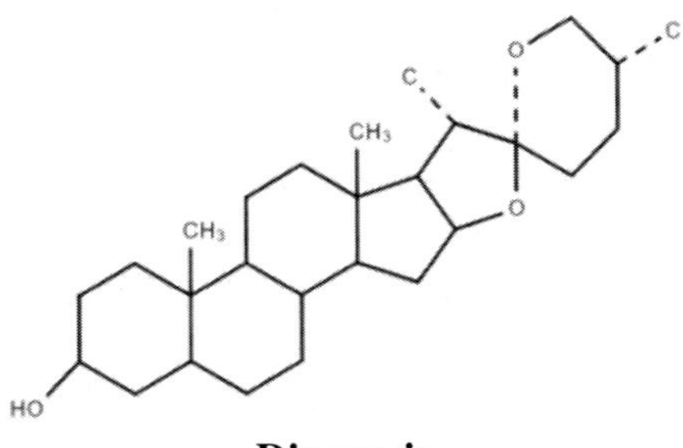

Diosgenin

Isolation steps:

You can isolate diosgenin by following the below-mentioned steps:

Method 1 (Alcoholic extraction process)

Step 1. Cut, dry, and grind the dried tubers into a fine powder, then extract them for 6 - 8 hours with alcohol (e.g., ethanol or methanol).

Step 2. Filter and concentrate the extract into a syrupy liquid.

Step 3. Hydrolyze by using hydrochloric acid or sulphuric acid for 2 - 12 h. You will get a precipitation of 85% crude diosgenin.

Step 4. Filter, wash with water, and purify with alcohol.

Method 2 (Acid hydrolysis process)

Step 1. Reflux or heat the fine powder in an autoclave with 2 - 4 N mineral acid for 2 - 6 h.

Step 2. Filter and wash the crude hydrolyte with water to a neutral pH.

Step 3. Dry and extract with a hydrocarbon solvent for 6 hours. Concentrate the liquid to about 25 mL.

Step 4. Allow to stand for a while in a refrigerator for 1 hour. It will give you diosgenin crystals that you can filter and wash with acetone.

Method 3 (Fermentation cum acid hydrolysis process)

Step 1. Collect fresh green roots and smash them in a hammer mill.

Step 2. Place the mesh in the fermentation bin and allow for fermentation for 2 days.

Step 3. Perform sun drying to reduce the moisture content to 7 - 8%.

Step 4. Subject to hydrolysis with a mineral acid at a reduced temperature. Extract with heptane to obtain diosgenin.

Method 2 (Incubation cum acid hydrolysis process)

Step 1. Incubate fresh plant material in water at 37 °C for a few days. Then it is subject to acid hydrolysis.

Step 2. Concentrate and extract with a hydrocarbon solvent to obtain diosgenin.

4.2.11. Emetine

Emetine is isolated from *Cephaells ipecacuanha* and *C. acuminate* (family: Rubiaceae).

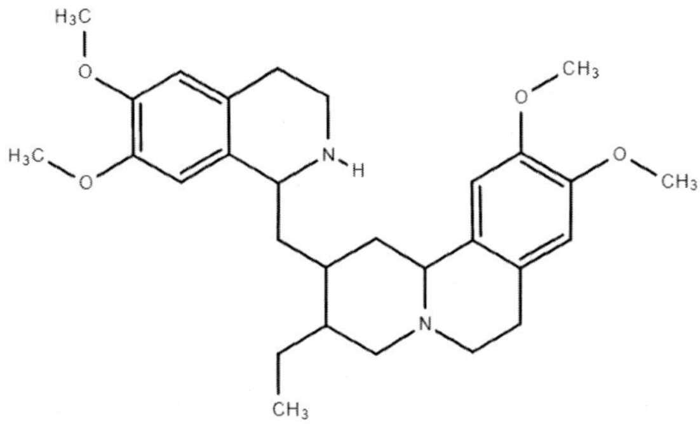

Emetin

Isolation steps:

Follow the below-mentioned steps for this purpose:

Step 1. Extract powdered materials with 70% alcohol (e.g., ethanol, methanol).

Step 2. Concentrate the extract, dissolve it in distilled water, add an excess amount of ammonia, and extract with di-isopropyl ether.

Step 3. Treat the extract with 10 - 15% aqueous potassium hydroxide. It will remove cephaeline. Further evaporate to obtain emetine. Purify via dihydrobromide or dihydroiodide salt.

Step 4. You can treat ipecac powder with ammonia and ether. Subject the extracts to dilute sulphuric acid to yield alkaloids.

Step 5. Neutralize, wash with ether, add strong alkali, and treat with ether. Separate the ether layer. It contains emetine, while the water layer contains cephaeline.

Step 6. Concentrate the ether extract, re-dissolve it in methanol, and convert it to emetine hydrobromide with a methanolic solution of hydrobromic acid.

4.2.12. Ergometrine

Ergometrine (ergonovine, a natural indol alkaloid) is isolated from *Claviceps purpurea* (family: Clavicipitaceae).

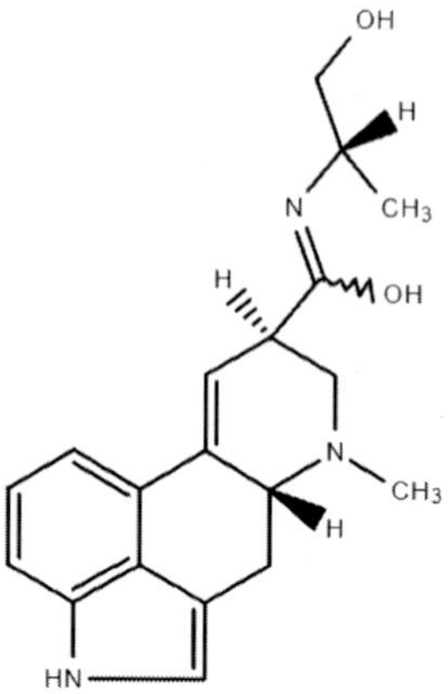

Ergometrine

Isolation steps:

Follow the below-mentioned steps for this purpose:

Step 1. Extract the powder with petroleum ether (60 – 80 °C) in a Soxhlet extractor. It will remove about 30% of the fat and color matter from the extract.

Step 2. Transfer the residue to a porcelain dish. Make it a semi-solid mass by adding sufficient ether and dilute ammonia with continuous stirring.

Step 3. Allow to dry and extract with ether for 5 hours; filter, add a few mL of acetone, and shake in a separating funnel with three volumes of 1% tartaric acid.

Step 4. Combine the total acidic extract and dry under reduced pressure. It will give you total ergot alkaloid.

Step 5. Dissolve this alkaloidal sample in dilute ammonia and extract it with four volumes of ether.

Step 6. Combine the total ether extract and wash thoroughly with sufficient distilled water. Now, the ether fraction contains water-insoluble ergotamine and ergotoxine alkaloids, while water-soluble ergometrine tartrate will be found in the aqueous portion.

Step 7. Add diluted ammonia to the aqueous extract and saturate with ether. It causes ergometrine-free base shifting to an ethereal solution. Then wash it with water. This will remove impurities from other alkaloids.

Step 8. Treat the ether extract with three volumes of 1% w/w tartaric acid in water. Concentrate the combined acid extract under reduced pressure to yield a water-soluble alkaloid. Then purify it by applying column chromatographic fractionation.

4.2.13. Eugenol

Eugenol (4-allyl-2-methoxyphenol) is isolated from the essential oils of *Eugenia caryophyllus* (family Myrtaceae) and *Cinnamomum zeylanicum* (family: Lauraceae).

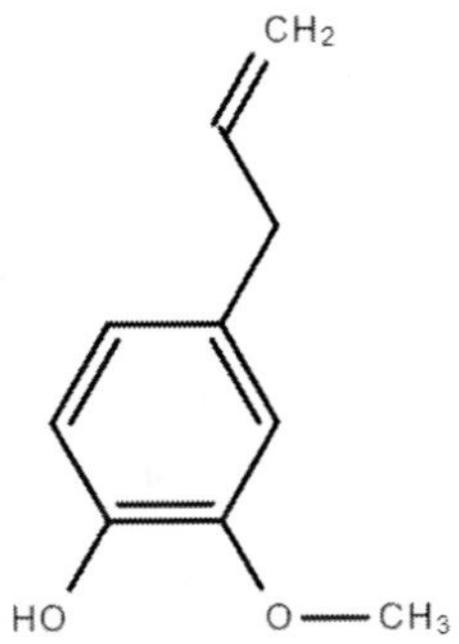

Eugenol

Isolation steps:

Follow the below-mentioned steps for this purpose:

Step 1. Hydrolyze dried clove buds to obtain clove oil. It will remain beneath the water layer due to its heavier nature.

Step 2. After separation, dissolve the oil in ether to make about a 10% solution. Shake with three successive volumes of 10% potassium hydroxide solution. Eugenol will convert to phenoxide and become soluble in water.

Step 3. Combine total aqueous alkaline extract with fresh ether to remove other impurities.

Step 4. Regenerate eugenol by acidifying the aqueous alkaline extract with an excess of sulphuric acid. Extract the mixture with three successive volumes of solvent ether and wash with water. Remove ether by distillation at a very low temperature to yield pure liquid eugenol.

4.2.14. Gingerols and Shogaols

Gingerols (oleoresin constituents) are isolated from *Zingiber officinalis* (family: Zingiberaceae).

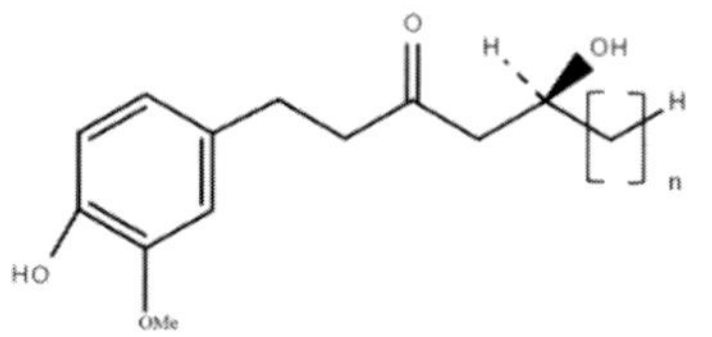

Gingerols
(n = 0, 2, 3, 4, 5, 7, 9)

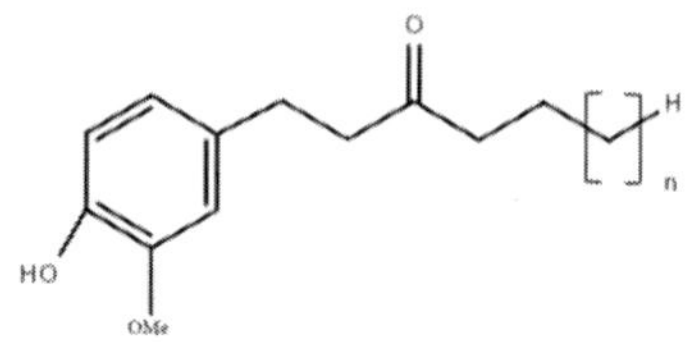

Shagoals
(n = 4, 5, 7, 9, 10)

Isolation steps:

Follow the below-mentioned steps for this purpose:

Step 1. Crush dry ginger, extract with 95% ethanol, and evaporate the solvent by distillation. It will produce a thick, pasty mass.

Step 2. Suspend the pasty mass in distilled water. You will see a precipitation of resin.

Step 3. Filter it and dry it under vacuum conditions. You can extract oleoresin with ether for this purpose.

Step 4. Add 5 mL of 70% sulphuric acid and 5 mg of vanillin to a small quantity of this extract. Keep it for 15 minutes, and add equal volumes of distilled water. Azure blue indicates the presence of gingerol.

4.2.15. Glycyrrhetinic Acid

Glycyrrhetinic acid (pentacyclic triterpenic acid) is isolated from *Glycyrrhiza glabra* (family: Leguminoseae).

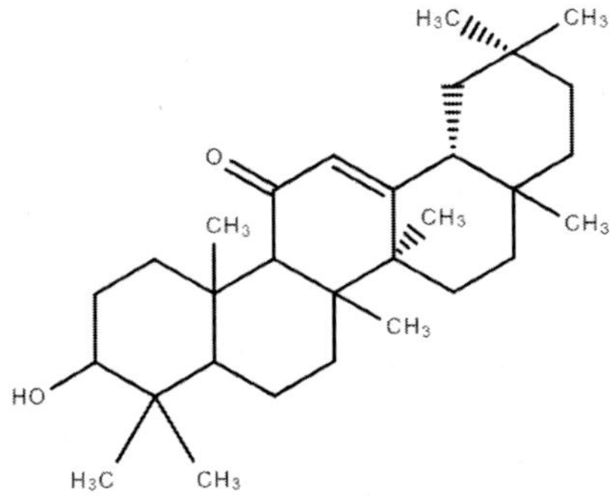

Glycyrrhetinic acid

Isolation steps:

Follow the below-mentioned steps for this purpose:

Method 1:

Step 1. Extract the crude powder with chloroform, evaporate to dryness, and add 0.5 M sulphuric acid to it.

Step 2. Cool and shake this extract with chloroform. Concentrate the combined chloroform extract and dry it to get a glycyrrhetinic acid yield. Hydrolyze glycyrrhizin into glycyrrhetinic acid during extraction with sulphuric acid.

Method 2:

Step 1. Extract the powder with boiling water and concentrate until dry. Then add hydrochloric acid to attain pH 3 - 3.4. This will precipitate glycyrrhetinic acid.

Step 2. Filter, wash with water to attain a neutral pH, and dry to get glycyrrhetinic acid.

4.2.16. Guggulsterone

Guggulsterone (gugulipid) is isolated from *Commiphora mukul* (family: Burseraceae). It is present in the form of stereoisomers, i.e., E-guggulsterone and Z- guggulsterone.

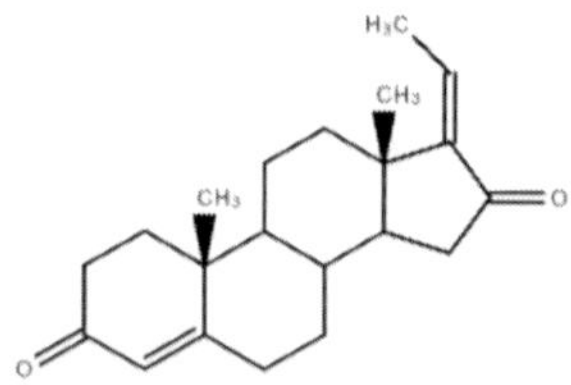

E-guggulsterone

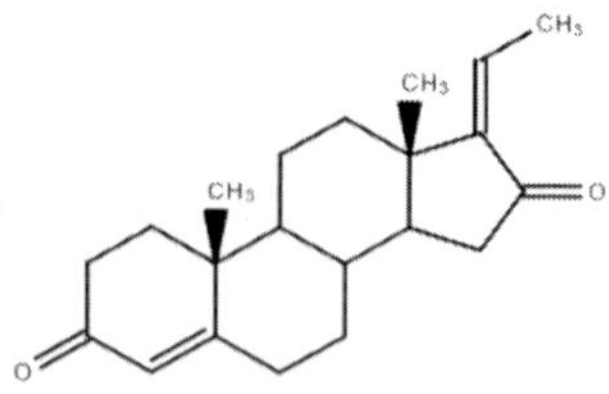

Z-guggulsterone

Isolation steps:

Follow the below-mentioned steps for this purpose:

Step 1. Extract the coarse powder with ethyl acelate and evaporate the solvent under vacuum at 50 °C. This will yield a dark, brownish gummy extract. Dissolve it in ethyl acetate and extract it with 3 N HCl.

Step 2. Divide the fraction into non-carbonyl and neutral ketonic parts. Mix 10% semi-carbazide on silica gel and toluene with the neutral fraction, stir and heat at 60 - 62 °C for 14 h, cool, and filter.

Step 3. Wash with toluene. It will result in a toluene-soluble non-carbonyl fraction. Mix it with aqueous 10% oxalic acid and toluene, stir and reflux for 2.5 hours, cool, and filter.

Step 4. Wash the extract three times with ethyl acetate. Combine ethyl acetate extract, wash with distilled water, and dry to concentrate. It will result in a neutral ketonic yield.

Step 5. Perform chromatography to get a mixture containing E-and Z-guggulsterone.

4.2.17. Hesperidin

Hesperidin is isolated from many species, including *Citrus mitis*, *C. aurantium*, and *C. sinensis* (family: Rutaceae).

Isolation steps:

Follow the below-mentioned steps for this purpose:

Method 1:

Step 1. Take approximately 200 g of powdered materials and add 1 L of petroleum ether (40 - 60 °C) to it.

Step 2. Apply heat to a water bath for 1 hour. Then filter the contents and allow them to dry at ambient temperature.

Step 3. Add 1 liter of methanol to it. Apply heat under reflux for 3 hours, filter, and wash with 200 mL of hot methanol.

Step 4. Concentrate the filtrate under reduced pressure. It will leave you with a syrupy residue. Crystallization converts it into white needles of hesperidin.

Method 2:

Step 1. Take approximately 200 g of powdered materials and add 750 mL of a 10% calcium hydroxide solution to them. Mix properly, and keep the mixture overnight at an ambient temperature.

Step 2. Filter the mixture. It will produce a yellow-orange colour. Then add conc. hydrochloric acid to attain pH 4 - 5.

Step 3. This will result in an amorphous powder. Then collect, wash with water, and re-crystallize the aqueous formamide.

4.2.18. Levodopa

Levodopa, also called L-Dopa (dihydroxyphenyl alanine), is isolated from *Mucuna pruriens* (family: Fabaceae).

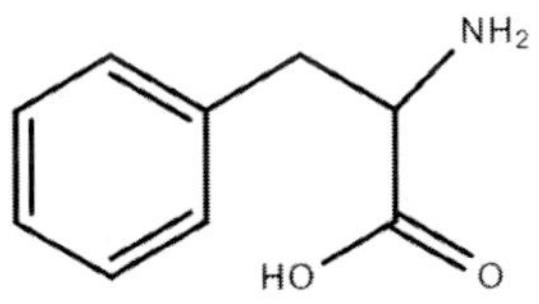

Levodopa

Isolation steps:

Follow the below-mentioned steps for this purpose:

Step 1. Extract the powder with demineralized water containing 1% v/v of acetic acid at 50 °C. Then filter the extract.

Step 2. Concentrate the extract by reverse osmosis and keep it at a low temperature (6 - 8 °C) for 1 day for crystallization of L-dopa.

Step 3. Filter the crystals through centrifugation. Then wash with cold water and dry under a vacuum at 50 °C. You can perform a second wash similarly. These two washing products contain a yield of about 2.0 - 2.5% of L-dopa. It also consists of amino acid impurities.

Step 4. Purify the contents either by re-crystallization or by using liquid ion exchangers.

4.2.19. Menthol

Menthol (a monoterpene alcohol) is isolated from many species, including *Mentha piperita Var. vulgaris*; *M. piperita Var. officinalis*; *M. arvensis*; *M. canadensis Var. piperascens* etc. In a laboratory, menthol is synthesized by hydrogenation of thymol.

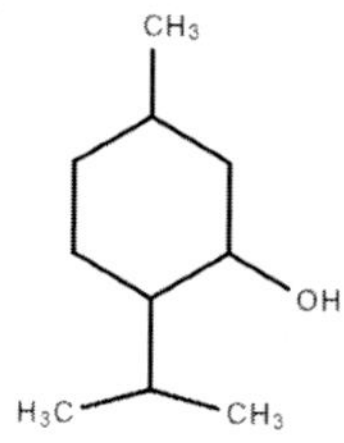

Menthol

Isolation steps:

Follow the below-mentioned steps for this purpose:

Step 1. You can get menthe oil by hydrodistillation or steam distillation of a crude sample. The cooling of peppermint oil results in (-) menthol. If you centrifuge the oil, you will get crystals of menthol.

Step 2. Steam distillation of cornmint oil results in about 70 - 80% free (-) menthol. You should cool the cornmint oil and centrifuge it to crystalize the menthol. It may contain a trace amount of cornmint oil.

Step 3. Re-crystallize the content to get pure (-) menthol. You should evaporate the solvent at this stage.

4.2.20. Nicotine

Nicotine (a pyridine alkaloid) is isolated from *Nicotiana tabacum* (family: Solanaceae).

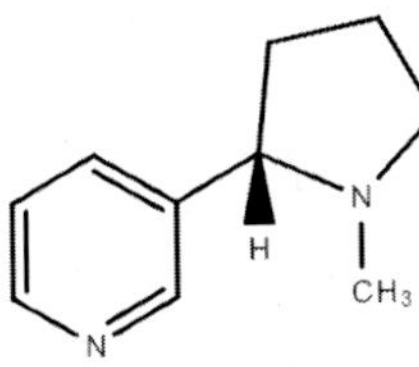

Nicotine

Isolation steps:

Follow the below-mentioned steps for this purpose:

Step 1. Mix tobacco waste with lime and extract with distilled water, followed by extracting with chloroform.

Step 2. Then treat the organic solvent extract with dilute sulphuric acid. It will give you a nicotine sulfate solution.

Step 3. Separate as a heavy layer, recover the solvent, and recycle the extraction process.

Step 4. Pass the extracted solution through a cation exchanger. If necessary, regenerate the exchanger by washing it with dilute acid and reusing it several times.

4.2.21. Opium Alkaloids

Opium alkaloids such as morphine and codeine are isolated from *Papaver somniferum* Linn (family: Papaveraceae).

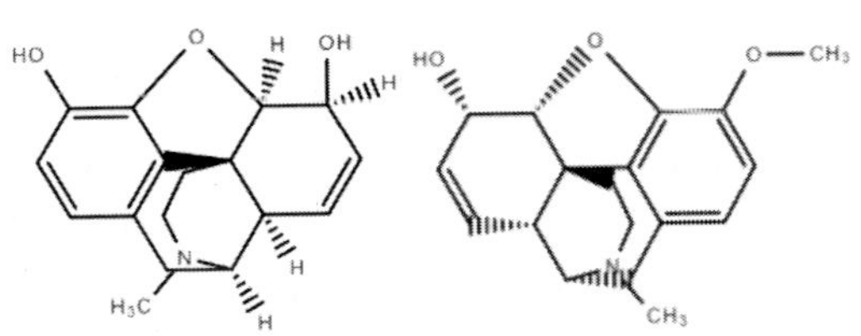

Morphine **Codeine**

Isolation steps:

Follow the below-mentioned steps for this purpose:

Step 1. Extract the powdered materials with boiling water, add calcium chloride, and concentrate the extract. You will find crystals of morphine and codeine. Then treat it with chloroform. The soluble portion consists of codeine, and the insoluble portion consists of morphine and narceine.

Step 2. You can shake the powered materials with calcium chloride. After filtration, add 10% sodium hydroxide solution. Then filter again. This filtrate consists of morphine and codeine.

Step 3. Extract the filtrate with chloroform and separate the chloroform layer. The soluble portion consists of codeine, and the insoluble portion consists of morphine and narceine.

Step 4. Acidify the aqueous layer and then add ammonia to basify. You will get morphine in the ammonia layer and narceine in the aqueous layer.

Step 5. Dissolve the marc consisting of narcotine, papaverine, and thebain in alcohol. Then acidify with acetic acid. Add 3 volumes of boiling water. It will precipitate narcotine and papaverine. However, thebain will remain in the aqueous solution. Add a 0.3% oxalic acid solution and cool the extract to separate papaverine from narcotine. If you cool the solution, it will give you papaverine crystals.

Step 6. Add ammonia to the aqueous layer. It will precipitate narcapine. Crystalize it by adding water.

4.2.22. Piperine

Piperine is obtained from many plant species, including *Piper nigrum, P. clusii, P. longum, P. fainechotti, P. chaba,* and *Cubeba censii.*

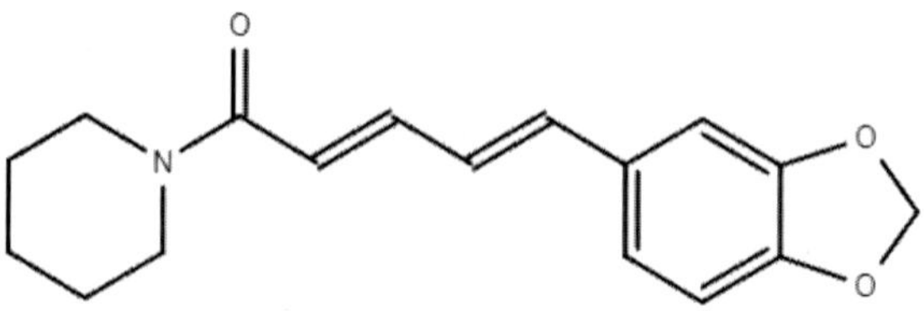

Piperine

Isolation steps:

Follow the below-mentioned steps for this purpose:

Step 1. Take approximately 20 g of fine powder materials and extract them with 300 mL of 95% ethanol in a Soxhlet extractor for 2 h.

Step 2. Filter the solution and concentrate it in a vacuum evaporator at 60 °C.

Step 3. Add 20 mL of alcoholic potassium hydroxide to the filtrate residue and keep it for a while. Then decant the insoluble residue.

Step 4. Keep the alcoholic solution overnight. You will obtain yellow-coloured, needle-shaped piperine crystals.

4.2.23. Podophyllotoxin

It is a tetrahydronapthalin derivative with OH and lactone groups. It is isolated from *Podophyllum hexandrum* Royle (family: Berberidaceae).

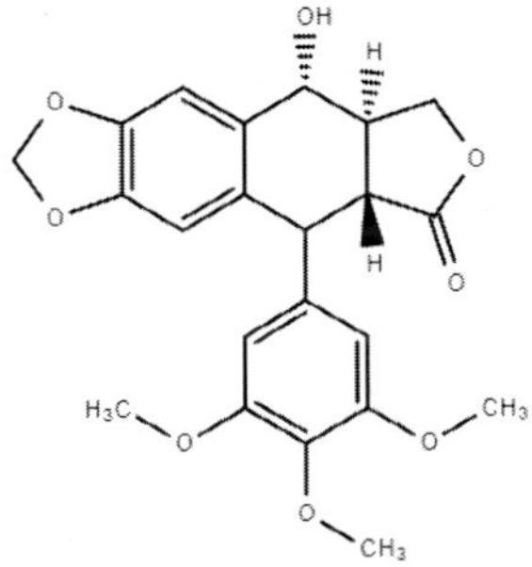

Podophyllotoxin

Isolation steps:

Follow the below-mentioned steps for this purpose:

Method 1:

Step 1. Extract the powdered materials with methanol and evaporate the solvent to get a semi-solid mass.

Step 2. Add acidulated water (10 mL of HCl to 100 mL of water) to it. It will cause precipitation. After a while, filter, decant, and wash with cold water. You will get resin.

Step 3. Dry it. It gives a dark brown amorphous powder called podophyllin.

Step 4. Extract the powder with chloroform, re-crystallize from benzene alone or with an alcohol-benzene mixture, followed by washing with petroleum ether/hexane, yielding podophyllotoxin.

Method 2:

Step 1. Extract with $CHCl_3$ and add alcohol to it.

Step 2. Reflux with neutral aluminum oxide. It results in a light yellow solution.

Step 3. Add benzene. You will get approximately 95–98% podophyllotoxin.

Method 3:

Step 1. Extract the crude sample powder over a bed of neutral alumina with benzene, toluene, or xylene for 1.5 - 4 h.

Step 2. Re-crystallization from organic solvents such as hot benzene, toluene, and xylene yields pure podophyllotoxin (95 - 97%).

4.2.24. Quinine and Quinidine

Quinine is laevorotatory, while quinidine is a dextrorotatory stereoisomer. These are isolated from *Cinchona calisaya* Wedd, *C. ledgeriana* Moens, *C. officinalis* Linn, and *C. sucirubra* Pavon or their hybrid species (family: Rubiaceae).

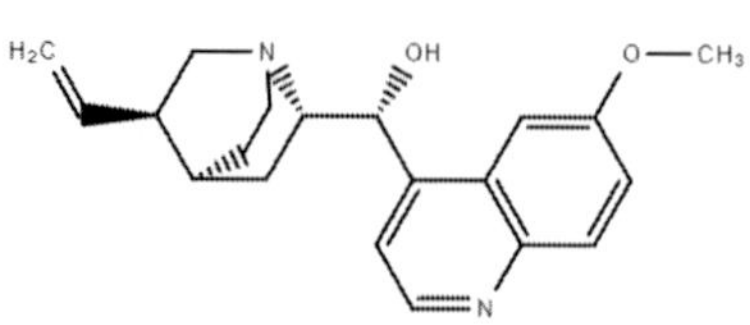

Quinine

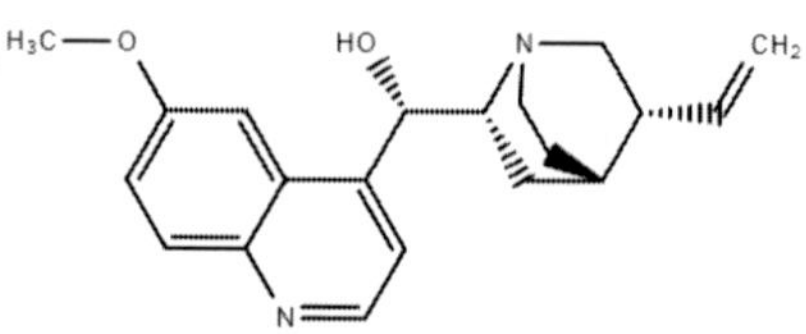

Quinidine

Isolation steps:

Follow the below-mentioned steps for this purpose:

Step 1. Mix the powdered materials with about 30% of their weight in calcium hydroxide or calcium oxide.

Step 2. Add a sufficient quantity of 5% sodium hydroxide solution to this mixture.

Step 3. Make a paste. Wait for a few hours.

Step 4. Transfer the mass into a Soxhlet extractor and extract with benzene.

Step 5. Add 5% sulphuric acid to the extract solution and mix properly.

Step 6. Separate the benzene layer and discard it.

Step 7. Add sodium hydroxide to the aqueous layer and adjust the pH to 6.5.

Step 8. Cool the solution. You will have quinine sulfate precipitation.

Step 9. Filter and separate the precipitates. Then re-crystallize the precipitates with hot water to free the salts from cinchonine and cinchonidine.

Step 10. Treat it with activated charcoal to remove color matter.

Step 11. Add dilute sulfuric acid to dissolve quinine sulphate. Then add ammonia.

Step 12. Quinine will crystallize, wash, and dry at 45 - 55 °C.

Step 13. Add ammonia to the mother liquor (consisting of quinidine, cinchonine, and cinchonidine). It will result in precipitation. Then extract with ether.

Step 14. The ether insoluble portion consists of cinchonine crystals, while the ether soluble portion consists of quinidine and cinchonidine.

Step 15. Add diluted hydrochloric acid to the ether-soluble fraction and stir. Then add 25% sodium potassium tartrate solution to it.

Step 16. Allow to stand. It will precipitate cinchonidine tartarate. Then re-crystallize the cinchonidine with alcohol.

Step 17. Add a potassium iodide solution to it. It will cause the precipitation of quinidine hydroiodide. Upon treatment with an alkali (ammonia), it liberates a base, which is dissolved in acetic acid.

Step 18. Remove the coloring matter as mentioned above. Re-crystallize quinidine from alcohol.

Thalleioquin test (identification test): Add 1 drop of dilute sulphuric acid and 1 mL of water to the sample. Add bromine water dropwise till the solution acquires a permanent yellow colour and add 1 mL of dilute ammonia solution. Quinine will attain a green color.

4.2.25. Reserpine

Reserpine (an indole alkaloid) is isolated from various species of Rauwolfia, including *Rauwolfia serpentina*, *R. micrantha*, *R. vomiforia*, and *R. tetraphylla* (family: Apocyanaeae).

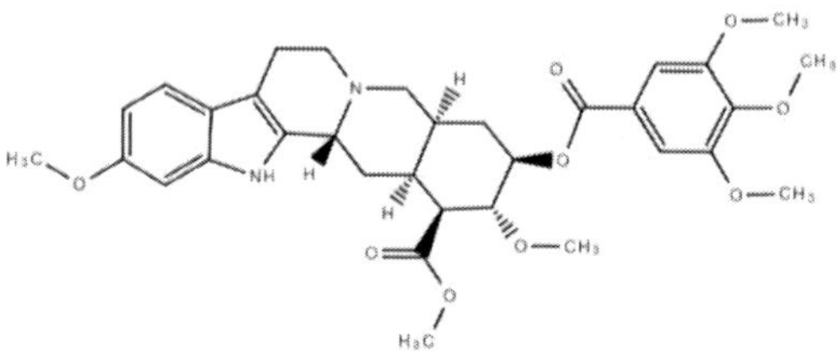

Reserpine

Isolation steps:

Follow the below-mentioned steps for this purpose:

Step 1. Extract the powder with 90% alcohol (percolation method).

Step 2. Concentrate the extract under reduced pressure and below 60 °C.

Step 3. Extract further with proportions of ether, chloroform, and 90% alcohol (20:8:2.5).

Step 4. Add diluted ammonia and shake the mixture.

Step 5. Add water, shake vigorously, and allow it to stand.

Step 6. Filter the solution and extract the residue with 4 volumes of 0.5 N H_2SO_4.

Step 7. Combine the total acid extract, filter, and add diluted ammonia. This will liberate alkaloids.

Step 8. Then extract with chloroform.

Step 9. Filter the total chloroform extract, remove the solvent by distillation, and dry under vacuum. This will give you a total of 30 different Rauwolfia alkaloids.

Step 10. Perform column chromatographic fractionation to separate reserpine.

4.2.26. Sennosides

Sennosides are isolated from *Tinnevelley senna* and *Cassia angustifolia* Vahl (family: Leguminosae).

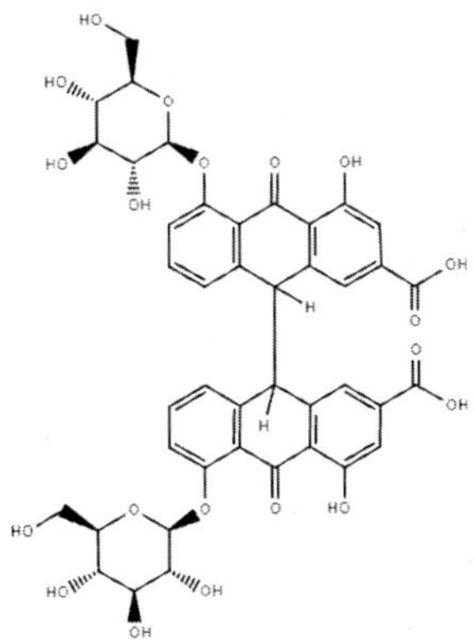

Sennosoid A (trans)

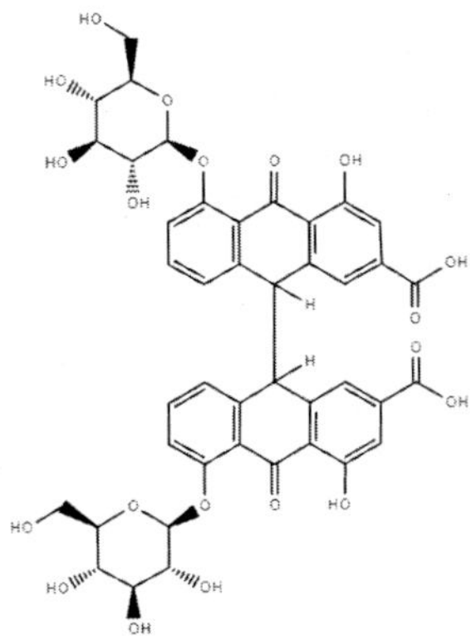

Sennoside B (Meso)

Isolation steps:

Follow the below-mentioned steps for this purpose:

Method 1:

Step 1. Extract the powdered materials with benzene and shake for 2 hours on an electronic shaker.

Step 2. Filter and extract with 70% methanol for 4 - 6 h. Filter it under a vacuum and transfer it to a separate vessel.

Step 3. Re-extract the marc with 70% methanol for 2 hours and filter.

Step 4. Combine the alcoholic extract and concentrate to $1/8^{th}$ of its original volume.

Step 5. Add hydrochloric acid to attain a pH of 3.2.

Step 6. Keep this solution for 2 hours at a temperature of 5 °C. Filter the solution and add anhydrous calcium chloride (dissolved in 25 ml of denatured spirit) to this filtrate with constant and vigorous stirring.

Step 7. Adjust the pH to 8 by adding ammonia and allowing it to stand for 2 h.

Step 8. Filter the solution. You will get precipitation. Dry it over P_2O_5 in a desiccator.

Method 2:

Step 1. Extract the powdered materials with ethanolic chloroform (93 parts chloroform and 7 parts ethanol) for 30 minutes with continuous shaking.

Step 2. Filter it. Add acidic methanol (1.2 g of oxalic acid per liter of methanol) to the marc and extract again.

Step 3. Combine the extracts and concentrate.

Step 4. Keep it overnight at room temperature.

Step 5. Sennoside A will precipitate out while sennoside B will remain in the solution.

Step 6. Add trimethylamine to the solution. It will re-crystallize sennoside A.

Step 7. Add a 10% methanolic solution of $CaCl_2$. It will precipitate sennoside B.

Step 8. You can use a methanolic ammonia solution (40 mL ammonia + 60 mL methanol) for further separation.

Step 9. Dry, wash with water, and keep for one day. Re-crystallize using glycolmonoethylether.

Identification tests: Add benzene, ether, or chloroform to the crude extract and shake. Separate the organic layer and add the ammonia solution. The ammoniacal layer will produce a pink to red color, indicating the presence of anthraquinone glycosides.

4.2.27. Solasodine

Solasodine (an aglycone of steroidal glycoalkaloid) is isolated from many species of the Solanaceae family, including *Solanum incanum* (1.8–2%), *S. khasianum* (1–1.75%), and *S. xanthocarpum*. Hydrolysis yields an aglycone, solasodine, and sugars such as mannose, glucose, and galactose.

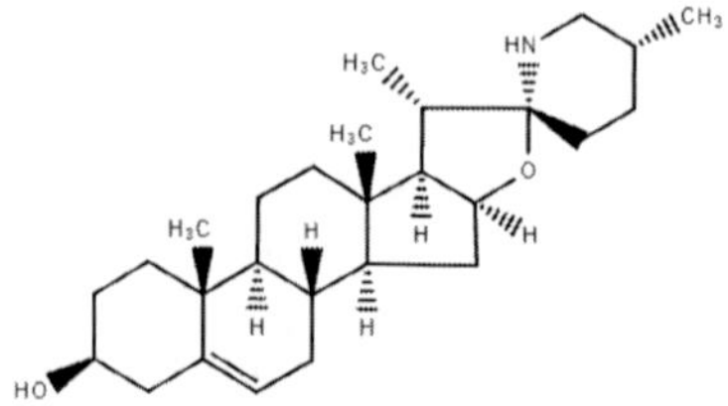

Solasodine

Isolation steps:

Follow the below-mentioned steps for this purpose:

Step 1. Powder the materials and subject them to degrading with petroleum ether. This will provide a greenish-yellow oil. Discard it, as it contains other substances.

Step 2. Extract the defatted material three times with ethyl alcohol and concentrate it to 1/10th of its volume.

Step 3. Add conc. hydrochloric acid to attain a final concentration of about 5-6%.

Step 4. Reflux the whole mass for 6 h to hydrolyze the glycoalkoloid.

Step 5. Add ammonia and re-reflux for 60 minutes; cool; filter and wash with distilled water till neutral pH; and dry the filtrate.

Step 6. Dissolve in chloroform, filter, and evaporate to dryness. It will provide solasodine. Further purify it by crystallizing it from methanol or by sublimation in a high vacuum.

4.2.28. Strychnine and Brucine

Strychnine and brucine are the derivatives of *Strychnos nuxvomica* (family: Loganiaceae).

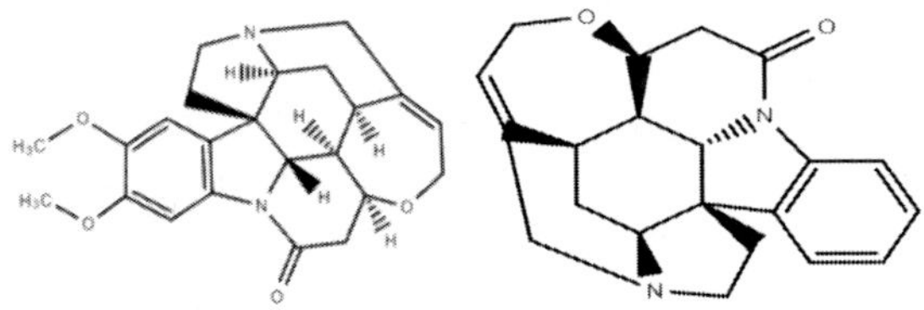

Brucine **Strychnine**

Isolation steps:

Follow the below-mentioned steps for this purpose:

First compound:

Step 1. Take approximately 100 g of powdered materials and mix them with 100 mL of 10% calcium hydroxide in water. Keep it overnight at an ambient temperature.

Step 2. Extract with chloroform in a Soxhlet extractor for 3 hours.

Step 3. Ten extract this extract with 5% sulphuric acid solution several times.

Step 4. Add a 10% aqueous sodium hydroxide solution.

Step 5. Cool and filter the crystals.

Step 6. Add 50% ethanol. Reflux the mixture until most of the solids are dissolved.

Step 7. Add charcoal and filter the solution.

Step 8. Wash it with a small amount of 50% ethanol. This will give you strychnine.

Step 9. (You can use the mother liquor and washings to isolate brucine.) Dissolve the crude strychnine in 9 volumes of boiling water, add a 15% sulphuric acid solution, and stir slowly. It will attain a slightly acidic to Congo-red condition.

Step 10. Add activated charcoal and reflux the solution for 1 hour. Filter the mixture.

Step 11. Cool the solution off. It will give you strychnine sulfate crystals. Filter and wash with cold water.

Step 12. Dissolve the crystals in 15 volumes of water, heat to 80 °C, and neutralize with 10% aqueous sodium carbonate.

Step 13. Add charcoal and filter the hot solution.

Step 14. Add an aqueous sodium carbonate solution. This will precipitate strychnine on cooling.

Step 15. Filter the precipitates, wash with cold water, and re-crystallize using ethanol.

Second compound:

Step 1. Concentrate the mother liquor remaining after the separation of strychnine in vacuo in a water bath. Carry out the process until most of the alcohol is removed.

Step 2. Add dilute sulphuric acid to the residue to attain pH 6.

Step 3. Concentrate the solution to a volume of 3 - 4 mL overnight.

Step 4. Keep it in a refrigerator with the filter off and wash it with cold water.

Step 5. Add 4.5 volumes of hot distilled water and boil with a little charcoal for 1 hour. This will purify brucine sulfate.

Step 6. Filter and keep it in a refrigerator for several days.

Step 7. Recover brucine from the sulfate using the same procedure used for strychnine.

Step 8. Re-crystallize by using an aqueous acetone solution.

Identification tests:

- Treat the sample with sulphovanadic acid. If it contains strychnine, it will produce a purple-red colour.
- Treat with sulphuric acid and crystals of potassium dichromate. If it contains strychnine, it will produce a purple colour. But it will slowly change to red. And brucine gives an immediate red color.
- Treat with nitric acid. If it contains brucine, you will see a blood-red colour. It will be discharged by the addition of stannous chloride solution.

4.2.29. Vasicine

Vasicine (a pyrrolazoquinazoline alkaloid) is isolated form *Adhatoda vasica* leaf (family: Acanthaceae).

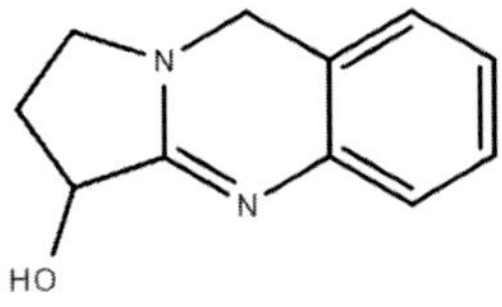

Vasicine

Isolation steps:

Follow the below-mentioned steps for this purpose:

Step 1. Dry leaves, coarsely powder, and basify to pH 9 with an ammonia solution.

Step 2. Extract with chloroform. Combine the chloroform extract, wash with water, and dry over anhydrous sodium sulfate.

Step 3. Evaporate the solvent to get the total alkaloid extract. It contains vasicine as a major alkaloid.

Step 4. Further purification by crystallization.

4.2.30. Vinca Alkaloids

Vinblastine is isolated from *Catharanthus roseus* Linn (family: Apocynaceae).

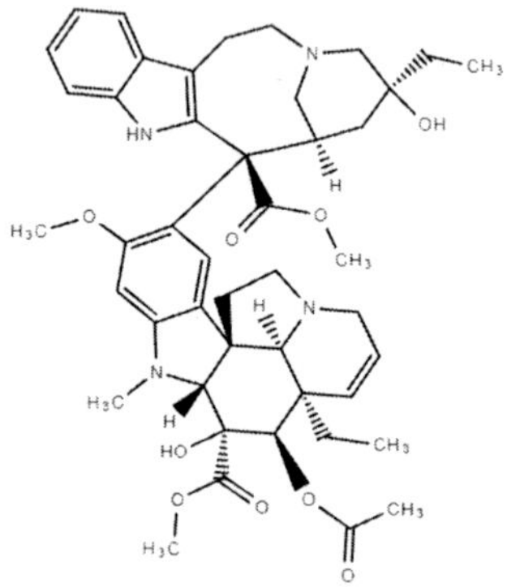

Vinblastine

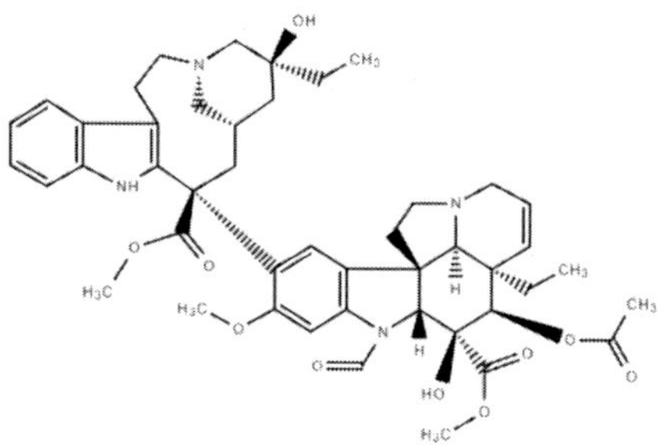

Vincristine

Isolation steps:

Follow the below-mentioned steps for this purpose:

Step 1. Prepare a coarse powder of dried leaf material and extract the hot ethanol-water-acetic acid (9:1:1) mixture.

Step 2. Remove the solvent, add 2% hot hydrochloric acid to the residue, and adjust the pH to 4. This will precipitate non-alkaloidal components.

Step 3. Filter the mixture, adjust the pH to 7, and extract with benzene.

Step 4. Evaporate the benzene layer to obtain vinblastine and other alkaloids.

Step 5. Remove the phenolic materials by washing the extract with dilute alkali.

Step 6. Run chromatography on alumina and carry out elution in 18 fractions, starting with the benzene-methylene chloride (65:35) mixture and ending with pure methylene chloride. This will recover vinblastine in the ninth fraction. Further elution will give you vincristine.

References

Balunas, M. J., & Kinghorn, A. D. (2005). Drug discovery from medicinal plants. *Life sciences*, *78*(5), 431-441.

Chaachouay, N., & Zidane, L. (2021). The practice of herbal medicine to prevent Sars-CoV-2 in Salé, Morocco.

Cheng, R. (1984). Chinese herbalism. *Canadian Family Physician*, *30*, 119.

De Smet, P. A. (2002). Herbal remedies. *New England Journal of Medicine*, *347*(25), 2046-2056.

Ernst, E. (2005). The efficacy of herbal medicine–an overview. *Fundamental & clinical pharmacology*, *19*(4), 405-409.

Wachtel-Galor, S., & Benzie, I. F. (2011). Herbal medicine. *Lester Packer, Ph. D.*, 1.

Wan, Z. L., Guo, J., & Yang, X. Q. (2015). Plant protein-based delivery systems for bioactive ingredients in foods. *Food & Function*, *6*(9), 2876-2889.

Chapter 5

Management of Experimental Animals

5.1. Animal Experimentation

Currently, we use approximately 50 - 100 million animals every year for various experiments. These animals range from zebra fish to non-human primates. These animals are not only used for experimentation; we also use them for higher education and training purposes. Although they have diverse connotations, the terms "animal testing," "animal experiments," "animal study," "*in vivo* studies," and "vivisection" are frequently used synonymously. Dissecting a live animal is known as "vivisection," a term favored by individuals who disagree with using animals for research purposes. "Animal experiments" is the phrase that researchers choose to use (Arrington, 1978).

Animal testing allowed for the biggest drug breakthroughs of the 19 and 20th centuries. Every medical research Nobel Prize awarded during the past century has indeed been based on animal studies. For serum therapy and studies involving the use of horses, the first Nobel Prize in medicine was awarded in 1901. Rapid advancements in animal experimentation and advances in clinical therapy are strongly correlated. Behring utilized horses in the 1880s to produce diphtheria antitoxin and create a diphtheria and tetanus vaccine, which helped him win the first Noble Prize in physiology or medicine in 1901. The discovery of canine insulin in 1922 completely changed how diabetes was treated. Leprosy vaccines and antibiotic treatments were created using armadillos in the 1970s. Prontosil's antibacterial properties were first demonstrated by Domagk in 1939 through tests on chickens (Olfert et al. 1993). Experimental animals used for the discovery of lifesaving drugs are shown in Table 5.1.

Ethical issues are the major concern when conducting an experiment using laboratory animals. So how do we judge the ethical issues of animal experimentation? Thus, you should critically analyze the following ethical issues while using laboratory animals for your studies:

- Suitability of the selected animal for your experiment.
- The need for your study problem to be solved.

Table 5.1. Lifesaving drug discoveries from animals

Drug	Animals used	Scientist	Year
Diphtheria/tetanus antitoxin	Horse	Emil Adlof von Behring	1901
Insulin	Dogs	Frederick, Banting, Macleod	1922
Prontosil	Mice	Gerhard Domagk	1939
Penicillin	Rats	Alexander Fleming	1941
Streptomycin	Chicken	Selman Waksman	1952

- Maximum level you will be able to attain to minimize pain and discomfort for the selected animal for your study.

The laws and regulations applied worldwide for the use of laboratory animals are shown in Table 5.2.

Table 5.2. Laws and regulations worldwide for the use of laboratory animals

Law/Regulation	Year
An act to prevent the cruel and improper treatment of cattle – Martin's act or The act of 1822, UK	1822
Society for the prevention of cruelty to animals (SPCA), UK	1824
America's first animal protection act, outlawing cruelty against cattle, sheep and horses, USA	1828
Royal society for the prevention of cruelty to animals (RSPCA), UK	1840
The society protectrice des animaux (Animal protection society), France	1846
American society for the prevention of cruelty to animals (ASPCA)	1866
Cruelty to animals act of 1876, UK	1876
Victoria street society for the protection of animals from vivisection, UK	1875
American humane association (AHA)	1877
American antivivisection society (AAVS)	1883
British union for the abolition of vivisection (BUAV)	1898
Humane society of the United States (HSUS)	1954
National catholic society for animal rights (International society for animal rights or ISAR)	1954-57
Animal welfare act (Laboratory animal welfare act)	1966
Congress enacts the animal enterprise protection act, USA	1992

5.2. Selection of Laboratory Animals

It is one of the most important steps for animal studies. An animal model must be able to produce a similar disease and response profile as humans. In this case, you should consider the following three objects:

1. Animals should be phylogenetically closer to humans.
2. The process under investigation should be similar to that in humans.
3. The anatomy, physiology, and biochemistry of animals should be closer to humans.

5.3. Most Frequently Used Laboratory Animals

5.3.1. Rodents: Mouse, rat, guinea pig, gerbil, hamster etc.
5.3.2. Non-rodents: Rabbit, monkey, dog, cat, pig etc.
5.3.3. Miscellaneous: Frog, pigeon, zebra fish, chicken etc.

5.3.1. Rodents

Mouse (Mus musculus):

- Smallest rodent used in laboratory studies.
- Easy to maintain and handle.
- Invaluable resource in identifying the several alleles which have further developed in the research of mutagenesis.
- Only known species in that it is possible to grow totipotent embryonic stem cells *in vitro* and form germ lines once reinjected into a developing embryo.

Table 5.3 presents some species of laboratory mice, and Table 5.4 shows the discovery year of some mouse species.

Table 5.3. Some species of lab mice

Region	Species
Asian	Mus cervicolar, Mus cookee, Mus caroli, Mus famulus (India) and Mus fragilicauda (Thailand)
Western Mediterranean	Mus spretus
Eastern Mediterranean and Central Europe	Mus spicilegus, Mus macedonicus
Western Europe and Africa	Mus domesticus
India, Eastern Europe, japan, Russia, Northern China	Mus musculus (common strain Swiss albino mice)

Table 5.4. Discovery of some mice species

Laboratory species	Discoverer (discovery year)
DBA/2	CC Little in 1909
C57BL/6	Miss Lathrop 1919
C3H, CBA and A	LC Strong

- Mice have a high genome similarity to the human genome (>99% conserved). Thus, mice provide a good model for research not only on mammalian biology but also on a wide variety of human diseases like cancer, diabetes, ageing, atherosclerosis, immunological diseases, autoimmune disorders, neurological dysfunction, and other endocrine diseases, as well as several other diseases and disorders.
- Knockout and knock-in mice have been developed for selective study at the genetic level.
- *Nude* mice are hairless genetic mutants that lack a thymus gland.
- *Biege* mice lack natural killer cells and are susceptible to cancer.
- Mice use their tails for thermoregulation.
- Common diseases in mice include salmonellosis, mouse typhoid, small pox, and *streptobacillus* infection.

Rat (Rattus norvegicus):

- These also provide handling and maintenance facilities. But not as economical as the mice.
- Wistar (wide head and long ears, small tail) and Sprague-Dawley (longer and narrower head, long tail) rats are commonly used in biomedical research.
- Albino rat (Pink-eyed White, or PEW) is most likely the very first mutation to be discovered and purposely bred.
- *Nude* rats resemble *nude* mice, lack a thymus and functional T cells, and are phenotypically hairless with possible fine-sparse hair growth. They are the most preferred model in immunological research.
- Rats are preferred for use in behavioral, pharmacology, physiology, neuroscience, immunogenetics, histopathology, transplantation, cancer risk assessment, cardiovascular diseases, and ageing studies. Moreover, these are also used for the evaluation of psychopharmacological agents, toxicity studies, anti-ulcer agents,

liver physiological studies, anti-hypertensive effects, hormonal assays, etc.

- Do not vomit (due to a strong sphincter between the stomach and the esophagus and a lack of vomiting centers).
- Do not have tonsils or a gallbladder.
- Diffuse pancreas, thus not suitable for type 1 diabetes research.
- Coprophagy (eating their own stool).
- Tail helps in body thermoregulation.
- Baby rat has a blunt and broad large head relative to its body, whereas mice have a tringular, small head relative to their body.
- Baby rat has small ears relative to their heads, whereas mice have large ears. Baby rats also have larger hind paws and body ratios than baby mice.
- Tail is thick and shorter than the body length in a baby rat, while mice have a thin, larger, or the same length tail as compared to the body.

Guinea pig (Cava porcellus):

- We use three major varieties in research.
- Herbivorous and eats green foods, seeds, and roots.
- Unable to synthesize the required vitamin C daily; therefore, this vitamin (200 mg to 1 gm/L of drinking water) should be added to their chow.
- Duration of the estrous cycle ranges from 13 - 20 days. Thus, the other 16 days can be further divided into the other stages, such as proestrus, estrus, metestrus, and diestrus.
- Sensitive to various diseases and infections, which makes it suitable for diagnostic research.
- Ideal model for enteric amoebiasis and used for testing hypersensitivity, immune responses, anaphylactic shock, encephalomyelitis, tuberculosis, and ascorbic acid metabolism.
- It is also used to screen local anesthetics, bronchial asthma or bronchodilatory COPD, sensitization studies like egg albumin and horse serum, bioassays of digitalis, histamine, and acetylcholine, and screening of spasmodic and antispasmodic compounds.
- It has high sensitivity to histamin (1000 times more).
- Serum contains asparaginase, which shows antileukemic action.
- Very susceptible to tuberculosis and anaphylactic shock.

- Highly sensitive to penicillin (100 - 1000 times more sensitive than rats).

Gerbil (Meriones unguiculatus):

- One of the few species that were originally developed in Japan as laboratory animals.
- Mongolian gerbil is a small laboratory rodent (length between mice and rats).
- Phenotypically related to rats and also known as 'jirds' or 'sand rats.
- Small size and ease of handling; quite in nature.
- Gerbils require a different type of housing. 5 gallons (1 gallon = 231 cubic inches) are required for each gerbil (USA standard). 15×12×10 tank is ideal for each pair of gerbils (UK standard).
- Gerbils are used in stroke, epilepsy, auditory studies, parasite and bacterial infections, lipid metabolism, and heart disease research.

Hamster (Mesocricetus auratus):

- Brown to gold in color, the third most commonly used biomedical research animal are Syrian hamsters (golden, most commonly used in research), Chinese hamsters (striped back), and European and American hamsters (gray).
- Relatively free from spontaneous disease and susceptible to many introduced pathogenic agents.
- European hamsters are quite larger than other hamsters (300–400 g) and are more suitable for high-concentrated and prolonged smoke inhalation studies than Syrian hamsters.
- American hamsters are used in mutagenic, carcinogenic, and meiosis research.
- Chinese hamsters have the lowest number of chromosomes and are used in cytogenic research.
- Hamsters are used in many studies, such as those on diabetes melitus, dystrophy (e.g., autosomal recessive skeletal muscle degeneration, cardiomyopathy, cardiohypertrophy, and congestive heart failure), cholesterol cholelithiasis or gall stones, polycystic diseases, dental caries, etc.
- A suitable model for the physiology and pathogenesis of Duchenne's dystrophy includes variable sizes of muscle, fibers, and

centrally located nuclei, with fatty infiltration and fibrous connective tissue replacement.

- Suitable model for slow virus (e.g., scrape, chronic measles) type C, oncovirus, influenza virus, respiratory syncytial virus (RSV) research, and vaccine production (e.g., foot and mouth).
- Do not have intact lymphatic drainage, thus can be used in tissue transplants such as tumors and gratis research.
- Allow *in vitro* and *in vivo* studies for the diagnosis of many infectious agents, including *Clostridum* spp., *Leptospirosis* spp., etc.
- They have a characteristic cheek pouch, which is used to collect or transport food materials or any nesting materials.
- They have *whiskers* (also called *vibrissae*) on their faces and sides of their bodies to navigate the surroundings and objects around them, especially at night.

5.3.2. Non-rodents (Mammalians)

Rabbit (Oryctolagus cuniculus):

- Commonly used species are New Zealand white (albinism due to lack of melanin), Dutch, Flemish giant, and so on.
- Rabbits are used in biomedical research, including genetics, nutrition, toxicology, physiology, immunology, and reproduction. New Zealand rabbits are used in diabetes, diphtheria, tuberculosis, cancer, and heart disease research.
- Rabbits are used in human pregnancy tests (by injecting the serum from the patient into the rabbit and thereby inducing ovulation in the doe).
- Rabbits are also used in the evaluation of skin creams, cosmetics, special diets, and food additives.
- Standard animal for pyrogen testing and other toxicological research. Also used in antibodies and antiserum production.
- More homology to humans to inspect diseases and medications.
- A female rabbit (doe) is fertile all year.
- The gestation period ranges from 28 - 31 days.
- Not possible for cervical dislocation as these have short necks.
- It has very simple cardiac connective tissue, free of connective tissue. Thus, it can be used frequently in cardiac research.
- Very sensitive to histamine.

- Do not vomit (like rats and horses).
- Lack of cytochrome 3A4.
- Has atropinesterase that degrades atropine.
- Has ability to taste water (absent in humans and rats).
- Only mammal from which tubules of the kidney can be dissected with the basement membrane intact.
- Lack of vasomoter reversal phenomenon (absence of adrenergic vasodilator nerve).

Monkey (Macaca mulatta):

- More frequently used than dogs and cats.
- Rhesus monkey is commonly found in South Asia.
- Adult body weight: 10 - 12 kg (male) and 8 - 10 kg (female).
- In lab, they are maintained in the gang cages (24 × 30 × 30 for single; 28 × 10 ft for group; 8 females and 1 male can be maintained).
- Diet: 18 - 20% protein, 65 - 70% carbohydrates, 4 - 6% fat, 4 - 5% crude fiber, minerals, and vitamins.
- Widely used as primate models (for pharmacokinetic studies) for the study of drug metabolism as they have a similar pattern to the human metabolic profile.
- Their uterus resembles humans, and they exhibit regular menstrual periods.
- Suitable for studying drugs acting on the CNS (e.g., memory, anxiety, and depression), CVS (e.g., antihypertensive, antianginal), GIT, and fertility.
- Require routine checkups for rabies and tuberculosis and timely immunization.

Dog (Canic familiaris):

- Mongrels and Beagles are the most commonly used types of dogs in research. It has a small gastrointestinal tract and can be trained easily.
- Allow cardiovascular, diabetes melitus, ulcerative colitis, open heart surgery, organ transplantation, CNS, reproduction, and safety pharmacology and toxicology research.
- Stomach and intestinal tract resemble humans.

- Distinct structure of the pancreas.
- May develop spontaneous hypertension resembling humans.
- Cervical sympathetic and vagal nerves are run together; hence, stimulation of the nictitating membrane through preganglionic sympathetic is complicated by central vagal stimulation, causing reflex variations in blood pressure.

Cat (Felis catus):

- Has similar human physiological features and can be used in cardiovascular, behavioral, nerve impulse transmission, toxicology, oncology, and chromosomal abnormality research.
- Allow study of the transmission of vitamins and minerals to the fetus and newborn.
- Have a distinct nictiating membrane and thus can be used in the screening of ganglion-blocking agents.
- It regains its righting reflex even after falling from a high altitude. Therefore, you will not be able to study the loss of the righting reflex by using a cat model.

Pig (Sus scrofa domestica):

- Allows isolated organ tests, skin permeation tests, cardiovascular research (e.g., atherosclerosis, MI), digestive tract studies, etc.
- Suitable for R&D studies in pharmaceutical research.
- Dissimilarities are that they have poorer vascularization than humans and fewer sebaceous glands (only apocrine glands).
- Small size lungs and are susceptible to bronchitis and pneumonia.
- Alimentary tract resembles humans.

5.3.3. Miscellaneous

Zebra fish (Danio rerio):

- In the 1970s, Dr. George Streisinger was considered the "*Father of Zebra Fish Research*" as he invented this model.
- Vertibrates have a backbone like humans.

Table 5.5. Important features of some experimental animals

Character	Experimental animals					
	Mus musculus	*Rattus norvegius*	*Cavia porcellus*	*Mesocricetus auratus*	*Meriones unguiculatus*	*Oryctolagus cuniculus*
BW (g)	18 - 40	150 - 400	600 - 1200	85 - 150	55 - 100	1000 - 3500
Life span (yr)	1.5 - 3	2 - 4	4 - 8	1 - 3	2 - 4	6 - 12
Gestation period (days)	19 - 21	21 - 23	59 - 72	15 - 16	24 - 26	31 - 32
Estrous cycle (days)	4 - 5	4 - 5	15 - 19	4	4 - 6	5 - 14
Rectal temperature (oC)	38 - 39	36 - 40	37 - 40	37 - 38	37 - 38	38 - 40
Heart rate (min)	310 - 840	250 - 450	230 - 380	250 - 500	360	130 - 325
BP (S/D)	133 - 160/ 90 - 110	84 - 134/60	80 - 94/ 55 - 58	150/100	-	90 - 130/ 60 - 90
Blood volume (mL/kg)	58.5	54 - 70	69 - 75	78	66 - 78	57 - 65
Respiratory rate	60 - 220	70 - 115	42 - 104	35 - 135	90	30 - 60
Mating age (weeks)	6 - 8	10 - 12	12 - 20	6 - 8	12	24 - 36

Ref: Medhi B & Prakash A. Practical manual of experimental and clinical pharmacology. Jaypee Brothers Medical Publishers, 2010.

- Allow study of embryo development and genetics.
- Allow it to hatch its eggs outside of the mother's body within 2 - 4 days. A single spawning produces 100 - 200 eggs that are easily collectible.
- Long lifespan (approximately 5 years).
- Length of an adult fish is about 6 cm. Thus, many animals can be accommodated in a single tank.
- Requires aquarium maintenance.
- Not closely related to humans or other experimental animals like mice, rats, etc.
- Genetic modification has yet to be done.

Important features of some experimental animals have been shown in Table 5.5.

5.4. Caring of Laboratory Animals

Rats and mice make up over 95% of all laboratory animals, with mice being utilized in biology and medicine the most frequently. Dogs, cats, nonhuman primates, rabbits, hamsters, guinea pigs, and marine mammals are some other types of laboratory animals. This section will discuss the care of the mice and rats. The personnel responsible for animal care and studies must be diligent in carrying out their responsibilities; responsible; mindful of the health and welfare of the animals; knowledgeable about the proper handling and use of laboratory animals; and highly motivated. Training and supervision are crucial to ensuring that standard operating protocols are constantly followed and that a high standard of animal care is provided. Environmental factors must be carefully managed within research facilities in order to provide the optimal circumstances for performing research, combined with well-implemented systems of animal care and utilization. Proper handling of your laboratory animals can reduce animal pain and distress and improve their welfare. Programs for disease monitoring in colony-maintained mice and rats include any or all of the following:

- Surveillance;
- Assessment of isolation and quarantine;
- Continuous postmortem and clinical evaluation while conducting investigations;

- Perform live sentinel animals and environmental sampling;
- Assessment after the study is finished.

Besides these, you should consider the following important facilities:

5.4.1. Housing

Setting an appropriate micro- or macro-environment for your lab animals requires careful thought. This is because macro-environment facilities and certain types of caging may have quite different micro-environments. The area in cages, pens, or runs should be sufficient to accommodate animals' regular physiological needs, allow for postural modifications, and satisfy the needs of species-specific activity. Social animals that get along well with one another can live together. Primary enclosures ought to be made of sturdy materials, be simple to clean and disinfect, and be fashioned for convenience and security. Transmission of infectious organisms from cage to cage is prevented using static micro-isolation (filter-top) cages and individually ventilated cage (IVC) systems. Avoid contaminated environments, shared feeding or watering equipment, research apparatus, and other similar things to prevent the horizontal or vertical transmission of infection. Figure 5.1 presents a typical standard animal cage.

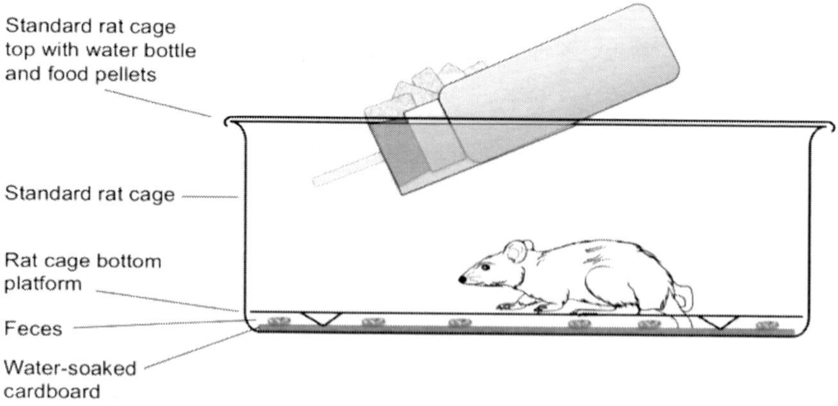

Figure 5.1. A typical standard animal cage

To reduce the amount of heat, dust, allergens, and foul odors that are emitted into the wider area, make sure that each person gets clean ventilation. Unless prohibited by experimental or behavioral requirements, some larger laboratory animals, like dogs, need to exercise frequently and should have sensory contact with other dogs. Nonhuman primates need enriched social and environmental environments in order to maintain psychological health that is compatible with experimental and real-world housing requirements.

The following factors should always be properly adjusted and monitored as needed: temperature, relative humidity, ventilation rates, lighting conditions (spectrum, intensity, and photoperiod), gaseous contaminants (such as ammonia), and noise. The comfort, health, and metabolism of animals can all be significantly impacted by unstable environmental conditions, which can also have an impact on the accuracy of the results of experiments. In general, the air temperature should be set to +/-2°F from the set point and should be in the 64 to 73°F (18 to 22°C) comfort zone where human workers perform best. For the majority of species, relative humidity should be kept between 30 and 70%, ideally within 10% of the target point. On the other hand, ventilation rates of between 10 and 15 fresh air changes per hour are ideal. Recirculating air is generally discouraged unless it has been cleaned to remove particles and gaseous impurities.

Animal welfare and circadian rhythmicity are supported by evenly distributed, suitably powerful lighting, which also enables staff to view the animals and carry out all maintenance and husbandry tasks in a secure manner.

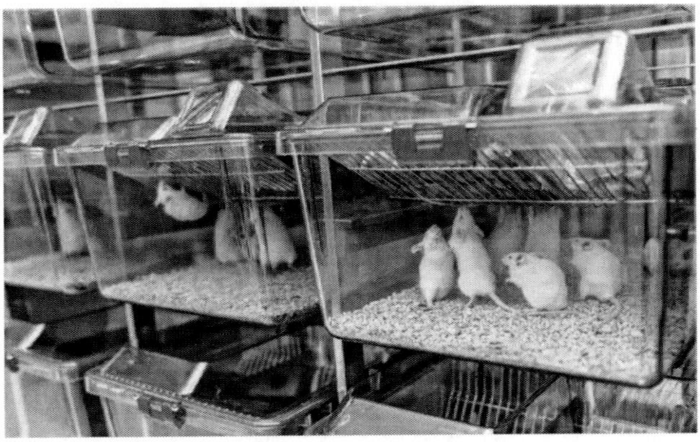

Figure 5.2. Laboratory animal housing cages

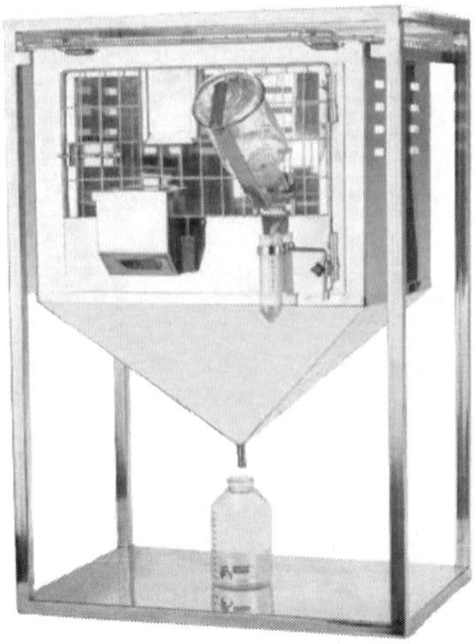

Figure 5.3. A typical single metabolic cage for animal studies

To sustain circadian and neuroendocrine regulation, diurnal or day-night cycles should be managed by automatic timers, depending on the needs of the species. Although cool, white fluorescent lighting has been used for decades and offers many benefits to consumers, the advent of LED lighting may have the greatest impact on experiments involving circadian rhythms since the decades-old removal of windows and seasonal sunshine exposure from institutions used for animal research. Figure 5.2 shows laboratory animal housing cages, and Figure 5.3 shows a typical metabolic cage for animal studies.

5.4.2. Bedding

Animal bedding is a modifiable environmental component that may affect the results of experiments and the welfare of the animals. Materials for bedding should be non-irritating, absorbent, free of infections and chemicals, and unappealing enough to inhibit digestion. A sufficient quantity is necessary to keep animals dry and clean between bedding and crate changes.

Rodents are the group of mammals that are kept most frequently in contact bedding, which is typically made of virgin cellulose, recycled paper, heat-treated softwood shavings, hardwood chips, or pulverized corncobs. Untreated softwoods are not recommended because they contain volatile oils that may alter hepatic enzyme systems and affect various types of investigations. The microbiome, the tactile sense, the reproduction process, behavior, physiology, mucosal immunity, nutritional research, and environmental microbes are all impacted by bedding.

The potential of bedding materials to inhibit the production of ammonia, the most prevalent and harmful gas in the micro-environment which is a consequence of the fecal bacterial urease catalysis of urea, also varies depending on their vitamin C and phytoestrogen content. Bedding can either be used as-is or sanitized before use using an autoclave or radiation, depending on the needs of the research. Mice are kept in the greatest numbers on contact bedding; they favor soft materials and those that may be used for nesting and burrowing in large quantities. These materials are supplemented with enrichment that supports these and other typical behaviors. Figure 5.4 shows how a mother *Swiss* mouse and her newborns are using standard bedding materials.

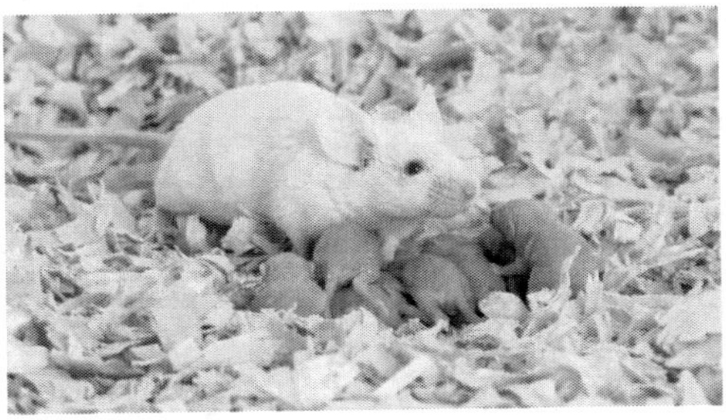

Figure 5.4. A mother *Swiss* mouse with her newborns

5.4.3. Feeding

Your animal feed (Figure 5.5: A typical standard animal feed) must have a fresh and adequate shelf life, be palatable, contamination-free, uniformly constituted, or have a balanced diet, be easily accessible, and be manufactured specifically for research animals. The shelf life of diets should be 9 months (if kept at or below 70 °F (21 °C) and 50% relative humidity). Certain vitamins, including vitamin C, can be added to diets as supplements. To prevent obesity and reduce waste, feed levels for rabbits, laboratory carnivores, swine, aquatic amphibians, and monkeys may be capped at measured amounts each day. Animals used in laboratories often consume 4 - 6% of their body weight in food each day. If you are using professionally produced food for your lab animals, quality control reports might be useful.

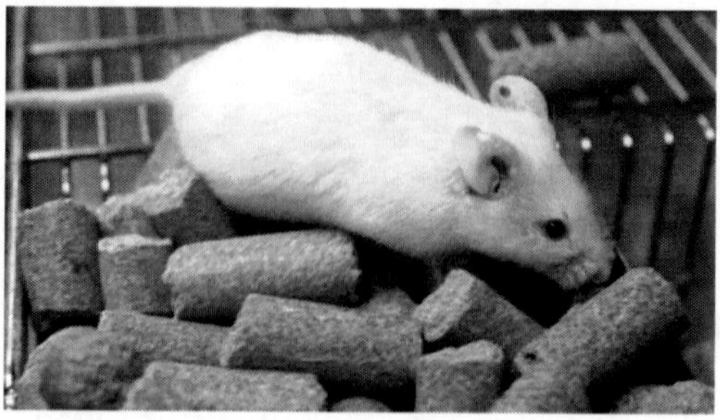

Figure 5.5. A *Swiss* mouse having standard food

5.4.4. Water

Water from a local or home source should be sufficient, potable, and uncontaminated and meet broad guidelines suitable for human consumption. Keep in mind that variations in regular drinking water have a significant impact on research findings. A typical water treatment plant should feature high-quality recycling, storage, and distribution facilities in addition to well-designed softening, deionization, and extra purification systems. The water used for laboratory animals should be tested for pH, hardness, chemical content, and microbial load. Water that has been acidified, chlorinated, or sterilized may be necessary in some experimental or husbandry situations.

Water is typically made available on demand (*ad libitum*) in bottles, plastic pouches, automated delivery systems, and, in some cases, nonwetting, and sterile gels. The risk of hypothermia, drowning, or dehydration for cage occupants as a result of the in-cage water delivery valve failing is the disadvantage of using an automatic drinking water supply for rodents.

Water quality is the most significant environmental factor for aquatic animals and a major factor in determining health. Poor water quality or temperature swings are physiologic stresses that have an effect on food intake, digestion, and utilization, change the immune system, and increase the risk of opportunistic infection. Nitrite, ammonia, and chlorine should not be present in water used for aquatic vertebrates, and the total coliform count should not be more than 200/mL. The pH of this kind of water should range from 6.5 to 8.5. Figure 5.6 presents a typical standard water feder (supply) for laboratory animals.

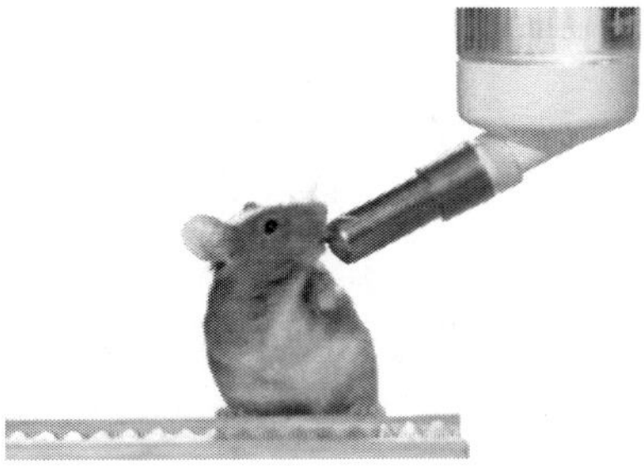

Figure 5.6. Water feeder for laboratory animals

5.4.5. Sanitation

Maintain clean, appropriate facilities for your experimental animals. Typically, one to three changes per week are sufficient for rodents kept in solid-bottom cages; every other week should be sufficient for mice kept in vented cage systems; and rodents, rabbits, and nonhuman primates kept in suspended cages over excreta pans. Excreta and filthy bedding should be removed daily from larger animals' primary enclosures, which should also be cleaned and sterilized at least once every two weeks. Water bottles and other feeding supplies must be cleaned and sterilized at least once a week. Robotic watering techniques can be designed and set up to flush constantly or often, but only if they are manually drained, cleaned, and disinfected at regular, frequent intervals. By heating cages and other equipment to 180 °F (82.2 °C), hazardous nonspore-forming microorganisms (e.g., bacteria and viruses) can be destroyed. They can also be destroyed by using the appropriate chemical disinfectants, such as hypochlorite solutions. All cages and other equipment need to be properly rinsed after using detergents or disinfectants. Regular evaluations of the sanitation programs' efficacy should be conducted using the appropriate microbiologic, organic material detection systems, or other techniques.

5.4.6. Vermin Control

Take the required actions to detect, avoid, and control escaped, feral, or wild rodents (Figure 5.7). Use no insecticides on the bedding of animals. Use relatively inert compounds to manage crawling insects, such as cockroaches such as silica aerogel or boric acid powder.

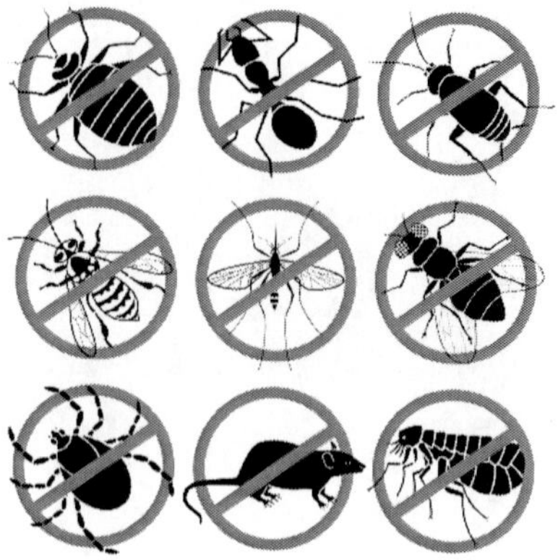

Figure 5.7. Some common enemies for laboratory animals

References

Arrington, L. R. (1978). Introductory laboratory animal science. The breeding, care and management of experimental animals. *Introductory Laboratory Animal Science. The Breeding, Care and Management of Experimental Animals.*, (2nd edition).

Olfert, E. D., Cross, B. M., & McWilliam, A. A. (Eds.). (1993). *Guide to the care and use of experimental animals* (Vol. 1, No. 2). Ottawa: Canadian Council on Animal Care.

Chapter 6

Acute Toxicity Study and Dose Determination

6.1. Acute Toxicity Study

Oral administration of basic plant medicine formulations has long been practiced. According to OECD guidelines, acute oral toxicity is assessed using a limit dose of 5 g/kg for experimental animals (such as mice or rats), while the control animal receives distilled water. At the first, second, fourth, and sixth hours after treatment, the animals are examined for toxicity and deaths. Each group's observed 24-hour mortality is noted (Robinson et al. 2008).

Following that, animals in groups of five are given doses that are either less than the limit dosage if the limit dose is not effectively tolerated or larger than the limit dose if it is effectively tolerated. For an extra seven days, they are monitored every day for any signs of delayed toxicity. By reading the associated probit units, the percentage death values are transformed into probit values, which are then plotted versus log dosage. As a result, the probit value that matches probit 5 or 50% is used to graphically determine the median lethal dose (LD_{50}). Prior to the treatment phase, during the treatment course, and following the treatment course, the animals' body weights are noted. The average body weights of the group are also computed. After fasting for 16–18 hours, all remaining animals that have received at least three doses are killed; two out of each group are sacrificed for necropsy analysis. The internal organs are excised and weighed.

Histopathological analysis carries out gross pathological examinations of the tissues. A solution of 1% chlorose in 25% urethrane (w/v) (5 mL/kg) is administered to induce anesthesia. The heart is used to draw blood for hematological and biochemical examinations. Utilizing a computerized weighing balance from Mettler-Toledo GmbH, internal organs are removed, prepared, and weighed. The organs (e.g., liver, kidney, and heart) of the animals are fixed in a 10% formalin solution in clearly labeled bottles and processed routinely for histopathological evaluation. Using a conventional light microscope, tissues fixed in paraffin wax are sectioned into 5 μm-thick pieces, stained with hematoxylin and eosin, and mounted on glass slides. See the *toxicity analysis* section for more details.

6.2. Hippocratic Analysis

This is the symptomatologic analysis of experimental animals after receiving the test sample, especially at an acute dose. It is frequently performed during the LD_{50} determination of crude extracts in the field of drug discovery and development. A gross physical analysis is done in this case, as shown in Table 6.1.

Table 6.1. Hippocratic parameters for animal studies (Molone and Robichaud 1962)

Symptoms	Animals				
	1	2	3	4	5
Motor activity					
Body tremors					
Ataxia					
Analgesia					
Anesthesia					
Pupil size					
Lacrimation					
Corneal reflex					
Pineal reflex					
Screen grip loss					
Paralysis neck					
Paralysis front legs					
Paralysis hind legs					
Respiratory rate					
Dyspnea (shortness of breath)					
Respiratory depth					
Startle sensitivity (towards bursts of noise or tones)					
Convulsions					
Fasciculation					
Ptosis					
Body motions					
Cyanosis					
Chromodacryorrhea (red tears)					
Salivation					
Tail erection					
Micturition					
Diarrhea					
Abdominal grip					
Hyperemia					
Body temperature					

(+): Present; (-): Absent.

6.3. Lethal Dose Fifty (LD_{50}) Calculation

LD_{50} means the dose that causes fifty percent (50%) of experimental animals' deaths. In an acute toxicity study, if the animals at the limit dose do not display obvious poisoning symptoms, including weariness, paw licking, loose stools, salivation, writhing, and decreased appetite, as well as noticeable changes in physical activity (See *Hippocratic analysis* section), there is a substantial difference between the LD_{50} of your extract in animals and the percentage of deaths up to 3 days after treatment. The different extracts are then given additional doses up to a maximum of 1920 mg/kg (p.o.).

6.4. Selection of Test Dose/Concentration

For study dose selection, see the *LD_{50} calculation* section (OECD, 2008; Ogbuehi et al. 2015). In most cases, for intraperitoneal doses, medicinal scientists use one tenth (1/10) of the orally used dose. For the *in vitro* studies, you can convert the dose (i.e., mg/kg) to a test concentration (i.e., μM or μg/mL).

6.5. Conversion of Human Dose to Experimental Animal Dose

A series of studies, including animal studies, are conducted during the development of new drugs. In this case, dose conversion from humans to animals or vice versa is done. In this regard, researchers face trouble figuring out the right dose for their study due to misunderstandings of dose conversion for a target route of administration, particularly when they estimate the initial dose in clinical or animal investigations to look into efficacy, toxicity, and causes. Therefore, a better understanding of the appropriate dose calculation is crucial. The animal dose should not be extrapolated to humans by a simple conversion method based only on body weight (BW), because many studies suggest the normalization method is based mainly on body surface area (BSA). In general, the BSA seems to have a good correlation among species with several parameters, including oxygen utilization, caloric expenditure, basal metabolism, blood volume, and circulating plasma protein. Likewise, a safety factor should be taken into consideration while deciding the high dose in an animal toxicology study (Shin et al. 2010). The aim of this section is to depict the dose conversion of test drugs from humans to other animals or vice versa.

6.5.1. Human Equivalent Dose (HED) Calculation Based on Body Surface Area

The dose of a drug depends on some crucial factors, including the administration route, differences between metabolisms, the volume of distribution, clearance, basal metabolic rate, etc. Therefore, before converting a human dose to an experimental animal dose, it is important to know the pathophysiology and above-mentioned matters of that animal.

The accurate conversion of a mg/kg dose to a mg/m^2 dose depends on the actual BW of the species. Surface area has generally been calculated in formulae for converting doses as mg/m^2 = km × mg/kg. The km factor is not constant for any species but increases as BW increases. The km factor was calculated for a range of BW using km = 100/K × $W^{0.33}$, where K is a value unique to each species). HED can be calculated using the following formula.

HED (mg/kg) = Animal dose (mg/kg) × (Animal km ÷ Human km)

For *example*, suppose the effective dose in mice is 1000 mg/kg. HED (mg/kg) = 1000 mg/kg × (3/37) = 81.1 mg/kg (4.866 g/day = for an adult human weighing 60 kg) in humans. Suppose the clinically effective dose is 200 mg/kg. Animal dose (mg/kg) = 200 mg/kg × (37/3) = 2466 mg/kg in rats.

This can be calculated simply using the conversion factor in following table.

Animal dose (mg/kg) = HED (mg/kg) × Conversion factor

Example, suppose clinical effective dose is 200 mg/kg in human

Dose for mice = 200 × 12.33 = 2466 mg/kg

For a X gm mouse, dose = {Animal dose (mg/kg) × X} ÷ 1000

Example: If animal dose is 2466 mg/kg, for a 30 gm mouse, dose = (2466 × 30) ÷ 1000 = 73.98 mg

HED (mg/kg) = Animal dose (mg/kg) ÷ Conversion factor

For *example*, suppose effective dose in mice is 1000 mg/kg

HED (mg/kg) = 1000 ÷ 12.33 = 81.1 mg/kg

For a X kg human, dose = {HED (mg/kg) × X kg}

Example: If HED is 81.1 mg/kg, an adult human (60 kg), dose = 81.1 × 60 = 4866 mg

HED can be calculated from the formula as follows.

HED (mg/kg) = Animal dose (mg/kg) × {Animal weight (kg) ÷ Human weight (kg)}$^{0.33}$

Table 6.2 presents conversion factors for dose calculation for some animals.

Table 6.2. Conversion factors for dose calculation of some animals

Species	Body weight (kg)	Working weight range (kg)	Body surface area (m^2)	km factor	Conversion factor
Human adult	60		1.6	37	-
Human child	20		0.8	25	1.48
Baboon	12	7 - 23	0.06	20	1.85
Dog	10	5 - 17	0.5	20	1.85
Monkey	3	1.4 - 4.9	0.24	12	3.08
Rabbit	1.8	0.9 - 3.0	0.15	12	3.08
Guinea pig	0.4	0.208 - 0.7	0.05	8	4.63
Rat	0.15	0.08 - 0.27	0.025	6	6.17
Hamster	0.08	0.047 - 0.157	0.02	5	7.40
Mouse	0.02	0.011 - 0.034	0.007	3	12.33

In practice, the maximum recommended starting dose for a clinical trial should be determined by dividing the HED derived from the animal's NOAEL (No observed adverse effect level determination) by the safety factor. The historically accepted *default safety factor* value is 10. However, a safety factor of 10 may not be appropriate for all cases.

1. Maximum recommended starting dose for clinical trails = HED/Safety factor
2. Estimating a high dose in animal toxicity study = Animal dose × Safety factor

6.6. Drug, Dose and Route of Administration for Chicken/Poultry

Chicks or chickens are also sometimes used for drug screening studies. Examples of some drugs and their doses and routes of administration are shown in the following table. Many studies suggest that a mouse dose can be used for 3–7-day-old chicks in drug screenings. Table 6.3 shows examples of some drugs with their doses and routes of administration.

The most common method to calculate the dose for chickens is based on BSA. This is calculated by using the following formula:

BSA (cm^2) = (weight (kg)^(0.67)) × 7,500

Once the BSA has been calculated, the dose can be determined by multiplying the human dose by the BSA ratio of a chicken to a human. For example, if the human dose is 100 mg and the BSA ratio is 0.06, the dose for chicken should be 100 × 0.06 = 6 mg.

6.7. Test Dose/Concentration Related Ques

Q1. What is a dilution factor?

Ans.

It is the total volume of solution per aliquot volume.

DF = (Aliquot volume + Diluent volume) ÷ Aliquot volume

i.e., DF = Vf ÷ Vi or Cf ÷ Ci

For example, DF 10 stands for a 1:10 dilution, i.e., 1 part solute is dissolved in 9 parts of diluent to attain a total of 10 parts.

Q2. How would you make 400 mL of a 1:200 dilution?

Ans.
In this case, your total volume is 400 mL and your DF is 200.
We know that, DF = Vf ÷ Vi
Therefore, 200 = 400 ÷ Vi or Vi = 400 ÷ 200 = 2

It means you should start with a diluent of 398 mL and add 2 mL of aliquot to it to attain the final volume of 400 mL.

Q3. How to prepare a vehicle containing 0.05% Tween-80 in a 0.9% NaCl solution?

Ans.
Step 1: Dissolve 0.9 g (900 mg) NaCl solid crystals in 100 mL distilled water.
Step 2: Remove 500 μL of this solution's aliquot. Then add 500 μL of Tween-80 to your 100 mL NaCl solution.

Q4. How to make 1000 mL of PBS?

Ans.
PBS means phosphate-buffered saline. This isotonic solution is used in many biological investigations. It contains NaCl (137 mM), KCl (2.7 mM), Na_2HPO_4 (10 mM), and KH_2PO_4 (1.8 mM). Typically, you may need to maintain its pH at 7.4. To make 1000 mL of PBS, you should mix 100 mL of 10× PBS with 900 mL of distilled water.

Q5. How to make 10 mL of a 250 μg/mL suspension of a crude extract?

Ans.
Step 1. Take/select an appropriate vehicle for your extract. Most often, we use DMSO, Tween-20, or 80 for preparing suspensions or emulsions of organic extracts.
Step 2. 250 μg/mL means 1 mL should have 250 μg extract. Therefore, add 250 × 10 μg of your crude extract to 10 mL of vehicle.

Q6. How to prepare 10 mL of a 500 mg/kg oral dose? Consider that you have been recommended to administer a 10 mL/kg dose to your laboratory animals.

Ans.

For a 10 mL/kg oral (p.o.) dose, you will be able to administer 10 mL volume to 1 kg or 1000 g of body weight (b.w.) of your experimental animals. Therefore, 0.01 mL should be given to 1 g b.w. of animals.

On the other hand, a 500 mg/kg (p.o.) dose means that you will need to administer 0.5 mg of drug to 1 g bw of animals.

In this case, 0.01 mL ≡ 1 g b.w. ≡ 0.5 mg

Thus, you should add 0.5 mg to 0.01 mL of vehicle, i.e., 50 mg in 10 mL.

Q7. Suppose you have a 2 mL ampule containing 10 mg of diazepam. You have been recommended to administer a 10 mL/kg dose at a dose of 2 mg/kg to your laboratory animals. How can you prepare a stock solution for your study?

Ans.

In this case, each mL consists of 5 mg of diazepam.

2 mg can be administered to 1000 g b.w.

Therefore, 0.01 mL ≡ 1 g (b.w.) ≡ 2 μg

Assume that you have a total animal weight of 500 g.

Thus, you should prepare a 500 × 0.01 = 5 mL sample solution, which should contain 500 × 2 = 1000 μg of diazepam. Thus, add 200 μL of diazepam from the ampule to 4.8 mL of WFI or sterile distilled water.

Table 6.3. Examples of some drugs with their dose and route of administration

Drug	Dose (mg)	Route	Drug	Dose (mg)	Route
Acyclovir	10/kg	IM	Metoclopramide	50/kg	IP
Amikacin sulphate	20/kg	IM	Methotrexate	0.2/kg	PO
Amoxicillin	16/kg	PO	Methohexital sodium	5 - 10/kg	IV
Amoxicillin Sodium + Clavulanate potassium	500/L	Drink	Metronidazole	30 - 110/kg	PO
Amprolium	40 - 250/kg	Feed	Monensin Sodium	100/kg	Feed
Apramycin	500/L	Drink	Narasin	60 - 80/kg	Feed
Bambermycin	3.3/kg	Feed	Neomycin Sulfate	11/kg	Drink
Ceftiofur sodium	0.16/kg	IM	Nicarbazin	20 - 50/kg	Feed
Chloramphenicol	50/kg	IM	Nitrofurazone	55/kg	Feed
Chlordiazepoxide	2.5 - 15/kg	IM	Nitromide	250/kg	Feed
Chlortetracycline HCl	1500/2500/L	Drink/Feed	Norfloxacin	8 - 10/kg	PO
Chlortetracycline HCl	20-60/kg	PO	Nosiheptide	5 - 10/kg	Feed
Chlortetracycline HCl	220/kg	Feed	Oxytetracycline	25000/L	Drink
Ciprofloxacin HC	5/kg	PO	Penicillin	44 KIU	PO
Clonidine	0.10 - 0.25/kg	IM	Pentobarbital Sodium	16.2/kg	IM
Clopidol	125 - 250/kg	Feed	Paracetamol	150/kg	PO
Decoquinate	30/kg	Feed	Propolis	30/kg	NL
Detomidine HC	0.3/kg	IM	Robenidine HCl	33/kg	Feed
Dibutyltin Dilaurate	200/kg	Feed	Salinomycin	0.006 - 60/kg	Feed
Diclazuril	0.5 - 1.0/kg	Feed	Sarafloxacin HCl	8-10/kg	PO
Dimethyl Sulfoxide	Mix: 50:50/kg	Topical	Semduramycin	NL	PO
Dinitolmide	40 - 187/kg	Feed	Spectinomycin HCl	5/500 - 2000/L	SC/Drink
Doxycycline	20/kg	PO	Streptomycin Sulfate	25 - 50/ 50 - 100/kg	IM/PO
Enrofloxacin	10/kg	Drink	Sulfadimethoxine	500/L	Drink
Erythromycin	100 - 200/L	Drink	Sulfamethazine	1000/L	Drink
Fluconazole	100/kg	PO	Sulfanitran	300/kg	Feed

Table 6.3. (Continued)

Drug	Dose (mg)	Route	Drug	Dose (mg)	Route
Fluoxetine	1 - 15/kg	IM	Sulfaquinoxaline	170/L	Drink
Halofuginon HBr	3000/Ton	Feed	Sulfaquinoxaline + Diaveridine	500 - 550/kg	Feed
Imipramine	1 - 15/kg	IM	Thiabendazole	44/kg	PO
Itraconazole	10/kg	PO	Thiopental Sodium	16.2/kg	IM
Ketamine HC	20 - 100/kg	IM	Tiamulin	250/L	Drink
Ketorolac	20/kg	IM	Tiletamine + Zolazepam	30/kg	IM
Lasalocid	75/kg	Feed	Tilmicosin	75/L	Drink
Lincomycin HCl + Spectinomycin HCl	50/kg	PO	Toltrazuril	6/kg	PO
Maduramicin	5/53/kg	Feed/IM	Trimethoprim + Sulfadiazine	44 - 62/kg	Drink
Maprotiline	2.5 - 20/kg	IM	Tylosin	250 - 500/L	Drink
Medetomidine HCl	0.06 - 0.08/kg	Parenteral	Valnemulin	500/L	Drink

IM: Intra-muscular; IP: Intra-peritoneal; IV: Intra-venous; PO: Per-oral; NL: Not listed; L: Liter.

References

Molone, M. H., & Robichaud, R. C. A. (1962). Hippocratic screen for pure or crude drug. *Lloydia*, *25*, 320-332.

OECD: Guidelines for the testing of chemicals; Acute oral toxicity: up and down procedures. OECD Publishing; 2008. http://www.oecdbookshop.org, No 425.

Ogbuehi, I. H., Ebong, O. O., & Obianime, A. W. (2015). Oral acute toxicity (LD50) study of different solvent extracts of Abrus precatorius Linn leaves in wistar rats. *European Journal of Experimental Biology*, *5*(1), 18-25.

Robinson, S., Delongeas, J. L., Donald, E., Dreher, D., Festag, M., Kervyn, S., Lampo, A., Nahas, K., Nogues, V., Ockert, D., Quinn, K., Old, S., Pickersgill, N., Somers, K., Stark, C., Stei, P., Waterson, L., & Chapman, K. (2008). A European pharmaceutical company initiative challenging the regulatory requirement for acute toxicity studies in pharmaceutical drug development. *Regulatory Toxicology and Pharmacology*, *50*(3), 345-352.

Shin, J. W., Seol, I. C., & Son, C. G. (2010). Interpretation of animal dose and human equivalent dose for drug development. *Journal of Korean Oriental Medicine*, *31*(3), 1-7.

Chapter 7

Administration Route Selection

7.1. Route of Administration and Its Impacts on Drug Screening

Route of administration refers to the method by which a drug is introduced into the body. Different routes of administration can have varying impacts on drug screening and how drugs are detected in the body (Ator et al. 2006). The route of administration can influence drug screening in several ways:

1. *Detection time*: The time it takes for a drug or its metabolites to be detectable in body fluids or tissues can vary depending on the route of administration. Some routes may lead to faster detection, while others may have a delayed appearance in drug screening tests.
2. *Metabolism*: Different routes of administration can affect how a drug is metabolized in the body. The metabolism can influence the detectability of the parent drug and its metabolites in drug screening tests.
3. *Drug concentration*: The route of administration can impact the peak concentration of the drug in the body. Drugs administered intravenously or inhaled may reach higher concentrations quickly, making them easier to detect in drug screening.
4. *Sensitivity of drug tests*: The sensitivity of drug screening tests can vary for different routes of administration. Some tests may be more suitable for detecting certain drugs or their metabolites depending on how they are administered.

Therefore, it is important to consider the route of administration when interpreting drug screening results and understanding the potential impacts on detection windows and test sensitivity. Additionally, individual variations in drug metabolism and other factors can also influence drug screening outcomes.

7.2. Different Routes of Drug Administration

Additional care should be taken while administering test samples to experimental animals (e.g., rodents and mammals) to minimize potential adverse events and the loss of drug samples (Turner et al. 2011).

7.2.1. Oral Route

In general, we choose the oral route for plant-based crude sample analysis in animals because traditional practitioners use it for the folk administration of crude drugs in animals, including humans. Although non-sterile and large volumes (10 - 20 mL/kg) of drugs can be administered orally, they may suffer from first-pass effects, reducing efficacy; slower onset of action due to polarity differences; palatability complications or local irritation; interference or degradation of digestive tract environment substances; inapplicability for unconscious conditions; or produce diarrhea or emesis. On the other hand, the intravenous route is efficient for drug absorption as it makes drugs available directly into the systemic circulation without resulting in first-pass effects or enzymatic interferences caused by organs. However, only very small volumes (2 to 3 mL/kg) are possible to administer via this route.

7.2.2. Intraperitoneal and Intravenous Routes

It is another commonly used route in laboratory rodents other than larger mammals in preclinical studies. For small species, it is difficult to administer drugs via an intravenous route. In this regard, we use the intraperitoneal route to administer slightly larger volumes of fluid safely. However, the intravenous approach usually results in a slower rate of drug absorption. Despite the fact that this route is regarded as a parenteral route, in pre-clinical studies, we can use non-sterilized drug samples via this route. The hepatic metabolism of an intraperitoneally injected sample could occur before it reaches the vascular system. Additionally, an intraperitoneal injectate could pass in very small amounts through tiny lacunae in the diaphragm and into the thoracic lymph node.

7.2.3. Topical Route

The absorption rate of a drug sample topically applied on skin depends on: the surface area occupied by the test sample; the dose applied; the lipid solubility profile of the sample or the vehicle used; the contact period of the applied drug; and the nature of the skin surface (e.g., intact, thickness, degree of hydration, surface occlusion). For example, the specialized skin layers of fish may restrict or reduce the penetration capacity of a test sample. Irritation, sensitivity, or allergic phenomena are commonly observed adverse events on this route. Moreover, it also limits the volume of administration and the rapid onset of action of drugs. The transdermal or percutaneous method, in contrast, could be a desirable substitute for the other parenteral routes because it offers continuous serum levels of the chemical being supplied, eliminating the need for recurrent animal restraint, uncomfortable injections, and sharp dangers. Irritation and skin sensitization may occur in this case.

7.2.4. Subcutaneous Route

Nonirritating substances are given subcutaneously to animals. This approach provides a quick, low-cost, and straightforward way to administer parenteral medication. However, compared to other parenteral methods, drugs given subcutaneously are frequently absorbed more slowly, producing a persistent impact. Subcutaneous administration may involve injections into adequately sized osmotic minipumps and perhaps other implanted pumps that are thereafter surgically placed into such a subcutaneous pocket, depots of oily substances for slow absorption, solid pellets, or aqueous or oily fluids. Large volumes can be administered through this delivery route. It is because the kidneys quickly eliminate extra subcutaneous fluid. Before administering an injection, filling a syringe with a small-gauge needle via a thick rubber stopper may dull the needle's sharpness and make the procedure more painful. Subcutaneous injection of contaminated chemicals frequently causes abscess development.

7.2.5. Intramuscular Route

In small animals, administering test samples intramuscularly is a rare parenteral route. However, it results in the uniform and rapid absorption of drugs due to the rich vascular supply. Compared to subcutaneous delivery, smaller quantities are given intramuscularly. In contrast to subcutaneous injection, this approach requires greater skill and should only be used by professionals. Paresis, paralysis, muscle necrosis, and localized muscle sloughing can occur as a result of irritating drugs injected intramuscularly or accidental nerve injections. Repeated injections may cause muscular necrosis and inflammation.

7.2.6. Intrathecal Route

Substances may be injected into the spinal cord's epidural or subarachnoid (intrathecal) area for quick effects on the cerebrospinal tissues or meninges. With this method, the blood-brain barrier's absorptive issues are avoided. This route is not used for small animals. It is frequently employed to provide contrast media or induce spinal anesthesia in order to visualize larger animals' vertebral bodies or the spinal cord. Large volumes cannot be administered via this delivery strategy.

7.2.6. Intranasal and Intratracheal Routes

To reduce struggle and sneezing during intranasal and intratracheal delivery, animals are typically sedated or anesthetized in research settings. To reduce the risk of asphyxia and death, intranasal doses are typically smaller than those given via other routes. In animals displaying symptoms of conjunctivitis or rhinitis, the approach might not be effective. In a sedated animal, intranasal delivery is straightforward to learn and execute. In order to reduce sneezing, post-treatment rhinitis, and epistaxis, medications given through this mode of administration should be non-irritating. Both local (such as vaccinations or decongestant sprays) and systemic drug delivery can be accomplished using intranasal approaches. Due to its rich vascularization and the lining of the nasal cavity, its mucosa promotes quick drug absorption and consequent systemic effects while avoiding the hepatic first-pass impact related to oral drug delivery. Medicines delivered intranasally may have blood drug levels that are similar to those reported after systemic administration because small, lipophilic compounds are absorbed quicker by this route than big, highly polar molecules. Since the lung has a huge surface area and a rich capillary network, absorption from this area occurs quickly. The most frequent method for giving drugs to fish is intrapulmonary administration. Table 7.1 shows recommended doses according to route of administration for some lab animals.

Table 7.1. Recommended dosages according to route of administration for some lab animals

Route	Species	Dose
Oral	Mammals	5 - 20 mL/kg
	Fish	2 g/kg
Intravenous	Rodents, rabbits	Up to 5 mL/kg (bolus)
	Fish	2 - 4 mL/kg/h (continuous infusion)
Subcutaneous	Mammals	5 mL/kg
	Fish	1 mL/kg
Intradermal	All	0.05 - 0.1 mL
Intramuscular	All	Up to 0.05 mL/kg
Epidural	Mammals	0.15 - 0.2 mL/kg/day
Intraperitoneal	All	Up to 10 mL/kg
Intranasal	Rodents	At least 35 μL per animal
	Dog, cats, non-human primates, rabbits	200 to 500 μL per animal

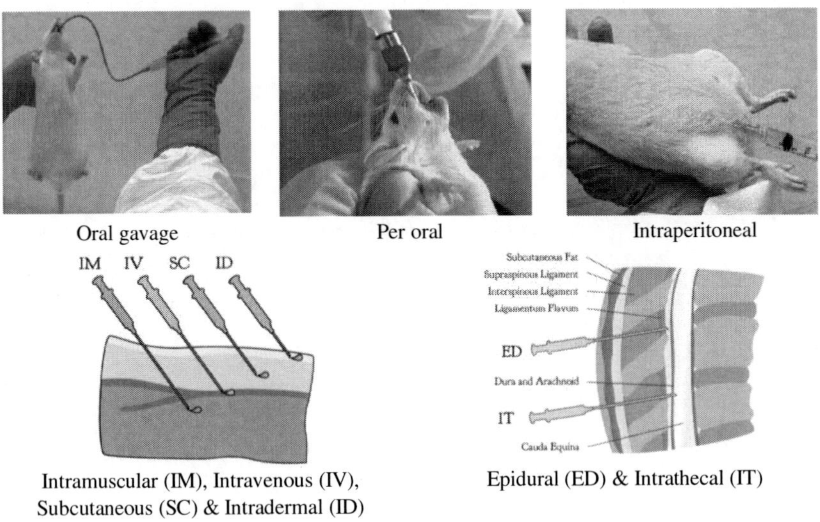

Figure 7.1. Some commonly used routes in experimental animals

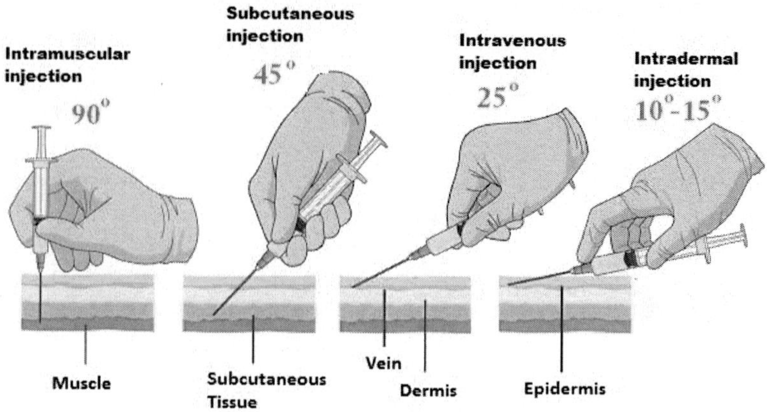

Figure 7.2. Angle of injection for some commonly used routes in animals

Therefore, adverse effects associated with the dosing route should be considered along with administration volumes, temperature of the test substances during administration, feeding and fasting effects before substance delivery, and the age or maturity of your experimental animals. Figure 7.1 shows some commonly used routes in experimental animals.

The angles of administration of the injection are shown in Figure 7.2.

References

Ator, M. A., Mallamo, J. P., & Williams, M. (2006). Overview of drug discovery and development. *Current Protocols in Pharmacology*, *35*(1), 9-9.

Turner, P. V., Brabb, T., Pekow, C., & Vasbinder, M. A. (2011). Administration of substances to laboratory animals: routes of administration and factors to consider. *Journal of the American Association for Laboratory Animal Science*, *50*(5), 600-613.

Chapter 8

Nanotechnology: Interaction of Metal Ions with Extracts

8.1 Nanosynthesize from Medicinal Plants

The introduction of nanotechnology (green synthesis) has evolved into an important branch of drug discovery, development, and therapeutic approaches. Besides the health sciences, nanomaterials are also applied in physics, chemistry, and biology. Many techniques of nanoparticle (NP) synthesis have been introduced to date, such as thermal decomposition of organic solvents, the chemical reduction and photo-reduction of reverse micelles, the chemical reduction of metal ions in aqueous systems with or without compatibilizer, and so on. NPs can be synthesized by using microorganisms, enzymes, fungi, plants, or plant extracts by applying diverse biological methods. These are eco-friendly and are alternatives to chemical and physical methods (Mittal et al. 2013). For example, NPs synthesized from medicinal plants or parts of plants appear to prove advantageous over raw extracts or other biological processes. It is because these NPs can eliminate additional steps in maintaining microbial cultures. The use of plant-mediated synthesized NPs is economic, rapid, sustainable, and biocompatible for human therapeutic uses.

8.2. Why Do You Use Plant Extracts to Synthesize NPs?

Plant-derived reducing ingredients such as flavonoids and phenols have reduction capacity. These can reduce metal cations to MNPs. Additionally, these MNP complexes prevent the aggregation of MNPs due to their stabilizing power. The presence of MNPs in a typical extract might be helpful to protect other readily oxidizable components present in the extract.

MNP synthesis from plant extracts generally consists of three phases: reduction, growth, and termination.

- *Reduction phase*: Phytoactives have reducing power by transferring electrons to decrease metal ions (to zero-valent metal atoms).
- *Growth phase*: Subsequently, zero-valent metal atoms aggregate to form NPs of different forms (e.g., linear, rod-shaped, triangular, hexagonal, or cubic).
- *Termination phase*: Antioxidant phytoactives surround the MNPs to protect them.

Although antioxidants are considered reducing agents, they can act in diverse ways. Extracts of medicinal plants possess both antioxidant and reducing properties. As a result, these plant-derived compounds can act as stabilizers to prevent MNP oxidation as well as reducing agents to prepare MNPs. For instance, through electrical interactions, flavonoids, tannins, and phenolic chemicals can bind to the surface of MNPs and maintain their stability. Figure 8.1 presents the general steps involved in a typical nanoparticle synthesis from plant extract.

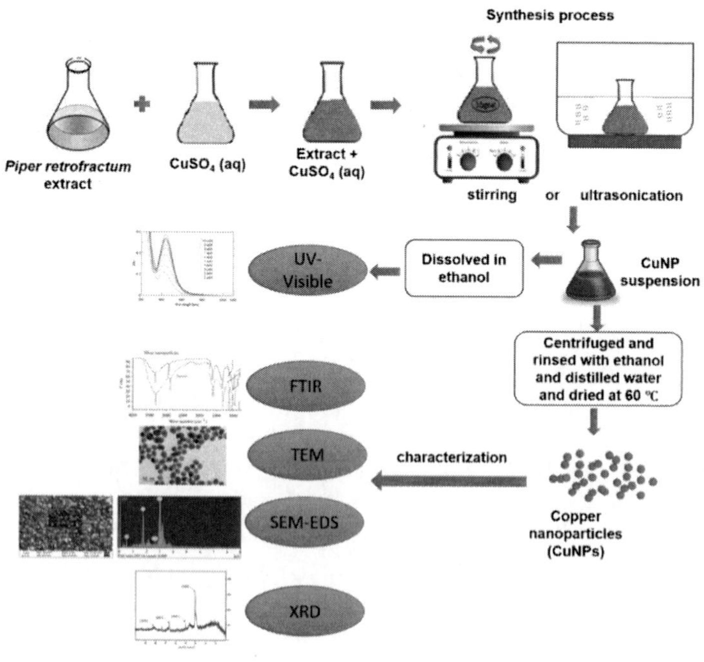

Figure 8.1. General steps involved in a typical nanoparticle synthesis from plant extract

8.3. Examples of Some Nanoparticle Synthesis Methods

8.3.1. AgNPs

According to Aritonang et al. (2019):

Step 1. Mix your plant extract (with the specified concentration) in sterile distilled water, heat it at 60 °C for 30 minutes in a water bath with occasional stirring, filter (0.45 μm polytetrafluoroethylene (PTFE) filter), and centrifuge at 2500 rpm for 15 minutes. Store at 4°C for further use.

Step 2. Prepare 5 mM of $AgNO_3$ in distilled water.

Step 3. Mix the $AgNO_3$ solutions with your plant extract (1:1 v/v ratio) in a beaker or conical flask. Wrap the reaction container (with aluminum foil) and heat in a water bath for 5 hours at 60 °C.

Step 4. Store the mixture in the refrigerator and perform the recommended biological and other studies, such as UV-Vis spectrophotometry and Transmission Electron Microscopy (TEM).

Step 5. To confirm AgNPs synthesis, monitor the Ag^+ ion reduction spectrophorometrically at 200 - 800 nm frequently (at 0, 1, 2, 3, 4, and after the 5th h of heating) of the extract-$AgNO_3$ mixture. Take an absorbance reading after mixing a small portion of the sample (200 L) with deionized water. Visually observe how the reaction combination (metal ion solution + extract) changes color.

Step 6. TEM at 120 V (an acceleration voltage of 15 kV) is helpful to analyze the morphology and size of AgNPs after separation (centrifuge) and drying (furnace at 300 - 400 °C) of the pellets. Extract samples containing AgNPs should be spread out on a copper grid for TEM examinations, then allowed to air dry. Measure AgNPs' particle size using a suitable particle size analyzer.

8.3.2. AuNPs

According to Aljabali et al. (2018):

Step 1. Prepare the plant sample similarly to that mentioned in the above procedure.

Step 2. Prepare 1 mM $HAuCl_4$ in sterile distilled water. Add 5 mL of extract to 45 mL of 1 mM $HAuCl_4$ aqueous solution (1:1 v/v ratio). Wrap it and heat it as mentioned above.

Step 3. Make observations and characterizations similarly.

8.3.3. CuNPs

According to Amaliyah et al. (2020):

Step 1. Prepare the plant sample similarly to that mentioned in the above procedure.

Step 2. Prepare a 0.1 M $CuSO_4$ solution in sterile distilled water.

Step 3. Mix 25 mL of a 0.1 M $CuSO_4$ solution with 50 mL of plant extract. Wrap it and heat it as mentioned above.

Step 4. Make observations and characterizations similarly.

8.3.4. PtNPs

According to Sundar et al. (2019):

Step 1. Dissolve 30.7 μL (0.5 mM) of H_2PtCl_6 in 10 mL of distilled water and stir for 10 minutes.

Step 2. Add your plant extract dropwise into the mixture (in a specified ratio).

Step 3. Verify the reduction of H_2PtCl_6 by seeing the colloidal sample's color change from yellow to brownish-black during the course of 30 minutes of stirring.

Step 4. Make observations and characterizations similarly.

8.3.5. PdNPs

According to Kanchana et al. (2010):

Step 1. Prepare the plant sample similarly to that mentioned in the above procedure.

Step 2. Mix 5 mL of this solution with 0.226 M $PdCl_2$ (100 mL). Wrap and heat it as mentioned above.

Step 3. Make observations and characterizations similarly.

8.3.6. NiNPs

According to Elango et al. (2016):

Step 1. Prepare your plant extract and 1 mM Nickel acetate ($C_4H_6NiO_4$) solution in sterile DDW.

Step 2. Mix 80 mL of plant extract with 20 mL of $C_4H_6NiO_4$ solution, stir, and heat at 60 °C for 7 hours in a water bath.

Step 3. Make observations and characterizations similarly.

8.3.7. FeNPs

According to Katata-Seru et al. (2018):

Step 1. Prepare an iron solution by dissolving $FeSO_4 \cdot 7H_2O$ (2.78 g) in sterile DDW (100 mL).

Step 2. Mix your aqueous plant extract (30 mL) with it in a 150 mL conical flask. Heat for 1 hour at 60 °C in a water bath.

Step 3. Wash the sample three times using anhydrous ethanol and deionized water, respectively.

Step 4. Make observations and characterizations as mentioned above.

8.3.8. Ag-PdNPs

According to Lu et al. (2014):

Step 1. Prepare your plant extract in sterile DDW and keep it in a sonicated water bath at 30 °C. Collect the clear extract after 120 minutes after filtering the mixture.

Step 2. Bimetallic Ag-PdNPs can be made by mixing and heating 10 mL of $AgNO_3$ (0.5 mM) with $Pd(NO_3)_2$ (0.5 mM) in an aqueous medium at

90°Cin an oil bath. You should keep the reaction temperature constant at a stirring rate of 600 rpm.

Step 3. Vigorously stir your sample for 120 minutes. Then, mix 10 mL of this test solution with an Ag-Pd (precursor) solution. By altering the ratio of the metal precursor ($AgNO_3/Pd(NO_3)_2$ ratios like 3:1, 1:1, and 1:3), you may regulate the content of Ag-Pd NPs.

Step 4. Make observations and characterizations as mentioned above.

8.3.9. Fe-PdNPs

According to Luo et al. (2016):

Step 1. Prepare your test extract in sterile distilled water, heat it at 60–100°C for 1 h, and filter it (0.45 μm PTFE filter).

Step 2. To create Fe-PdNPs, fully combine your extract (solution) with a 1:1:1 volume ratio of $FeCl_2$ (aqueous: 0.01 M/L) and $PdCl_2$ solution (diluted HCl). After 30 minutes of stirring at room temperature, look for the instant emergence of a deeply black precipitate.

Step 4. Make observations and characterizations as mentioned above.

8.4. Limitations and Challenges of Medicinal Plant-Based Nanoparticle Synthesis

Medicinal plant-based nanoparticle synthesis is a promising approach that combines the benefits of traditional medicine with the advantages of nanotechnology. However, like any emerging technology, it also faces several limitations and challenges that need to be addressed to fully harness its potential. Major limitations and challenges of medicinal plant-based nanoparticle synthesis include:

1. *Variability of plant material*: The composition and potency of bioactive compounds in medicinal plants can vary significantly depending on factors such as geographical location, climate, season, and harvesting methods. This variability can lead to inconsistent nanoparticle synthesis results and hinder standardization in terms of efficacy and safety.

2. *Contamination and impurities*: Plant extracts may contain various impurities and contaminants that can interfere with nanoparticle synthesis or compromise the quality and safety of the final product. Proper purification and quality control measures are essential to ensure the reliability of medicinal plant-based nanoparticles.
3. *Scalability and reproducibility*: The synthesis of nanoparticles using medicinal plants can be a laborious and time-consuming process, making it challenging to scale up production to meet commercial demands. Achieving consistent results on a large scale is also a significant hurdle.
4. *Characterization techniques*: Traditional methods for characterizing nanoparticles may not be suitable for plant-based nanoparticles due to their complex composition. Developing specialized characterization techniques to assess the size, morphology, stability, and other critical properties of these nanoparticles is essential.
5. *Biological interactions*: While plant-based nanoparticles hold promise for drug delivery and therapeutic applications, their interactions with biological systems are not yet fully understood. Issues such as bioavailability, biodistribution, and potential toxicity need thorough investigation.
6. *Stability and shelf-life*: Plant-based nanoparticles can be susceptible to degradation over time, affecting their stability and shelf-life. Ensuring long-term stability and preserving their therapeutic properties is crucial for practical applications.
7. *Regulatory considerations*: The use of medicinal plant-based nanoparticles may fall into a regulatory gray area, as it involves combining traditional medicine with nanotechnology. Navigating regulatory approvals and compliance with existing pharmaceutical guidelines can be challenging.
8. *Ethical and sustainability concerns*: The increasing demand for medicinal plants for nanoparticle synthesis could potentially lead to overharvesting and threaten the biodiversity of certain plant species. Sustainable sourcing and ethical considerations are crucial to prevent environmental degradation and preserve local traditions and knowledge.
9. *Cost implications*: The synthesis of plant-based nanoparticles can be more expensive compared to conventional synthetic methods. As a result, the final products might be less competitive in the market, limiting their accessibility to patients in need.

Addressing these limitations and challenges will require collaborative efforts between researchers, regulatory bodies, and industry stakeholders. As the field of medicinal plant-based nanoparticle synthesis advances, these challenges are likely to be overcome, leading to more effective and sustainable therapeutic applications.

References

Aljabali, A. A., Akkam, Y., Al Zoubi, M. S., Al-Batayneh, K. M., Al-Trad, B., Abo Alrob, O., Alkilany, A. M., Benamara, M., & Evans, D. J. (2018). Synthesis of gold nanoparticles using leaf extract of *Ziziphus zizyphus* and their antimicrobial activity. *Nanomaterials*, *8*(3), 174.

Amaliyah, S., Pangesti, D. P., Masruri, M., Sabarudin, A., & Sumitro, S. B. (2020). Green synthesis and characterization of copper nanoparticles using *Piper retrofractum* Vahl extract as bioreductor and capping agent. *Heliyon*, *6*(8).

Aritonang, H. F., Koleangan, H., & Wuntu, A. D. (2019). Synthesis of silver nanoparticles using aqueous extract of medicinal plants' (*Impatiens balsamina* and *Lantana camara*) fresh leaves and analysis of antimicrobial activity. *International Journal of Microbiology, 2019*.

Elango, G., Roopan, S. M., Dhamodaran, K. I., Elumalai, K., Al-Dhabi, N. A., & Arasu, M. V. (2016). Spectroscopic investigation of biosynthesized nickel nanoparticles and its larvicidal, pesticidal activities. *Journal of Photochemistry and Photobiology B: Biology*, *162*, 162-167.

Kanchana, A., Devarajan, S., & Ayyappan, S. R. (2010). Green synthesis and characterization of palladium nanoparticles and its conjugates from *Solanum trilobatum* leaf extract. *Nano-micro Letters*, *2*, 169-176.

Katata-Seru, L., Moremedi, T., Aremu, O. S., & Bahadur, I. (2018). Green synthesis of iron nanoparticles using *Moringa oleifera* extracts and their applications: Removal of nitrate from water and antibacterial activity against Escherichia coli. *Journal of Molecular Liquids*, *256*, 296-304.

Lu, F., Sun, D., Huang, J., Du, M., Yang, F., Chen, H., Hong, Y., & Li, Q. (2014). Plant-mediated synthesis of Ag–Pd alloy nanoparticles and their application as catalyst toward selective hydrogenation. *ACS Sustainable Chemistry & Engineering*, *2*(5), 1212-1218.

Luo, F., Yang, D., Chen, Z., Megharaj, M., & Naidu, R. (2016). Characterization of bimetallic Fe/Pd nanoparticles by grape leaf aqueous extract and identification of active biomolecules involved in the synthesis. *Science of the Total Environment*, *562*, 526-532.

Mittal, A. K., Chisti, Y., & Banerjee, U. C. (2013). Synthesis of metallic nanoparticles using plant extracts. *Biotechnology Advances*, *31*(2), 346-356.

Sundar, S., Kim, K. J., & Kwon, S. J. (2019). Observation of single nanoparticle collisions with green synthesized Pt, Au, and Ag nanoparticles using electrocatalytic signal amplification method. *Nanomaterials*, *9*(12), 1695.

Chapter 9

Biological Activity Studies

9.1. Biological Activity Study

Sometimes it is quite difficult to understand how and when a discovery is made about a natural product. For example, in general, drug discovery from a medicinal plant starts with traditional practice information. The non-clinical and pre-clinical studies in drug discovery programs aim to supply a significant number of clinical candidate moieties. Each lead having sufficient evidence of a target biologic activity along with an adequate safety and effectivity profile qualifies to enter human testing (Mohs and Greig 2017). Most often, drug discovery processes supply multiple candidate molecules to make the overall progress successful. It is because all molecules cannot enter clinical trials due to safety, potency, kinetics, protection, and so on. Unfortunately, we do not have a single step to produce a real clinical drug candidate. It is entirely dependent on the extensive collaboration of chemistry, biology, toxicology, and biopharmaceutics departments. Recently, the overall process has been boosted by a new approach called an *in silico* study. The overall cycle time and cost for a new drug candidate are shown below. However, it is applicable for regular and faster progress. We may wait a long time and invest a large amount to get a successful candidate outcome.

Time and cost	**Target to hit**	**Hit to lead**	**Lead optim**	**Before clinical phases**	**Phase I**	**Phase II**	**Phase III**	**Sub to launch**
Cycle time (yrs)	1	1.5	2	1	1.5	2.5	2.5	1.5
Cost ($mil)	94	166	414	150	273	319	314	48

It is clear that the discovery, design, and synthesis of potential drug candidates are dependent on well-designed and well-executed non-clinical and pre-clinical studies. As said before, drug discovery and development are complex processes that connect multiple disciplines. Therefore, multiple steps and models can be employed to obtain only a single outcome. It is to be mentioned that many established drug candidates also regularly undergo non-clinical and pre-clinical studies for many purposes.

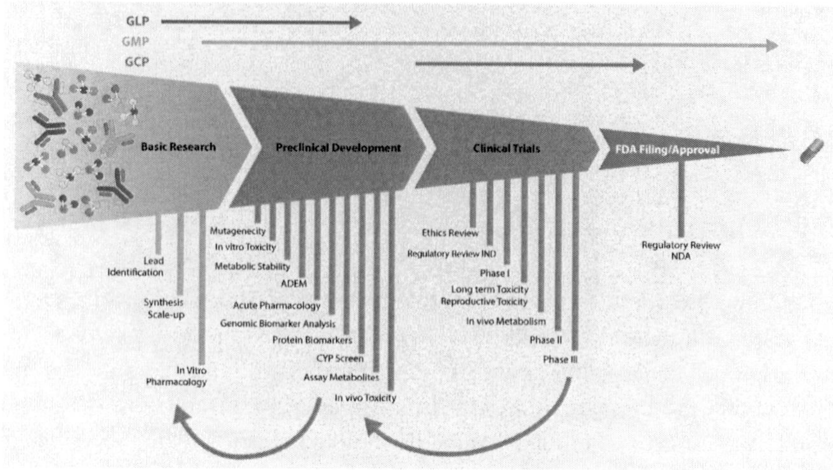

Figure 9.1. Scheme of the total activities involved in the drug discovery and development program

Figure 9.1 presents a scheme of the total activities involved in the drug discovery and development program.

This guide aims to depict some widely used non-clinical and pre-clinical strategies along with stepped models aiming to supply the freshers' and researchers' who are planning to do research for their academic, professional, and interest purposes. *Limitations* include this guide:

1. Limit discussion to the steps of each model used for biological activity testing rather than the causes and mechanisms of the effect.
2. Most of the time, it will not provide adequate information for the study outline regarding the steps involved in reagent preparation.
3. It will supply only the existing and currently available (possible) methods rather than theories for developing new models.
4. It will require time-to-time updates due to medicinal scientists' continuously developing new and newer biological test models.

9.2. Importance of Biological Activity Screening

Biological activity studies play a crucial role in drug discovery and development, as they are essential for identifying and characterizing potential drug candidates. These studies involve evaluating the effects of a compound on biological systems, such as cells, tissues, or whole organisms, to understand its pharmacological properties and therapeutic potential. Some *reasons* why biological activity studies are of great importance in the drug discovery and development process include:

1. *Target identification and validation*: Biological activity studies help researchers identify and validate potential drug targets. By testing a compound's effects on specific biological pathways or receptors, scientists can gain insights into the mechanisms of action and understand whether the target is suitable for therapeutic intervention.
2. *Lead compound selection*: In the early stages of drug discovery, researchers often screen thousands of compounds to find potential lead molecules. Biological activity studies help prioritize compounds based on their ability to interact with the target of interest and produce a desired biological response. This is critical for choosing the most promising lead candidates for further development.
3. *Structure-activity relationship (SAR) studies*: SAR studies involve evaluating different chemical modifications of a lead compound to understand how structural changes influence its biological activity. This iterative process guides medicinal chemists in optimizing the compound's potency, selectivity, and safety profile.
4. *Assessment of efficacy*: Biological activity studies assess a compound's effectiveness in producing the desired therapeutic effect. For example, in the case of antimicrobial agents, it involves evaluating the compound's ability to inhibit the growth of microorganisms or in the case of anticancer drugs, to kill cancer cells.
5. *Dose-response relationship*: Understanding the dose-response relationship is crucial for determining the appropriate dosage of a drug. Biological activity studies help establish the dose at which the compound produces the desired effect without causing significant adverse effects.
6. *Safety and toxicity evaluation*: While assessing biological activity, researchers also gain insights into a compound's safety profile. They can determine potential toxic effects and understand the compound's impact on healthy cells or tissues.

7. *Pharmacokinetic studies*: Biological activity studies often go hand-in-hand with pharmacokinetic studies, which assess how a drug is absorbed, distributed, metabolized, and excreted in the body. This information is vital for predicting how the drug will behave in humans and guiding dosage recommendations.
8. *In vivo studies*: Biological activity studies in animal models provide valuable preclinical data to support the decision-making process before advancing to human clinical trials. These studies help evaluate the drug's efficacy and safety in a more complex biological setting.
9. *Regulatory approval*: Robust biological activity data is a fundamental requirement for regulatory approval of new drugs. Regulatory agencies need evidence that a drug candidate exhibits the desired therapeutic effects and has an acceptable safety profile before allowing it to be tested in humans.

Thus, biological activity studies are a cornerstone of drug discovery and development. They provide critical information about a compound's effectiveness, safety, and mechanism of action, guiding the selection and optimization of potential drug candidates before they can be tested in human clinical trials.

Part I: Antioxidant Tests

This study aims to either claim antioxidant properties or identify antioxidants present in your test sample. Medicinal plants provide antioxidant capacity due to the presence of antioxidant substances in their parts or extracts. In general, antioxidants are protective in nature. They can protect our bodies from various damages caused by oxidative stress and the bad effects of free radicals. Certain plants are reported for their potential antioxidant capacities, including leeks, onions, garlic, eggplant, grapes, pumpkin, mangoes, apricots, carrots, spinach, parsley, berries, tea, seafood, lean meat, milk, and nuts. Natural antioxidants are quite impressive. It is due to their unique composition and variable chemical and biological properties. They have low volatility. Therefore, they are more heat-stable. As a result, these antioxidants are more effective at protecting the finished product throughout food preparation operations like frying, cooking, or baking. In fact, plants also use these biocompatible antioxidants for their own defense. Antioxidant assays are quite important due to free radicals and other oxidants that regularly affect humans (Antolovich et al. 2002).

Oxidative stress (results from free radicals and other oxidants) is associated with various diseases and disorders in humans, including cancer, cardiovascular diseases, neurological diseases and disorders, hepatic and renal diseases, ulcerative colitis, atherosclerosis, and aging. To date, a significant number of *in vitro*, *ex vivo*, and *in vivo* antioxidant test models have been introduced, aiming to investigate samples (e.g., crude extracts or their fractions, diets, isolated compounds, synthetic compounds, commercial antioxidants, etc.) for their antioxidant effects. Antioxidant assays are based on the claim or detection of the antioxidant capacity of your test substance or on the identification of antioxidant components present in your sample. The power of antioxidant molecules is determined in comparison to one or more reference antioxidants (Apak 2019). Some widely used antioxidant assay methods are given below.

In Vitro Models

DPPH Radical Scavenging Assay

Step 1. Take a 0.2 mL sample solution and add 2 mL (0.5 mM) DPPH (1,1-diphenyl-2-picrylhydrazyl or 2,2-diphenyl-1-picrylhydrazyl) solution to it.

Step 2. Keep the test tubes away from light for 30 min. Then use a spectrophotometer to measure the reaction mixture's absorbance at 517 nm.

Step 3. Calculate the %scavenging DPPH radical using the below equation.

$$\%\text{Scavenging DPPH radical} = [(A_{br} - A_{ar}) / A_{br}] \times 100$$

where, A_{br} and A_{ar} is the absorbance of before and after reaction, respectively.

Step 4. Also calculate the half-minimum inhibitory concentration (IC_{50}), confidence of intervals (CI), and coefficient of determination (r^2) values to compare your test value with the controls (Manzocco et al. 1998).

Hydrogen peroxide (H_2O_2) Scavenging Assay
According to Ruch et al. (1989):

Step 1. Prepare H_2O_2 (2 mM) and phosphate buffer (PBS: 50 mM, pH 7.4) solutions.

Step 2. Add a 0.1 mL sample aliquot to 0.3 mL of PBS and 0.6 mL of H_2O_2 solution.

Step 3. Vortex the mixture and keep it away from the light for 10 min.

Step 4. Stectrophotometrically measure the absorbance at 230 nm and determine the ability of H_2O_2 scavenging capacity by using the equation:

$$\%H_2O_2 \text{ scavenging capacity} = [(A_0 - A_1) / A_0] \times 100$$

where, A_0 and A_1 represent control and sample absorbance, respectively.

Peroxidase enzyme assay
According to Liu and Huang (1989):

Step 1. Add 50 mM PBS (pH 7.8), 20 mM guaiacol and 40 mM H_2O_2 to your test sample (100 μL). The final volume of the mixture will be 3 mL.

Step 2. Determine the absorbance changes of this mixture every 20 sec at 470 nm.

Step 3. One (1) unit of peroxidase activity equals the absorbance change of 0.01 units per 60 sec.

Nitric oxide (NO•) Radical Scavenging Assay
According to Marcocci et al. (1994):

Step 1. To a 0.5 mL sample, add 2 mL sodium nitroprusside (10 mM) and 0.5 mL PBS (pH 7.4) and mix the solutions.

Step 2. Incubate the mixture at 25 °C for 2.5 h.

Step 3. Take 0.5 mL of this mixture and add 0.5 mL of Griess reagent [(1.0 mL of sulfanilic acid reagent (0.33% in 20% glacial acetic acid at room temperature for 5 min with 1 mL of naphthylethylenediamine dichloride (0.1% w/v)].

Step 4. Keep this mixture at room temperature for 30 min. Then measure the absorbance at 546 nm.

Step 5. Determine NO• scavenging power using the below equation:

$$\%\text{Inhibition of NO}\bullet: [(A_0 - A_1) / A_0] \times 100$$

where, A_0 and A_1 are the absorbance before and after reaction with the Griess reagent, respectively.

Peroxynitrite (ONOO•) Radical Scavenging Assay

According to Kooy et al. (1994):

Step 1. Prepare dihydroxyrhodamine 123 (5 mM) solution in dimethylformamide and store at -80 °C.

Step 2. Prepare the working solution from the dihydroxyrhodamine 123 solution (5 μM) and place it on ice in the dark.

Step 3. Prepare a buffer solution (50 mM Na_3PO_4 (pH 7.4) + 90 mM NaCl + 5 mM KCl with 100 μM EDTA) and place it on an ice box.

Step 4. Measure the oxidation level at (excitation and emission state) at 485 and 530 nm by using a fluorescence spectroscopy at ambient temperature.

Step 5. Measure the intensities of basement and final fluorescent 5 min after post-treatment without 3-morpholino-sydnonimine or authentic (ONOO•).

$ABTS^+$ Decolorization Assay

According to Seeram et al. (2006):

Step 1. Prepare $ABTS^+$ radicals by mixing solid MnO_2 (80 mg) and 5 mM aqueous ABTS solution (20 mL with 75 mM Na/K buffer (pH 7.0)) and keep it in dark for 16 h.

Step 2. Add 40 μL sample to 1960 μL $ABTS^+$ solution and measure the absorbance spectrophotometerically at room temperature at a time of 6 min at 734 nm.

Step 3. Calculate the %scavenging of $ABTS^+$ as follows:

$$\%ABTS^+ \text{ scavenge} = [(A_{control} - A_{reaction\ mixture}) / A_{control}] \times 100$$

Total Radical-Trapping Antioxidant Parameter (TRAP) Assay

According to Ghiselli et al. (1995):

Step 1. Mix 120 μL sample with 2.4 mL PBS (pH 7.4). Add 375 μL of double distilled water (DDW), 30 μL of dil. R-Phycoerythrin and 75 μL of ABAP.

Step 2. Record the kinetics of this reaction for 45 min at 38 °C by using a spectrometer (luminescence).

Step 3. Determine TRAP values from the lag-phase's length.

Ferric reducing-antioxidant power (FRAP) assay

According to Benzie and Strain (1999):

Step 1. Prepare FRAP solution (25 mL 300 mM/L acetate buffer + 2.5 mL 10 mM/L 2,4,6-tri(2-pyridyl)-1,3,5-triazine (TPTZ) solution + 2.5 mL $FeCl_3$ (20 mM/L) solution in a ratio of 10:1:1).

Step 2. Mix 3 mL of FRAP solution with 100 μL of sample and incubate the mixture for 30 min at 37 °C.

Step 3. Measure absorbance at 593 nm using a diode-array spectrophotometer. Calculate mM of Fe^{2+} equiv./kg (solid sample) or per L (liquid sample).

Superoxide (O_2•-) Radical Scavenging Assay

According to Robak and Gryglewski (1988):

Step 1. Generate O_2•- by mixing 3.0 mL of Tris–HCl buffer (16 mM, pH 8.0) with 0.5 mL of nitroblue tetrazolium (NBT) (0.3 mM).

Step 2. Mix 0.5 mL of NADH (0.936 mM) solution with 1.0 mL of your test sample.

Step 3. Add 0.5 mL of Tris–HCl buffer to this mixture and mix the reaction mixture with 0.5 mL of phenazine methosulfate (PMS) solution (0.12 mM).

Step 4. Keep the mixture at room temerature (25 °C) for 300 sec.

Step 5. Measure the absorbance at 560 nm using a blank sample against it.

Hydroxyl (OH•) Radical Scavenging Assay

According to Kunchandy and Rao (1990):

Step 1. Mix 100 L of 2-deoxy-Dribose (28 mM) in 20 mM KH_2PO_4-KOH buffer (pH 7.4) with 500 μL of your test sample. Then add 200 μL EDTA (1.04 mM) to this mixture following the addition of 200 μL of $FeCl_3$

solution. Finally, add H_2O_2 (1.0 mM) and ascorbic acid (1.0 mM) to this mixture. The last two solutions should be added at 100 µL of each.

Step 2. Incubate the test tubes for 1 h at 37 °C.

Step 3. Prepare a 1% thiobarbituric acid and 2.8% trichloroacetic acid solution. Mix 1 mL of thiobarbituric acid with 1 mL of trichloroacetic acid and add this mixture to the reaction mixture. Finally, heat the reaction tubes for 20 min at 100 °C in a water bath.

Step 4. Cool the mixture and take the absorbance at 532 nm, using a blank sample against it.

Hydroxyl Radical Averting Capacity (HORAC) Assay

According to Ou et al. (2002):

Step 1. Prepare 0.55 M H_2O_2 solution (in distilled water).

Step 2. Prepare 4.6 mM Co (II): Mix 15.7 mg of $CoF_2.4H_2O$ with 20 mg of picolinic acid in 20 mL distilled water.

Step 3. Mix 170 µL of fluorescein (60 nM) with 10 µL of your test sample. Then incubate the reaction mixture at 37 °C for 10 min.

Step 4. Add 10 µL of H_2O_2 (27.5 mM) and 10 µL of Co (II) (230 µM) and measure the initial fluorescence in every 60 sec.

Step 5. Determine the HORAC values by applying a regression equation between the standard antioxidant concentration and the net AUC.

Oxygen Radical Absorbance Capacity (ORAC) Assay

According to Prior et al. (2003):

Step 1. Take AAPH (2,2-azobis 2-amidopropane dihydrochloride) in a place in a pre-heated (37 °C) multi-label counter.

Step 2. Shake the plate (orbitally) for 10 s and measure the fluorescence at 60 sec intervals for 35 min (excitation and emission) at 485 and 520 nm, respectively.

Step 3. Calculate the AUC for your test sample using Wallac Workout 1.5 software and express the results in µM of standard antioxidant equiv./g dry weight of the sample (µM StdE/g).

Reducing Power Assay

According to Oyaizu (1986):

Step 1. Mix 2.5 mL of 0.2 M PBS (pH 6.6) and 2.5 mL of $K_3Fe(CN)_6$ (1% w/v) with 1.0 mL of test sample (in distilled water).

Step 2. Incubate the reaction mixture at 50 °C for 20 min.

Step 3. Add 2.5 mL of trichloro acetic acid (10% (w/v)) and centrifuge at 3000×*g* for 10 min.

Step 4. Collect the supernatant (2.5 mL) and mix it with distilled water (2.5 mL) and $FeCl_3$ (0.5 mL of 0.1% (w/v)).

Step 5. Measure the absorbance at 700 nm using a blank against it.

Phosphomolybdenum Assay

According to Prieto et al. (1999):

Step 1. Add 0.1 mL of sample aliquot to 1 mL of reagent solution (0.6 M H_2SO_4, 28 mM Na_3PO_4 and 4 mM $(NH_4)_6Mo_7O_{24}$).

Step 2. Incubate the mixture at 95 °C for 1.5 h in a water bath.

Step 3. Cool the test tubes at ambient temperature and record the absorbance at 765 nm.

Step 4. Use the following equation to estimate the antioxidant capacity of the test sample:

$$\%\text{Antioxidant activity} = [(A_{control} - A_{sample})/A_{control}] \times 100.$$

Ferric Thiocyanate (FTC) Assay

According to Kikuzaki et al. (1991):

Step 1. Add 4 mg of your test sample to 4 mL of ethanol. Then add 4.1 mL of 2.51% linoleic acid (in ethanol) to 8.0 mL of 0.02 M PBS (pH 7.0). Finally, add 3.9 mL of distilled water and take this mixture in a screw cap vial.

Step 2. Incubate the mixture at 40 °C in a dark environment.

Step 3. Transfer 0.1 mL of this reaction mixture to a clean test tube. Add 9.7 mL of 75% ethanol to it. Then add 0.1 mL of 30% aqueous NH_4SCN and 0.1 mL of 0.02 M $FeSO_4$ in 3.5% HCl and keep the reaction mixture away from light for 180 sec.

Step 4. Re-add a few drops of $FeCl_2$ solution to the mixture and measure the absorbance at 500 nm every 24 h until the absorbance of the control reaches its maximum.

Thiobarbituric Acid (TBA) Assay
According to Ottolenghi (1959):

Step 1. Mix 2 mL of 20% trichloroacetic acid with 2 mL of 0.67% thiobarbituric acid. Add 1 mL of your test sample to this mixture.

Step 2. Boil the mixture in a water bath for 10 min and cool it at room temperature. Then centrifuge the mixture at 3000×*g* for 20 min.

Step 3. Measure the absorbance of the supernatant at 552 nm and determine the TBA reducing activity of your test sample in comparison to the controls.

N,N-dimethyl-p-phenylene diamine dihydrochloride (DMPD) Assay
According to Fogliano et al. (1999):

Step 1. Mix 1 mL of DMPD solution (200 mM) with 0.4 mL of $FeCl_3$ (0.05 M). Then add 100 mL of 0.1 M $NaCH_3COO$ buffer solution (pH 5.25) to this mixture.

Step 2. Keep the reaction mixture in dark at a low temperature (4-5 °C).

Step 3. After 10 min, take 50 μL of test sample (dissolved in distilled water) and add it to 950 μL of the $DMPD^+$ solution.

Step 4. Measure the absorbance after 10 min at 505 nm of this mixture with continuous stirring.

Beta-carotene-Linoleic Acid (conjugated diene) Assay
According to Kabouche et al. (2007):

Step 1. Take 0.5 mg of beta-carotene in a test tube. Then add 1 mL of $CHCl_3$ to it.

Step 2. Add 25 μL of linoleic acid and 200 mg of tween-80 to the mixture.

Step 3. Evaporate the chloroform at 40 °C and add 100 mL of distilled water (saturated with oxygen).

Step 4. Vigorously agitate the solution to form a stable emulsion.

Step 5. Take 4 mL of this mixture and add 200 μL of a methanolic test sample to it.

Step 6. Immediately measure the zero (0) time absorbance at 470 nm.

Step 7. Incubate the reaction tubes for 2 h at 50 °C and take final absorbance after 120 min.

Step 8. Calculate the antioxidant activity as %inhibition in comparison to the control using the below equation.

$$\%\text{Antioxidant capacity} = (A_s - A_{s120}) \div (A_c - A_{c120})$$

where, A_s and A_{s120} represent the initial absorbance and the absorbance after 120 min of the test sample, respectively, and A_c and A_{c120} represent the initial and the absorbance after 120 min of the test control, respectively.

Xanthine oxidase Assay

According to Noro et al. (1983):

Step 1. Add 500 µL of test sample to methanolic allopurinol (100 µg/mL) solution. Then add 1.3 mL of PBS (0.05 M, pH 7.5) and 0.2 mL of 0.2 units/mL xanthine oxidase solution to this mixture.

Step 2. Keep the mixture for 10 min at ambient temperature (25 °C) and add 1.5 mL of xanthine substrate (0.15 M) solution to it.

Step 3. Keep the mixture at ambient temperature for another 0.5 hours.

Step 4. Measure the absorbance spectrophotometrically at 293 nm against a blank (0.5 mL methanol + 1.3 mL phosphate buffer + 0.2 mL xanthine oxidase). As a control, add 1.5 mL of xanthine substrate to the blank and take the absorbance similarly.

Step 5. Calculate the %inhibition by using the following formula:

$$\%\text{Inhibition} = [1 - (A_s/A_c)] \times 100$$

where, A_s and A_c represent the absorbance of the test sample and control, respectively.

Cupric Ion Reducing Assay

According to Apak et al. (2008):

Step 1. Mix 1 mL (0.01 M) $CuCl_2$ with 1 mL (0.0075 M) neocuproine. Then add 1 mL (1 M) of NH_4CH_3COO solution to it.

Step 2. Add 400 µL of freshly prepared standard solution (diluted in 4.1 mL deionized water). Similarly, perform for the test sample.

Step 3. Mix the solutions and keep them at room temperature for 0.5 h.

Step 4. Take the absorbance spectrophotometrically at 450 nm.

Metal Chelating Assay

According to Chew et al. (2009):

Step 1. Add 0.2 mL of $FeSO_4$ (0.1 mM) to 0.4 mL of ferrozine (0.25 mM) and 0.2 mL of test sample.

Step 2. Keep the mixture at an ambient temperature for 10 min.

Step 3. Record absorbance spectrophotometrically at 562 nm and calculate the chelating activity using the below formula:

$$\text{Metal chelating activity} = (A_{control} - A_{sample})/A_{control} \times 100$$

where, $A_{control}$ and A_{sample} represent the absorbance of control reaction (without test sample), and the absorbance in the presence of a test sample, respectively.

Hemoglobin-Induced Linoleic Acid System Assay

According to Yuan et al. (2005):

Step 1. Add 50 μL test sample to 1 mM/L of linoleic acid emulsion. Then add 40 mM/L PBS (pH 6.5) and 0.0016% hemoglobin to this mixture. Incubate the mixture at 37 °C for 45 min.

Step 2. To stop the lipid peroxidation, add 2.5 mL of 0.6% HCl in ethanol.

Step 3. After coloring with 100 mL of 0.02 M/L $FeCl_2$ and 50 mL of NH_4SCN (0.3 g/mL), examine the absorbance at 480 nm to determine the peroxide value in triplicate using the thiocyanate method. Make use of vitamin C as a good control.

Total Alkaloid Assay

According to Shamsa et al. (2008):

Step 1. Dissolve 1 mg of your test sample in DMSO. Then add 1 mL (2 N) of HCl to this mixture. Filter the mixture.

Step 2. Transfer the solution to a separating funnel. Add 5 mL of bromocresol green solution to it. Then mix this reaction mixture with 5 mL of PBS.

Step 3. Shake the reaction mixture with 1, 2, 3 and 4 mL of $CHCl_3$ vigorously and collect it in a 10-mL volumetric flask and dilute it with $CHCl_3$.

Step 4. Prepare a set of concentrations of atropine (reference drug) (e.g., 20-100 μg/mL) similarly.

Step 5. Using a UV/Vis spectrophotometer, determine the absorbance of the test and standard solutions in comparison to the reagent blank at 470 nm. Total alkaloid content should be expressed as mg of AE/g of extract.

Total Phenolic Assay

According to Makkar (1999):

Step 1. Take 0.05 mL aliquots of your test sample into test tubes and adjust their volume to 1 mL by using distilled water.

Step 2. Add 500 μL of Folin–Ciocalteu reagent and 2.5 mL of Na_2CO_3 solution to it.

Step 3. Measure the absorbance of the solution at 725 nm after 40 min.

Step 4. Utilizing a standard curve, convert the total phenol levels to tannic acid equivalents and express them as a percentage.

Total flavonoid assay

According to Ndhlala et al. (2008):

Step 1. Take 50 μL aliquots of the crude extract and adjust the volume to 1 with methanol-HCl (2.5 mL) and vanillin reagent (2.5 mL).

Step 2. Measure the mixture's absorbance at 500 nm after 20 min of incubation at 30 °C. As a negative control, substitute a methanol-containing reaction mixture for your test sample.

Step 3. Determine flavonoids and express the concentration as catechin equiv./g of extract based on your predetermined standard curve.

Total Tannin Assay

According to Amorim et al. (2008):

Step 1. Add 0.1 mL of the extract to 0.5 mL of the Folin-Coilett-Phenol Reagent, 1 mL of the 35% Na_2CO_3 solution, and 10 mL of distilled water to dilute the mixture.

Step 2. Shake the mixture thoroughly, let it stand at ambient temperature for 30 min, and then take a 725 nm absorbance reading.

Step 3. Use only distilled water to create a blank. Check the blank against a collection of standard tannic acid solutions. Summarize the effects of tannins in terms of mg/g of your test sample (e.g., extract) tannic acid.

Step 4. An equation derived from a standard tannic acid calibration curve can be used to calculate the total tannin content as mg of tannic acid equiv./g.

Ex Vivo Assay(s)

Hemolysis Inhibition Capacity Assay

According to Girish et al. (2012):

Step 1. Collect blood from the retro-orbital plexus of an anesthetized (sodium pentobarbital 35 mg/kg; intraperitoneal) Wistar rat and prepare a 10% suspension of it in PBS (pH 7.4).

Step 2. Add 0.15 mL of H_2O_2 (200 mM in PBS; pH 7.4) to 0.2 mL of test sample and 0.5 mL of 10% RBC suspension.

Step 3. Incubate the reaction mixture at 37 °C for 0.5 h and immediately centrifuge at 2,500×*g* for 180 sec.

Step 4. Mix 0.2 mL of supernatant with 2.8 mL of PBS (pH 7.4) and measure the absorbance at 475 nm. Use a 0.2 mL vehicle as a control.

Step 5. Calculate the percentage of hemolysis inhibition using the below formula.

$$\%\text{inhibition of hemolysis} = [(A_{control} - A_{sample}) / A_{control} \times 100$$

where, $A_{control}$ and A_{sample} represent the control absorbance with 100% hemolysis induced by H_2O_2 and the absorbance of aliquots containing test sample, respectively.

In Vivo Assays

Ferric Reducing Ability of Plasma

According to Benzie and Strain (1996):

Step 1. Collect blood from the rat's retroorbital plexus and mix with heparin in a glass tube.

Step 2. Take 3 mL freshly prepared and warm (37 °C) FRAP reagent [1 mL (10 mM) of 2,4,6 tripyridyl-s-triazine (TPTZ) solution in 40 mM HCl,

1 mL 20 mM $FeCl_2.6H_2O$, 10 mL of 0.3 M acetate buffer (pH 3.6)] and mix with 0.375 mL distilled water and 0.025 mL of test sample.

Step 3. Keep the mixture at 37 °C for 180 sec. Measure the absorbance spectrophotometrically at 593 nm.

Reduced Glutathione (GSH) Assay

According to Ellman (1959):

Step 1. Sacrifice the treated animal and collect its liver.

Step 2. To precipitate the tissue proteins, prepare a tissue homogenate (in 0.1 M PBS, pH 7.4) and add an equal volume of 20% trichloroacetic acid (TCA) with 1 mM EDTA.

Step 3. Allow the mixture for 5 min. Then centrifuge it 10 min at 2000×*g*.

Step 4. Transfer 200 L of supernatant to a new test tube and add 1.8 mL of Ellman's reagent (5,50 -dithiobis-2- nitrobenzoic acid (0.1 mM) prepared in 0.3 M PBS with 1% of sodium citrate solution).

Step 5. Adjust the final volume of 2 mL with phosphate buffer and take the absorbance spectrophotometrically at 412 nm using a blank against it.

Step 6. Compared to a standard curve made from known GSH, the sample absorbance values are lower.

Glutathione Peroxidase (GPx) Assay

According to Wood (1970):

Step 1. Prepare the cytosolic fraction of the organ/tissue of the experimental animals by centrifugation at 20,000×*g* for 25 min. Then filter it.

Step 2. Mix 2.0 mL (75 mM/L) PBS (pH 7.0) with 50 μL (60 mM/L) glutathione reductase (30 U/mL) solution. Then add 50 μL (0.12 M/L) Na_3N, 0.10 (0.15 mM/L) Na_2EDTA, 100 μL (3.0 mM/L) NADPH, and 100 μL of the cytoplasmic fraction.

Step 3. Add distilled water to the final 2.9 mL amount as needed.

Step 4. Add 100 μL of 7.5 mM/L H_2O_2 to the mixture. Then monitor the conversion of NADPH to NADP at 340 nm at a 60-second interval for 5 min.

Step 5. Calculate the enzyme activity of GPx in mg of proteins.

Glutathione-S-transferase (GST) Assay

According to Jocelyn (1972):

Step 1. Take equal volumes of 0.1 N K_3PO_4 (pH 6.5) and 1 nM/L GST and add the required amount of cytosol (6 mg protein/mL) to it.

Step 2. After incubation at 37 °C for 5 min, add 1 M/L l-chloro-2, 4-dinitrobenzene (substrate) into the mixture.

Step 3. Spectrophotometrically measure the absorbance at 340 nm.

Superoxide Dismutase (SOD) Assay

According to McCord and Fridovich (1969):

Step 1. Prepare a 5% RBC suspension from the treated animal's blood.

Step 2. Add 75 mM of Tris-HCl buffer (pH 8.2), 30 mM EDTA, and 2 mM of pyrogallol to 50 μL of the lysate.

Step 3. Record in an increase in absorbance at 420 nm for 180 sec spectrophotometerically.

Step 4. Calculate the change in absorbance per minute at 420 nm. Finally, express SOD activity as units/mg of protein.

Catalase (CAT) Assay

According to Aebi (1984):

Step 1. Add 50 μL of lysate to 2 mL of PBS (pH 7.0) and mix this solution with 1 mL of 30 mM H_2O_2.

Step 2. Record the absorbance at 240 nm for 60 sec, spectrophotometerically.

Step 3. Use the molar extinction coefficient of H_2O_2, 43.6 M/cm, to estimate CAT activity. One unit CAT activity equals to 1 mM of H_2O_2 degraded per 60 sec. Express the effect as units/mg of protein.

Gamma-Glutamyl Transpeptidase (GGT) Assay

According to Singhal et al. (1982):

Step 1. Add serum sample to a substrate solution containing glycylglycine, $MgCl_2$ and γ-glutamyl-p-nitroanilide in 0.05 M Tris (free base) (pH 8.2).

Step 2. Incubate the reaction mixture at 37 °C for 60 sec.

Step 3. Record the absorbance spectrophotometerically at 405 nm at 1 min interval for 5 min. Calculate GGT activity from the absorbance values.

Glutathione Reductase (GR) Assay

According to Kakkar et al. (1984):

Step 1. Collect approximately 400 g liver from the sacrificed animals (e.g., rats). Cut the livers into small pieces and homogenize with 9 mL (0.25 M) of ice-cold sucrose per g of rat liver in a blender.

Step 2. Centrifuge the homogenate for 45 minutes at 14,000×*g*.

Step 3. Suspend the pellets in a minute volume of 0.25 M sucrose and re-centrifuge. Mix the supernatants with the previous centrifuges.

Step 4. Adjust the pooled materials to pH 5.5 with cold 0.2 M acetic acid. Re-centrifuge the mixture similarly.

Step 5. Use the rate of oxidation of NADPH by GSSG at 30 °C as a standard measure of enzymatic activity. The composition of the reaction system (1 mL) includes: 1.0 mM GSSG, 0.1 mM NADPH, 0.5 mM EDTA, 0.10 M sodium PBS (pH 7.6), and required amount of the GR sample to give a change in absorbance of 0.05-0.03/min.

Step 6. Use the oxidation of 1 μM of NADPH/min under these conditions as a unit of GR activity. Express the specific activity as units/mg of protein.

Lipid peroxidation (LPO) Assay

According to Ohkawa et al. (1979):

Step 1. Homogenize the liver tissues in 0.1 M PBS (pH 7.4) with a Teflonglass homogenizer.

Step 2. To the tissue homogenate (0.2 mL), add 0.2 mL of 8.1% sodium dodecyl sulfate (SDS), 1.5 mL of 20% acetic acid, and 1.5 mL of 8% TBA.

Step 3. Adjust the final volume of the mixture up to 4 mL with distilled water. Heat the mixture at 95 °C in a water bath for 1 h, using glass balls as condensers.

Step 4. Cool the tubes at room temperature and adjust the final volume to 5 mL in each tube.

Step 5. Add 5 mL of butanol: pyridine (ratio: 15:1) mixture to the contents and vortex thoroughly for 120 sec.

Step 6. Centrifuge at 3000×*g* for 10 min. Collect the organic portion from the upper layer and measure its optical density (OD) at 532 nm using a blank against it.

Step 7. Express the levels of lipid peroxides as nM of TBARS/mg protein using an extinction coefficient of 1.56×10^5 mL/cm.

Malondialdehyde (MDA) Content Assay

According to Zhang and Kirkham (1994):

Step 1. Add 2 mL of your test sample to 1 mL of 20% (v/v) trichloroacetic acid and 0.5% (v/v) thiobarbituric acid.

Step 2. Heat the mixture in a water bath at 95 °C for 0.5 h. Cool the mixture at ambient temperature and centrifuge it at 14,000×*g* for 10 min.

Step 3. Determine the absorbance of the supernatant at 532 nm and subtract the nonspecific absorbance at 600 nm from it.

Step 4. Calculate the MDA content by using an extinction coefficient of 155 mM/cm.

Low-Density Lipoprotein (LDL) Assay

According to El-Saadani et al. (1989):

Step 1. Wash and dialyze isolated LDL against 150 mM/L NaCl and 1 mM/L Na_2EDTA (pH 7.4) at 4 °C.

Step 2. Sterilize the LDL by filtration (0.45 μM) and keep it under nitrogen away from light (at 4°C).

Step 3. Incubate LDL (100 μg of protein/mL) for 10 min at ambient temperature with your test sample.

Step 4. Add 5 μM/L of $CuSO_4$ and incubate the tubes for 120 min at 37 °C.

Step 5. Add 10 μM butylated hydroxytoluene (BHT) to terminate Cu^{2+}-induced oxidation.

Step 6. Determine the extent of LDL oxidation by measuring the generated amount of lipid peroxides and also by the TBARS assay at 532 nm, using MDA as a standard curve.

Oxidative Damage/Antioxidant Assay in Saccharomyces Cerevisiae

According to Oliveira et al. (2014):

Step 1. Collect wild-type and some isogenic *S. cerevisiae* strains, for example, deficient strains in cytosolic (Sod1Δ) and mitochondrial superoxide dismutase (Sod2Δ), catalase (Cat1Δ), double mutants like Sod1ΔSod2Δ, and Cat1ΔSod1Δ and maintain in YEL (yeast extract 0.5%, 2% of Bacto-peptone and 2% of glucose) medium at 28 °C.

Step 2. Seed the cell suspension from the center to the edge of a sterile media containing Petri dish in a continuous cycle on both sides, containing in the center of the plate a sterile filter paper disk containing your test sample or controls.

Step 3. Incubate the discs at 30 °C for 2 days and measure the zones of inhibition linearly in millimeters (mm). Duplicate each test.

Part II: Anti-Inflammatory Tests

Inflammation is an important physiological process for our bodies' healing processes. Short-term inflammation is thought to be beneficial, while long-term inflammation may lead to chronic inflammation and inflammatory diseases that are considered major threats to human health worldwide. Inflammation is therefore a crucial therapeutic target for the design of creative therapeutic intervention strategies. It has been demonstrated that natural products, particularly a variety of medicinal plants, have strong anti-inflammatory and immunomodulatory properties. These properties include inhibiting effects on the suppression of cellular and humoral immunity, lymphocyte activation, and the spread of apoptosis. An anti-inflammatory agent is a medicine or other chemical that lessens bodily inflammation, including pain, swelling, and redness. These mainly block one or more pathways in the body that cause inflammation, such as pro-inflammatory and inflammatory markers. It is to be highlighted that many of the agents are being studied in the management of cancers. Research evidence suggests that natural products have promising antioxidative power that can protect body organs from oxidative stresses or the harmful effects of infectious agents and also have anti-inflammatory properties (Ge et al. 2022). Some widely used anti-inflammatory assay methods are given below.

In Vitro Assays

Protein Denaturation Inhibition Assay

According to Mizushima and Kobayashi (1968):

Step 1. Mix your sample solution with 1% BSA (aqueous solution).

Step 2. Adjust the pH of the reaction mixture with the addition of 1 N HCl. Then heat the mixture at 37 °C for 20 min and further 57 °C for 20 min. Cool the mixture at the ambient temperature.

Step 3. Measure the OD at 660 nm.

Step 4. Triplicate the experiment and calculate the %protein denaturation inhibition rate as follows:

$$\%\text{Inhibition} = [(A_S - A_C) \div A_C] \times 100$$

where, A_s and A_c are the absorbance of test sample and control, respectively.

Or, you can follow the following modified pathways:

Step 1. Mix 0.2 mL of egg albumin with 2.8 mL of PBS (pH 6.4). Add 2 mL of your test sample to it. Use a similar volume of PBS as control.

Step 2. Incubate the reaction mixture in a BOD incubator at 37 °C for 15 min. Heat at 70 °C for 5 min.

Step 3. Cool the contents at ambient temperature and measure the absorbance at 660 nm using the vehicle as a blank. Any anti-inflammatory drug such as diclofenac sodium can be used as a reference drug.

Step 4. Calculate the inhibition of protein denaturation by using the following formula:

$$\%\text{Inhibition} = [\{(C\text{-}B) - (A\text{-}B)\} \div (A\text{-}B)] \times 100$$

where, A, B and C stand for absorbance of control, blank and sample, respectively.

Human Red Blood Cell (HRBC) Membrane Stabilization Assay

According to Shinde et al. (1999):

Heat-Induced (Thermolytic) Model

Step 1. Collect fresh human blood (5 mL) in heparinized (dipotassium salt of EDTA: 2.2 mg/mL of blood). Centrifuge at 3000×*g* for 10 min. Wash 3 times with an equal volume of isosaline solution (154 mM NaCl) in 10 mM sodium PBS (pH 7.4).

Step 2. Prepare a 10% suspension with isosaline.

Step 3. Add 1 mL of your test sample solution to 1 mL of RBC suspension. For control, add saline only. You can use aspirin (one or more concentrations) as a positive control for this study.

Step 4. Incubate the mixtures at 56 °C for 0.5 h. Centrifuge at 2500×*g* for 300 sec.

Step 5. Determine the supernatant's absorbance at 560 nm. Triplicate the experiment.

Step 6. Calculate the %membrane stabilization activity using the following formula:

$$\%\text{Protection} = [(100 - A_S) \div A_C] \times 100$$

where, A_C and A_S are the absorbance of the control and sample, respectively.

Hypotonic solution induced model

After step 2, proceed as

Step 3. Add 0.5 mL of RBC suspension to 4.5 mL of hypotonic solution (50 mM NaCl) in 10 mM sodium PBS (pH 7.4) containing the test sample or standard solution (0.5 mL).

Step 4. Use 0.5 mL of RBC suspension as a control and mix it with hypotonic-buffered saline alone.

Step 5. Keep the mixture at room temperature for 10 minutes. Centrifuge for 10 min at 3000×*g* and measure the OD of the supernatant at 540 nm by using a UV-Vis spectrophotometer.

Step 6. Calculate %inhibition of hemolysis by using following equation:

$$\%\text{Inhibition of hemolysis} = \{(OD_{control} - OD_{test\ samples}) \div OD_{control}\} \times 100$$

Proteinase Inhibitory Assay

According to Oyedepo and Femurewa (1995):

Step 1. Mix 0.06 mg of trypsin with 1 mL of Tris-HCl buffer (20 mM, pH 7.4). Add 1 mL of your test sample.

Step 2. Incubate the reaction mixture at 37 °C for 300 sec. Add 1 mL of 0.8% (*w*/*v*) casein to it.

Step 3. Re-incubate the mixture for 20 minutes.

Step 4. To stop the reaction, add perchloric acid (2 mL of 70%).

Step 5. Then centrifuge the cloudy suspension. Measure the supernatant's absorbance at 210 nm against the Tris-HCl buffer as a blank. Triplicate the experiment.

Phagoburst Assay

According to Nemudzivhadi and Masoko (2014):

Step 1. Transfer 200 μL of Raw 264.7 macrophages to a coverslip in a multi-well plate.

Step 2. Incubate the cells at 37 °C, 5% CO_2 overnight, to allow cells to attach.

Step 3. Treat the cells with 100 μL of your test sample and 10 mg/mL of LPS for 1 day.

Step 4. Add 2 μL of PMA and re-incubate for 0.5 h and aspirate the medium.

Step 5. Stain the cells with 50 μL of 10^{-5} M of H_2DCF-DA and incubate for 20 min away from light.

Step 6. Re-stain the cells with 50 μL of 20 μg/mL, 4′,6-diamidine-2-phenylindole (DAPI) and further incubate for 20 min away from light.

Step 7. Remove the staining solutions and add 3.7% paraformaldehyde to a coverslip to fix the cells.

Step 8. Mount the coverslips to a microscope slide and examine them under a fluorescence microscope.

Elastase Assay Model

According to Stein (1985):

Step 1. For this assay, collect human leukocyte elastase.

Step 2. Mix 250 μL of substrate solution (700 μM MeO-Suc-Ala-Ala-Pro-Val-pNA in Tris-HCl-buffer, pH 7.5) with 100 μL of your test sample (solubilized in Tris-HCl-buffer, pH 7.5) and vortex.

Step 3. Add 250 μL enzyme solution (approximately 0.5 mU) to the mixture and incubate for 1 h at 37 °C.

Step 4. Stop the reaction by adding 500 μL of soybean trypsin inhibitor solution (2 mg/mL Tris-HCl-buffer, pH 7.5) and placing it in an ice bath. Then vortex the mixture and measure the absorbance at 405 nm. Triplicate the assay and calculate the inhibition rates in percent to controls without inhibitors. Also, determine IC_{50} values from concentration-effect curves by linear regression.

In Vivo Assays

Egg albumin induced paw edema mouse model

According to Akindele and Adeyemi (2007):

Step 1. Take *Swiss* albino fasted overnight mice and randomly group them for the controls and test groups with the required number of animals in each group.

Step 2. Give the animals' respective treatments via suitable routes.

Step 3. Induce edema after 60 minutes of treatment by injecting (into the subplantar tissue of the right hind paw) egg albumin (0.1 mL, 1% w/v in saline solution).

Carrageenan-Induced Paw Edema Mouse Model

According to Demsie (2019):

Step 1. Take *Swiss* albino fasted overnight mice and randomly group them for the controls and test groups with the required number of animals in each group.

Step 2. Give the animals' respective treatments via suitable routes.

Step 3. Use a digital plethysmometer to measure the basal volume of each mouse's right hind paw after marking the leg of each mouse on the skin over the lateral maleous.

Step 4. Inject 0.05 mL of 1% carrageenan in normal saline into the dorsal surface of the right hind paw of each animal (after 0.5 h of each treatment taken before).

Step 5. Measure the volume of the injected paw at 1, 2, 3 and 4th h after carrageenan injection.

Step 6. By determining the %inhibition using the following formula, compare the paw diameter prior to carrageenan injection with the same paw diameter following carrageenan administration:

$$\%\text{Inflammation inhibition} = [\{(Vt - V0)_{\text{control}} - (Vt - V0)_{\text{test}}\} \div (Vt - V0)_{\text{control}}] \times 100$$

where, V0 is the mean paw volume prior to the carrageenan injection in the test and negative control groups, and V*t* is the mean paw volume following the injection at time *t*.

Step 6. Express the increase in paw volume, i.e., %inflammation as:

$$\%\text{Inflammation} = [(Vf - Vi) \div Vi] \times 100$$

where, V*f* is the final volume and V*i* is the initial mean paw volume before the injection of carrageenan (after carrageenan injection).

N.B. – Histamine (0.1 ml of 1% w/v freshly prepared histamine) induced paw edema model can be also used for this purpose (Alemu et al. 2018).

Xylene-Induced Mouse Ear Edema Model

According to Tang et al. (1984) and Akindele and Adeyemi (2007):

Step 1. Treat the animals (randomly divided with a suitable number in each group) with a test sample, indomethacin as a standard at 10 mg/kg or vehicle (10 mL/kg), and apply 0.02 mL of xylene topically to the inner and outer surfaces of the right ear 15-60 minutes prior to inducing ear edema.

Step 2. Use the left ear as a control.

Step 3. Sacrifice the animals 15 - 60 minutes after under ether anesthesia (or by cervical dislocation) and cut off both ears, size and take weight.

Step 4. To determine the degree of ear edema, determine the weight differential between the right and left ear portions of the same animal.

Freund's Adjuvant-Induced Paw Edema Model in Mice

According to Milano et al. (2008):

Step 1. Distribute the animals' randomly in each group. Anesthetize the animals with a mixture of ketamine:xylazine (50:2 mg/kg) cocktail.

Step 2. Give 20 μL of complete Freund's adjuvant (CFA) subcutaneously on the plantar surface of the right hind paw to all groups (except vehicle group).

Step 3. After 1 day, treat the animals with the test drug and controls (indomethacin as standard at 10 mg/kg, or vehicle (10 mL/kg)).

Step 4. Calculate the level of inflammation of the right hind paw using a caliper at several time-points (0, 0.5, 1, 2, 4, 5, 6, and 7th h) and express in millimeters (mm).

Formalin-Induced Paw Edema Chick Model

According to Mousa et al. (2019):

Step 1. Collect broiler chicks 7 - 21 days old weighing between 48-125 g for this study.

Step 2. Group the chicks (n = 5/6) into controls and test sample.

Step 3. Treat the birds 30 min before to 0.05 mL (1%) formaldehyde injection in the right paw for inducing inflammation.

Step 4. Measure the right paw thickness with the digital caliber in millimeter (mm) both before and after 60 min of formaldehyde injection. Determine the delta change in paw thickness, which reveals the inflammation and compare the group results.

$$\%\text{Reduction of edema} = [(A\text{-}B)/A] \times 100$$

where, A and B stand for diameter of paw (mm) of control and test group, respectively.

Part III: Immunomodulatory Activity Tests

Immunological diseases and disorders can have significant impacts on various aspects of an individual's health and well-being. The immune system plays a crucial role in defending the body against infections, bacteria, viruses, and other harmful substances. When this system malfunctions or becomes imbalanced, it can lead to a wide range of conditions that can affect different organs and systems in the body (Pavlicevic et al. 2022). Some of the potential *impacts* of immunological diseases and disorders include:

1. *Increased susceptibility to infections*: One of the primary functions of the immune system is to protect the body from infections. Immunological disorders can weaken the immune response, making individuals more prone to recurrent and severe infections.
2. *Chronic inflammation*: Many immunological diseases are characterized by chronic inflammation, where the immune system is overactive and mistakenly attacks healthy tissues. This can lead to damage to organs and tissues over time, causing pain, swelling, and reduced organ function.
3. *Autoimmune disorders*: These occur when the immune system mistakenly attacks the body's own tissues as if they were foreign invaders. Autoimmune diseases can affect various organs, such as the thyroid (e.g., Hashimoto's thyroiditis), joints (e.g., rheumatoid arthritis), or the central nervous system (e.g., multiple sclerosis).

4. *Allergic reactions*: Allergies are caused by an overreaction of the immune system to harmless substances, triggering symptoms such as sneezing, itching, hives, and, in severe cases, anaphylaxis.
5. *Organ damage*: Some immunological diseases, like lupus and certain types of vasculitis, can cause damage to organs and tissues, leading to organ dysfunction and potential organ failure.
6. *Fatigue and reduced quality of life*: Chronic immunological diseases can cause persistent fatigue and a reduced quality of life due to the ongoing symptoms and limitations they impose on daily activities.
7. *Joint and muscle pain*: Inflammatory conditions such as rheumatoid arthritis and systemic lupus erythematosus can cause joint pain, stiffness, and muscle aches.
8. *Neurological symptoms*: Certain immunological disorders can affect the nervous system, leading to neurological symptoms such as numbness, tingling, muscle weakness, and cognitive difficulties.
9. *Infertility and reproductive issues*: Some immunological diseases can impact fertility and reproduction, affecting both men and women.
10. *Mental health impact*: Dealing with chronic conditions and their associated symptoms can take a toll on mental health, leading to anxiety, depression, and stress.
11. *Increased risk of other conditions*: Individuals with immunological disorders may have a higher risk of developing other health problems, such as cardiovascular diseases or certain types of cancer.

Managing immunological diseases often involves a combination of medication, lifestyle changes, and, in some cases, immunosuppressive therapies. Early diagnosis, proper medical care, and ongoing monitoring are essential to minimize the impacts of these conditions on an individual's health and quality of life. Additionally, ongoing research and advancements in immunology are continuously improving our understanding and treatment of these disorders. Immunomodulatory agents are substances that either stimulate or depress the immune system and may aid the body in fighting cancer, infections, or other disorders (Shi et al. 2021). The methods for determining the immunomodulatory effects of your test sample consist of a number of steps. Therefore, only two popularly used immunomodulatory assay methods are shown for this purpose.

Human Cell Model

According to Albrahim et al. (2020):

Step 1. The human cells (e.g., monocytic THP-1 cells) are grown in RPMI media supplemented with 10% FBS, 100 IU/mL penicillin, 100 µg/mL streptomycin, and 3.7 g/L $NaHCO_3$. Maintain the cells in 5% CO_2 at 37 °C.

Step 2. Phorbol 12-myristate 13-acetate 100 ng/mL is added to the cells and left to sit for 2 days. Undifferentiated cells should be removed from the cells by washing them in RPMI 1640 serum-free media.

Step 3. Treat differentiated cells with 100 ng/mL LPS, your test sample, or LPS + test sample for 4-6 h.

Step 4. Treat the cells at a density of cells/well and incubate them with the test sample for 1 to 8 days. Incubate with MTT reagent for 3 h and measure the absorbance using a microplate reader at 540 nm.

Step 5. Extract total RNA from the treated cells using a suitable Kit, and follow a double-stranded cDNA synthesis using a cDNA Synthesis system. Real-time PCR investigations using target-specific primers and probes should be performed using cDNA. The mRNA expression levels of the examined genes should be normalized to GAPDH.

Step 6. Collect supernatants and perform an ELISA approach to measure IL-1β, IL-8, CCL22, and CXCL10 levels. This involves adding supernatants to wells that have been pre-coated with protein-specific antibodies, incubating for 120 min, washing three times with PBS, and then incubating for 20 min with streptavidin-horseradish peroxidase (HRP). Once you've washed, add the tetramethylbenzidine substrate, wait 20 min, then halt the reaction and gauge the color intensity at 450 nm.

Step 7. Evaluate different markers like ERK5, Bax, Bcl2, Cyclin-D1, ERK1, MEK1, NF-κB, P-IKB-α, P-MAPK, P-NF-κB, and P-P38 in treated cells by applying Western blotting. Separate the cellular proteins using 12% SDS-polyacrylamide gel electrophoresis after lysing the treated cells in RIPA solution (PAGE). After transferring the proteins to PVDF membranes, add 5% nonfat dry milk to the mixture. Protein-specific primary antibodies should be used to probe the membranes overnight at 4 °C. After washing, secondary antibodies conjugated with HRP should be added. By including a chemiluminescent substrate, you can track the reaction. Utilize ImageJ software to quantify the proteins and observe the bands on an imager device.

Step 8. Utilize a cell migration test to assess cell migration. For this, incubate treated cells in an upper chamber of serum-free RPMI. Permit the cells to move into the RPMI and FBS-filled lower chamber. After a day of incubation, read the GR dye's fluorescence at a 480/520 nm excitation/ emission wavelength to determine the migratory capacity.

Step 9. Molecular Probes' Alexa Fluor 405-labeled Zymosan particles should be incubated with the treated cells for 60 min at 37 °C in a serum-free RPMI medium. To get rid of fluorescent beads that aren't absorbed, wash the cells three times in PBS. Measure the absorbance at an OD of 405 nm to analyze the cells. Also, determine cell apoptosis using flow cytometry using the Annexin V/propidium iodide double-staining technique.

Monkey Cell Model

According to Chan-Zapata et al. (2018):

Step 1. Collect experimental aniamls (e.g., Balb/c male mice; age: 6–8 weeks; average b.w.: 20-25 g) and ensure standard housing, feeding, and other conditions.

Step 2. Collect renal cell line of green monkey (Vero) and grow these cells in supplemented DMEM media consisting of 10% FBS and 1% penicillin–streptomycin. Maintain them in suitable condition (humidified incubator at 37 °C, 5% CO_2 atmosphere with 95% humidity).

Step 3. Sacrifice the mice through cervical dislocation. Isolate peritoneal macrophages by peritoneal lavage using cold PBS. Under a biological safety cabinet, they expose and clean their peritoneal cavities with 70% ethanol. Then inject 10 mL of cold PBS. Lavage fluid should be aspirated into a 10-mL plastic syringe to harvest the remaining macrophages, which should then be harvested by centrifugation for 15 min at 150×*g*, 4 °C. Re-suspend the cells in 10% FBS and 1% penicillin-streptomycin-supplemented DMEM medium. Ensure the cell viability (using a hemacytometer by trypan-blue dye exclusion) ≥95%. Use 1×10^4 cells/mL into each well of a 96-well plate for the cell viability assay, H_2O_2, NO, IL-6 and TNF-α production, while use 1×10^5 cells/mL per well of a 24-well plate for the assay of phagocytic activity. Maintain the plates in a humidified incubator for 48 h (37 °C, 5% CO_2). Treat the macrophages with the sample dissolved in supplemented DMEM media with 0.1% DMSO (200 μL for 96-well plates or 500 μL for 24-well plates). Incubate the plates for 24 h (37 °C, 5% CO_2). Activate the macrophages with LPS (1 μg/mL) and incubate during 48 h (37 °C, 5% CO_2). Use macrophages without treatment or stimuli as negative control and activated macrophages with LPS (1 μg/mL) without treatment employ as positive control in the H_2O_2, NO, IL-6 and TNF-α assays.

Step 4. Collect the supernatants of a 96-well plate with treated and activated macrophages and analyze them for nitrite production as an indicator of NO synthesis through the Griess reaction. For this, add 50 μL of the Griess reagent (0.1% N-(1-naphthyl) ethylenediamine dihydrochloride in H_2O and 1% sulphanilamide in 5% H_3PO_4) to 50 μL of each supernatant in 96-well plates. Measure the absorbance at 490 nm on the iMark Microplate Reader and determine nitrites concentration by comparison with a $NaNO_2$ standard curve (0-50 μM).

Step 5. Collect the supernatants of a 96-well plate with treated and activated macrophages and analyze them for H_2O_2 release. For this, mix cell culture supernatants (100 μL) with an equal volume of fresh phenol red solution (5.5 mM dextrose, 0.056 g phenol red, and 8.5 U/mL type I HRP in DPBS) in a 96-well plate and incubate for 3 h. Stop the reaction by adding 10 μL of NaOH 1 N solution. Measure the absorbance at 620 nm on the iMark Microplate Reader and determine the H_2O_2 concentration by the standard curve of H_2O_2 (0–50 μM).

Step 6. Analyze cytokines (e.g., IL-6, TNF-α) from the cell culture medium of treated and activated macrophages through the ELISA method. Use capture antibody at 2 μg/mL for IL-6 and 1 μg/mL for TNF-α. Use serial dilutions of recombinant IL-6 (0 - 4000 pg/mL) or TNF-α (0 - 2000 pg/mL) in diluent as standard curve. Detect the cytokines presented in the supernatants with a biotinylated avidin-HRP conjugated second antibody (0.5 μg/mL for IL-6 and 0.25 μg/mL for TNF-α). By extrapolating the absorbance from the standard curve, measure the absorbance at 490 nm similarly and calculate the cytokine concentration (pg/mL).

Step 7. Activated macrophages were co-cultured with yeasts of *Saccharomyces cerevisiae* (5×10^6 yeasts/well) labelled with PI (100 μg/mL) and incubated for 90 min (37 °C, 5% CO_2). Remove non-ingested labelling yeasts, and add 500 μL of separation buffer (0.5% BSA, 6.29 mM EDTA). Incubate the plate for 10 min (37 °C, 5% CO_2). Transfer the obtained cell suspension to 1.5-mL tube and centrifuge for 10 min at 150×*g*, 4 °C. Remove the supernatants by aspiration, and re-suspend the pellets in 1% formaldehyde. Determine the amount of *S. cerevisiae* yeasts phagocytosed by macrophages by measuring the cellular fluorescent intensity using a Cell Lab Quanta SC flow cytometer. Use macrophages with *S. cerevisiae* yeasts labelled with PI (1 μg/mL) as a negative control, and activated macrophages with LPS (1 μg/mL) and *S. cerevisiae* yeasts labelled with PI (1 μg/mL) as a positive control.

Step 8. Treat macrophages of 96-well plates (1×10^4 cells/well) with the test sample in supplemented DMEM media or DMSO (100%) as positive control. Treat pre-cultured Vero cells in 96-well plates (2.5×10^4 cells/well) with the test sample in supplemented DMEM media or CDDP (1 μg/mL) as a positive control. Use macrophages and Vero cells without treatment as a negative control. Remove the supernatants after 24 h and add 20 μL of the MTT solution (5 mg/mL in PBS) with 180 μL of supplemented DMEM media per well. Incubate the cells for 4 h (37 °C, 5% CO_2), remove the supernatants and add 100 μL of DMSO (100%) to each well, to dissolve produced-formazan crystals. Quantity the reduction of MTT by measurement of the absorbance at 490 nm similarly. Calculate %cell viability using the below-mentioned formula:

$$\%\text{Viability} = [(A_{TC} \div A_{NC}) \times 100$$

where, A_{TC} and A_{NC} stand for absorbance observed for treated cells and negative control, respectively.

Part IV: Anti-Arthritic Activity Tests

Rheumatoid arthritis (RA) affects 0.3 - 1% of the population worldwide. RA is a chronic and debilitating disease. It is the most common inflammatory rheumatic disease. Most frequently, RA appears in people aged 50–60 years old. It affects women more than men. It affects normal lives and limits the daily movement of humans. People with RA experience a marked decline in the quality of their daily life, which can cause depression. These people experience joint deformity with increased volume, loss of function, and bone and cartilage degeneration in their joints. This condition mostly affects the ankle joint, causing slow-moving painful swelling, exaggerated and aberrant synovial growth, pannus production, and morphological alterations to the joint. RA develops in three stages: swelling, warmth, pain, and redness around the joint caused by swelling of the synovial membrane; thickening of the synovial membrane caused by cell division and rapid growth, or pannus; and release of enzymes by inflamed cells that can digest bone and cartilage, leading to loss of shape and alignment of the involved joint, along with increased pain and loss of motion. The study of immunology is crucial to understanding rheumatic disorders. Monocytes, mast cells, macrophages, polymorphonuclear cells, and fibroblast synoviocytes are all present in rheumatoid synovium (Choudhary et al. 2015; Warriar et al. 2019). To date, a number of study models have been introduced to evaluate the anti-arthritic effects of a wide variety of test substances using *in vitro* and *in vivo* studies. Some important study models are given below.

In Vitro Assays

Preparation of Human Polymorpho Neutrophils (PMNs)

According to Zimmerman (1983):

Step 1. Aseptically collect 10 mL of venous blood from a healthy volunteer and mix it with heparin in a centrifuge tube. Use Ficoll hypaque density gradient centrifugation to isolate neutrophils.

Step 2. Mix whole blood, lymphocyte separation medium, and HBSS in equal volumes.

Step 3. Collect the supernatant after 30 min and slowly place it into empty centrifuge tubes of 15 mL containing 5 mL of lymphocyte separation medium and centrifuge (400×*g*, 20 min, room temperature).

Step 4. Discard the supernatant, add distilled water (1 mL) to the pellet for exactly 60 seconds for the lysis of RBCs, and add 1 mL of $HBSS^{--}$(2x) to stop the lysis.

Step 5. Add 5 mL of HBSS to the tubes and centrifuge the tubes (300×*g*, 10 min, 4 °C). Discard the supernatant and add $HBSS^{--}$ (1 mL) again and store it (on ice). Use the trypan blue exclusion method to check the viability and count the cells by hemocytometer. Use a cell concentration of 1×10^6 cells/mL for tests.

Peritoneal Macrophages Isolation from Rodents

According to Mahomoodally et al. (2007):

Step 1. Immunize animals (e.g., mice, rats) with FBS (1 mL) i.p. dose using sterile 1 mL syringe. Keep them 3 days in the animal house and kill by cervical dislocation.

Step 2. Inject 10 mL of 10% RPMI medium in the peritoneum cavity after sterilizing whole animal bodies by dipping into 70% ethanol.

Step 3. Massage the peritoneum cavity for 2 min and cut the abdominal skin from the lower side and retract to expose peritoneum cavity.

Step 4. Collect RPMI containing macrophage with the help of a sterile syringe from peritoneum. Centrifuge for 20 min (400×*g*, 4 °C).

Step 5. Wash the pellets after discarding the supernatant with RPMI media, then centrifuge for 10 min (300×*g*, 4 °C), then add 1 mL of RPMI media/HBSS. Use the trypan blue exclusion method to check the viability and count the cells by hemocytometer. Use a cell concentration of 1×10^6 cells/mL for tests.

Chemiluminescence Assay

According to Mahomoodally et al. (2007):

Step 1. Use white plates 96 wells for this test.

Step 2. Mix 25 μL of your test sample or standard drug ibuprofen with 25 μL of whole blood (diluted in $HBSS^{++}$ (1:50)) or PMNs (1×10^6) or macrophages (2×10^6) cells, except for control wells that receive only the $HBSS^{++}$ and cells without test sample.

Step 3. Incubate the plates for 20 min at 37 °C (thermostated chamber of Luminometer) to reach 100 μL volume/well, add 25 μL of Serum Opsonized Zymosan/PMA and/or 25 μL of luminol/lucigenin (7×10^5 M).

Step 4. Measure the results as relative light units (RLU). Use the following formula to calculate %inhibition for each treatemnt:

$$\%\text{Inhibition} = [(\text{RLU}_{\text{control}} - \text{RLU}_{\text{sample}}) \div \text{RLU}_{\text{control}}] \times 100$$

Cytokine Assay

According to Singh et al. (2005):

Step 1. Collect THP-1 (Human monocytic leukemia) cells and maintain them in endotoxin free RPMI1640 media.

Step 2. Introduce cultivated cells (2.5×10^5 cells/mL) in flasks up to 70% confluence into 24 wells tissue culture plates. Use PMA for differentiated cells into macrophage like cells (20 ng/mL) and incubate for 24 h at 37 °C in 5% CO_2.

Step 3. Use *E. coli* Lipopolysacchride B to stimulate cells (50 ng/mL).

Step 4. Treat the cells with your test sample or controls and incubate (4 h, 37 °C) in 5% CO_2.

Step 5. Collect the supernatants and analyze the level cytokines using human TNF-α and IL-1β ELISA Kit.

T-Cell proliferation assay

According to Rita et al. (2014):

Step 1. Introduce your test sample (50 μL) or prednisolone diluted in 5% RPMI to white 96 wells round bottom plates. Triplicate each dilution.

Step 2. Add 50 μL of isolated T-cells (2×10^6 cells/mL) and stimulate them with 50 μL of phytohemagglutinin-L (PHAL) (7.5 μg/mL). Prepare a negative control only with cells (50 μL) and 5% RPMI (150 μL) and a positive control with cells (50 μL) and PHAL (50 μL) and 5% RPMI (100 μL).

Step 3. Incubate the plates for 72 h at 37 °C in a 5% CO_2 incubator. 25 μL of 0.5 μCi/well (methyl 7 3H) thymidine is used to pulse the cultures, then the plates are further incubated (18 h) and a glass fiber filter is used to harvest the cells.

Step 4. Use an LS65000 liquid scintillation counter to determine the level of the thymidine integrated into the cells.

Step 5. Determine %inhibition by using the counts per minute (CPM) of each well according to the formula:

$$\%\text{Inhibition} = [(\text{CPM}_{\text{control}} - \text{CPM}_{\text{sample}}) \div \text{CPM}_{\text{control}}] \times 100$$

MTT Cytotoxicity Assay

Follow the cytotoxic assay for this and calculate the %inhibition or decrease in cell viability by using the formula (Scholz et al. 1999):

$$\%\text{Inhibition} = 100 - [(\text{OD}_{\text{test group}} - \text{OD}_{\text{blank}}) \div (\text{OD}_{\text{control}} - \text{OD}_{\text{blank}})] \times 100$$

In Vivo Assays

Formaldehyde-Induced Arthritis Inflammation Model

According to Akindele and Adeyemi (2007):

Step 1. Inject 0.1 mL of formaldehyde solution in the plantar aponeurosis of the left foot of mice or rats, on the 1st and 3rd day of the study.

Step 2. Administer your test sample, control and positive control (e.g., indomethacin at 10 mg/kg) orally once daily for 7-10 days.

Step 3. Measure the animals' paw circumference daily for 7-10 days and determine the percent inhibition paw edema of each treatment group on the last day and compared your data with the control group.

Type II Collagen-Induced Arthritis Model

Type II collagen (CII) is purified from chicken sternal cartilage (Sabino et al. 1999).

Step 1. At day 0, immunize the animals (e.g., mice) by an intradermal (i.d.) injection (0.1 mL) at the base of the tail with 200 μg CII in 50 mM acetic acid emulsified in Complete Freund's Adjuvant (CII:CFA; 1:2 (v/v)). Three weeks later, boost the animals with an intraperitoneal (i.p.) injection of 400 μg CII in 50 mM acetic acid.

Step 2. Monitor CIA throughout the experiment by measuring the hind paw oedema with a plethysmometer.

Step 3. Calculate the Arthritis Index (AI) as:

%AI = (hind paw volume day X-hind paw volume day 0) × 100/hind paw volume day 0

Step 4. Take the weight of animals weekly and determine the changes in body weight. Orally treat the animals with gavage (100 μL), daily, from day 21 until the end of the 6th week. Use methotrexate (0.2 mg/kg, p.o.) as a standard drug.

Cell Counting Model

According to Pereira et al. (2018):

Step 1. Collect blood from the orbital plexus (under anaesthesia). Place aliquots on slides, stain with a panotic haematological dye, and after drying, and examine the stained smears under light microscopy for a differential count of leucocytes.

Step 2. Process the lymph node and spleen in 1 or 5 mL of PBS (pH 7.4), respectively, for manual tissue dissociation.

Step 3. Perfuse the femur with 1 mL of PBS to obtain the bone marrow cells.

Step 4. Dilute the cells (10×) with 0.05% crystal violet in 30% acetic acid and count them by light microscopy in a Neubauer chamber.

Ref: Pereira WS, et al. Anti-arthritic properties of crude extract from *Chenopodium ambrosioides* L. leaves. *J Pharm Pharmacol.* 2018; pp. 1-14.

7-Ethoxyresorufin-O-deethylase and glutathione S-transferase Assay Model

According to Habig et al. (1974) and Peterson (1983):

Step 1. The liver 7-ethoxyresorufin-O-deethylase (EROD) activity is assayed on 2.5 μM of ethoxyresorufin in DMSO, 5 mM $MgCl_2$ and 0.25 mM NADPH in PPB (0.1 M, pH 7.8). The production of resorufin is determined using a standard curve, with a fluorometer excitation wavelength of 550 nm and emission at 582 nm at 27 °C.

Step 2. Also assay activity of glutathione S-transferase (GST) towards CDNB (several classes). Determine the activity of GST in the cytosolic fraction (100000 g supernatant) in 0.1 M sodium phosphate buffer containing 1 mM EDTA, pH 6.5. This solution contains 10 μg of protein, 2 mM of CDNB in ethanol 4%, and 5 mM of reduced glutathione (GSH). Duplicate each assay with correction for non-enzymatic conjugation using a complete assay mixture without enzyme.

Step 3. Ascertain protein concentration using BSA as a standard (10-100 μg). Measurement of conjugate formation continuously for 3 min at 340 nm at 25 °C.

Cytokine Determination by Cytometric Bead Array Model

Quantification of IL-6, IFN-γ, TNF-α, and IL-17 in an animal's serum by using this method, using kits Th1/Th17 cytokines kit according to the manufacturer's instructions. Express each cytokine in pg/mL (Pereira et al. 2018).

Tomographic Scan and Bone Density

Take 3D imaging of animal joints by using computerized tomography (CT), with cuts of 0.8 mm (Pereira et al. 2018).

Histopathology

According to Pereira et al. (2018):

Step 1. Remove the soft tissues and patella of the left joint of each animal.

Step 2. Fix the tissues in 4% neutral-buffered formalin for 1 day. Then place them under running water for 2 h to remove excess fixative and then store them in 10% EDTA, pH 7.4, with changes on a 48 /48 /72 h cycle for approximately 10 weeks, until satisfactory bone decalcification.

Step 3. Place the tissues in formalin, dehydrate in a graded series of ethanol and xylol, embed in paraffin, cut into 6-µm-thick serial sections and stained with haematoxylin and eosin.

Freund's complete adjuvant-induced arthritis model

Freund's complete adjuvant contains heat-killed dead *Mycobacterium tuberculosis* in liquid paraffin in the concentration of 10 mg/mL (Newbold, 1963).

Step 1. Inject intradermally with 0.1 mL of FCA into the left hind paw on day '0' all the animals (e.g., rats) (except normal control group).

Step 2. Give an interval of 7 days for arthritis to develop.

Step 3. All the animals will develop the signs of arthritis such as swelling, redness, and restricted movement during this period.

Step 4. On day 8, collect 3 mL of blood by retro-orbital puncture for baseline biochemical assays and treatment. Stop the treatment on day 28.

Step 5. Measure body weight, temperature, spontaneous activity, and measure paw volume of animals once every 7 days from day '0' to '28'.

Step 6. On day 28, perform an X-ray of the hind paw and collect blood samples for biochemical assays.

Step 7. Sacrifice the rats by administering a high dose of halothane and dissecting the ankle joints for histological studies.

Induction of AIA (adjuvant induced arthritis)

To induce arthritis, anesthetize animals with a small amount of ether vapor. Inject 100 µL of freshly prepared CFA (10 mg/mL) dissolved in mineral oil (sterile) into the hindpaw. Normal animals receive 100 µL of sterile mineral oil (Taniguchi et al. 2004).

Treatment Regimen

After classifying and grouping animals according to their weight, each animal is marked by the tail with a number and placed in a cage with a letter identifying the cage. Randomly divide the animals (e.g., rats) into the required groups (with the required number of animals in each group). Group 1 (healthy control) receives no treatment and no injection of CFA. Group 2 (arthritis control) receives a vehicle with CFA injected in the paw. Group 3 (positive control) receives indomethacin (5 mg/kg) with CFA injected in the paw. Test groups receive a test sample with CFA injected in the paw. Give all treatments orally 0.5 h before CFA induction (day 0), then the animals are treated daily for up to 19 days (Gabriella et al. 2007).

Paw Volume, Joint Diameter, Arthritic Score, Pain Threshold, Thermal Hyperalgesia and Body Weight Measurement

Step 1. Evaluate the severity of arthritis on days 0, 1, 3, 5, 7, 9, 11, 13, 15, 17, and 19. Use a plethysmometer to measure paw volume. Use a digital vernier caliper to measure the joint diameter. Use the Randall Selitto analgesiometer to measure mechanical pain threshold, while the plantar test apparatus measures thermal hyperalgesia.

Step 2. Express % values relative to the pre-administration value (100%) for each animal; variation of edema; joint diameter; paw withdrawal latency responses (pain threshold) and paw withdrawal latencies (thermal hyperalgesia).

Step 3. Assess the degree of arthritis daily by visual observation. Use a score scale of 0 - 4 to distinguish the different disease stages, with a maximum value of 8 for each animal.

Step 4. Scores are attributed according to the parameters such as edema, erythema, malformation and incapacity to use the limb. Record your body weight with the aid of a balance (Gabriella et al. 2007; Foyet et al. 2015).

Organs Weight Measurement and Biochemical Analysis

According to Mythilypriya et al. (2008) and Metha et al. (2012):

Step 1. On day 20, after anesthesia (using anesthetic ether), use cardiac puncture to draw blood and introduce it into a tube containing EDTA as an anticoagulant and into another tube without anticoagulant.

Step 2. Remove the liver, kidney, thymus, and spleen and take weight.

Step 3. Determine hematological parameters such as erythrocytes (RBC) and leukocytes (WBC) counts, hemoglobin (Hb), Hematocrit and platelets (PLT).

Step 4. Centrifuge blood without anti-coagulant for 5 min (4900×*g*) and collect the serum. Analyze serum AST, ALT, ALP, total protein, C-reactive protein (CRP) and rheumatoid factor (RF) levels.

Histopathological Analysis of Ankle Joints
Sacrifice the animals and separate the knee joints. Preserve in 10% formalin + PBS. After fixation and decalcification, cut the sample into 45 μm pieces, then use hematoxylin and eosin (H&E) for microscopic evaluation (Patil and Suryavanshi, 2007).

Part V: Hypoglycemic/Anti-Diabetic Test

Low blood sugar (also called hypoglycemia) is commonly found in people with type 1 diabetes. It can be dangerous if left untreated. Because our brains primarily rely on blood sugar for energy, hypoglycemia interferes with the brain's capacity to operate normally. This may result in neurological symptoms such as lightheadedness, headaches, blurred vision, difficulty focusing, and others. On the other hand, it is clear that hyperglycemia can become severe and cause major problems that need emergency care, including a diabetic coma. Even mild continuous hyperglycemia over the long run can cause problems with your eyes, kidneys, nerves, and heart. Consequently, accurate blood glucose level identification is a crucial concern. Generally speaking, a blood glucose test determines if your blood sugar levels are within a healthy weight range and is frequently used to assist in the diagnosis and monitoring of diabetes. Basic principles of oral hypoglycemic or anti-diabetic assays include: inhibition capacity of diabetogenic enzymes or factors; measurement of blood glucose levels in different stages; biomarkers present in diabetic conditions etc. (Tran et al. 2020). Some popularly used methods are given below.

In Vitro Assay

Alpha-glucosidase inhibition assay
According to Sancheti et al. (2011):

Step 1. Mix 250 μL PPB (100 mM, pH 7.0) with 150 μL of 0.5 mM 4-nitrophenyl-α-D-glucopyranoside. Add 50 μL of your test sample and 150 μL of α-glucosidase (0.1 unit/mL in 10 mM PPB) to it.

Step 2. Incubate the mixture at 37 ºC for 0.5 hours.

Step 3. Stop the reaction by adding 600 μL of 200 mM Na_2CO_3.

Step 4. Record the absorbance at 400 nm.

Step 5. Calculate the glucosidase inhibition activity by using the following formula:

$$\%\text{Inhibitory effect} = (A_{control} - A_{sample})/A_{control} \times 100$$

where, $A_{control}$ and A_{sample} represent the absorbance of control reaction (without test sample), and the absorbance in the presence of a test sample, respectively.

Alpha-Amylase Inhibition Assay

According to Khadayat et al. (2020):

Step 1. Prepare test concentrations and 50 mM PBS (pH 7.0) with 0.9% NaCl.

Step 2. Prepare p-nitroaniline (1.5 units/mL) in PBS and add it with test/controls.

Step 3. Incubate the tubes at 37 °C for 15 min.

Step 4. Add alpha-amylase (375 μM) to the all tubes. Adjust final volume up to 3 mL.

Step 5. Monitor the optical density by release of p-nitroaniline continuously at 405 nm and calculate the amylase inhibition activity by using the following formula:

$$\%\text{Inhibitory effect} = 100\text{-} (OD/min_{sample} \div OD/min_{control}) \times 100$$

where, $OD/min_{control}$ and OD/min_{sample} represent the optical density of control reaction (without test sample), and the optical density in the presence of a test sample, respectively.

In Vivo Assays

Acute hypoglycemic test in mice

According to Joy and Kuttan (1999):

Step 1. Randomly distribute overnight fasted mice into control, test, and standard groups, each having the required number of animals. Measure the fasting blood sugar (glucose) levels of all animals from the tail vein by using a glucometer.

Step 2. Give distilled water or the vehicle (10 mL/kg, p.o.) to the control group animals and glibenclamide (10 mg/kg, p.o.) to the standard group. Treat the test group animals with a suitable dose(s) similarly.

Step 3. Measure blood glucose levels similarly after 1 h of administration of your test sample or controls.

Step 4. Administer dextrose (2 g/kg, p.o.) solution to all groups and measure blood glucose levels similarly after 1st, 2nd and 3rd h by using same glucometer.

Ref: Joy K & Kuttan R. Anti-diabetic activity of *Picrorrhiza kurroa* extract. *J Ethnopharmacol.* 1999; 67(2): 143-148.

Alloxan-Induced Anti-Diabetic Test in Mice

According to Kameswara Rao et al. (1999) and Kumar et al. (2008):

Step 1. Estimate the base-line glucose levels in normal 12 h fasting animals and inject a freshly prepared alloxan solution (dissolved in PBS, 75 mg/kg, i.p.). Give the same volume of saline solution to the control animals.

Step 2. Collect blood samples from the tail vein after 8 days and measure the blood glucose levels with a glucometer.

Step 3. Distribute the diabetic mice (n = required number) to the standard and test groups. Use any suitable oral hypoglycemic drug, such as glibenclamide (10 mg/kg, p.o.) as a reference drug.

Step 4. Collect blood samples (approx. 0.3 mL) from the mouse tail vein before and at 2, 4, and 6 h after giving treatments by using the same glucometer and compare the obtained results with your control groups.

N.B. - For Wistar rats use alloxan monohydrate (100 mg/kg), dissolved in citrate buffer (pH = 4.5).

Maltose and Sucrose Tolerance Tests in Wistar Rats
According to Andrade-Cetto et al. (2008):

Step 1. Randomly distribute overnight fasted animals in control (distilled water/normal saline/vehicle), standard (e.g., acarbose 3 mg/kg) and test group(s) each having required number of animals.

Step 2. Treat all animals with 3 g/kg maltose solution 5 min after administration of controls and test drug.

Step 3. Collect blood samples from the tail vein and measure blood glucose levels by using a glucometer.

Rat Intestinal Sucrase Inhibition Assay
According to Nishioka et al. (1998):

Step 1. A number of normal animals' (e.g., rats') small intestines are removed. Wash the intestines 3 times with ice-cold isosaline, once with 0.1 M PPB (pH 7.0), and once with 5 mM EDTA. Scrap the mucosa, homogenize in a PPB, and centrifuge at 21,000×*g* for 1 h. Re-suspend the precipitate and incubate for 0.5 h in PPB containing 1% Triton X-100 and centrifuge at 100,000×*g* for 1.5 h. Dialyze the supernatant against PPB for 1 day. Lyophilize the dialysate and store at -20°Cuntil the test commenced.

Step 2. Mix 0.2 mL of 56 mM sucrose (enzyme substrate) and PPB (0.2 mL) with 0.1 mL of your test sample.

Step 3. Incubation the mixture at 37 °C for 5 min and add 0.2 mL of rat intestinal α-glucosidase solution. Use the vehicle, such as 0.1 mL of DMSO as a control (blank). Thoroughly mix respective samples (controls/test sample) and incubate at 37 °C for 15 min.

Step 4. By placing test tubes in boiling water for 4 minutes, the process can be stopped.

Step 5. To remove phenolic or acidic chemicals and measure the amount of freed glucose using a commercial test kit, run the reaction liquid over a basic alumina column (6 × 35 mm h).

Step 6. Measure the OD of the wells at 505 nm. Calculate the inhibitory activities of your test sample using the below-mentioned equation:

$$\%\text{Inhibition} = 100\,[1 - (OD_{\text{test sample}}/OD_{\text{control}})]$$

Rat Intestinal Maltase Inhibition Assay

The assay is conducted in the same way as the previous one, with the exception that 3.5 mM maltose is used as the enzyme substrate in 0.1 M PPB (pH 7, 0.35 mL) (Toda et al. 2000).

(Streptozotocin-induced) Diabetes Mellitus Test

According to Vianna et al. (2003) and Baquer et al. (2011):

Step 1. To induce type 1 diabetes in animals that have been fasting overnight, provide a single i.p. injection of STZ (65 or 150 mg/kg) dissolved in 100 μL of sterile PBS (pH 7.4). Before beginning a diabetic mellitus induction, weigh each individual animal and check their blood glucose level (BGL).

Step 2. Measure the glucose concentration in the tail or retroorbital sinus blood after 4 days of hyperglycemia using a glucometer. Animals having a BGL >20 mM or >200 mg/dL after 4 days of STZ treatment are included in this study. Give 5% glucose to all groups of animals after 6 hours of the STZ solution administration (to avoid death secondary to hypoglycemic shock).

Step 3. 72 h after fixing the groups (for controls and test samples), treat the animals respectively. Use metformin as a positive control at 500 mg/kg (p.o.) and vehicle (10 mL/kg, p.o.) as a control group.

Step 4. After 14 days of isoflurane anesthesia, sacrifice the animals, and on the day of termination, draw blood from the dorsal vena cava by opening the abdomen. Use an automatic biochemistry analyzer to collect serum and do estimations of glucose, cholesterol, triglycerides, LDL, SGOT, SGPT, ALP, creatinine, and total protein.

Step 5. Along with a histopathological investigation, effects of test sample/controls on variables including body weight, feed intake, and water consumption can be identified and recorded over the study time.

Insulin Resistance Test in Rats

According to Rees and Alcolado (2005):

Step 1. Give normal chow for 42 days and a 10% D-glucose solution as drinking water to animals that have been fasting overnight. During this period, control animals should be given a regular chow diet and tap water.

Step 2. After this period, collect blood to subsequently measure the glucose (by using a glucometer) and insulin (by the radioimmunoassay method) levels in animals fasted for 16 h.

Step 3. Use the Homeostasis Model Assessment (HOMA) as an index of insulin resistance and calculate it using the formula insulin (U/mL) × glucose (mol/L)/22.5 to determine the extent of insulin resistance. Only those animals (about 80% of the treated animals) that show a significant level of insulin resistance after 28 days of the 10% glucose water treatment are chosen for this investigation. Use metformin as a positive control at 150 mg/kg. Follow steps 4 and 5 of the previous model.

Insulin Tolerance Test in Rats

According to Yuan et al. (2013):

Step 1. Give an i.p. dose of 0.75 U/kg insulin to the 4 h fasted animals.

Step 2. Utilize a glucometer to measure your blood sugar levels instantly at 0, 0.5, and 2nd h. As a proportion of the starting plasma glucose level, present the value.

Step 3. Give the respective treatment and measure the blood glucose level similarly.

Step 4. Calculate the AUC to represent the insulin tolerance. AUC (mM/L-min) is calculated using the formula $AUC_{glucose} = 0.5 \times (G_0+G_{30})/2 + 0.5 \times (G_{30}+G_{60})/2 + 1 \times (G_{60} + G_{120})/2$, where G_0, G_{30}, G_{60}, G_{90}, and G_{120} are blood glucose values at different time points.

KK-A^y - Genetic Model of Type 2 Diabetes

The KK-A^y mice are a congenic yellow-obese KK mouse strain created by the introduction of the yellow agouti gene (Ay) into the KK mouse strain. It is a genetic representation of type 2 diabetes that displays extreme obesity, hyperinsulinemia, and insulin resistance—all characteristics that are essential to the disease (Matsuo et al. 1970).

Streptozotocin-Induced Chick Embryo Model

According to Yoshiyama (2005):

Step 1. Dissolve streptozotocin (STZ) in physiological saline and sterilize through a membrane filter. Dissolve regular human insulin to desired concentrations with sterilized physiological saline. Also, prepare your test sample with a suitable solvent.

Step 2. Collect fertile eggs (control group, n = 5) and incubate the eggs for 17 days at 37.5 ± 0.2 °C (relative humidity: 65%).

Step 3. Select large vitelline veins of an egg and mark them with a pencil under the fluorescent lamp (150-lux). Remove the eggshell of a marked range of 10 × 5 mm by electric drill and fill a drop of water to project clearly an artery (see the following Figure 9.2).

Step 4. Collect whole blood from a vein of an egg by means of a tuberculin syringe with a 0.55 × 32-mm needle.

Step 5. Measure the blood glucose level immediately (by the enzyme-electrode method or by using a suitable glucometer).

Step 6. Centrifuge the remaining blood sample at 3000 rpm for 10 min, collect the serum and store at -20°C until analysis. Measure the serum insulin level using the ELISA Insulin kit.

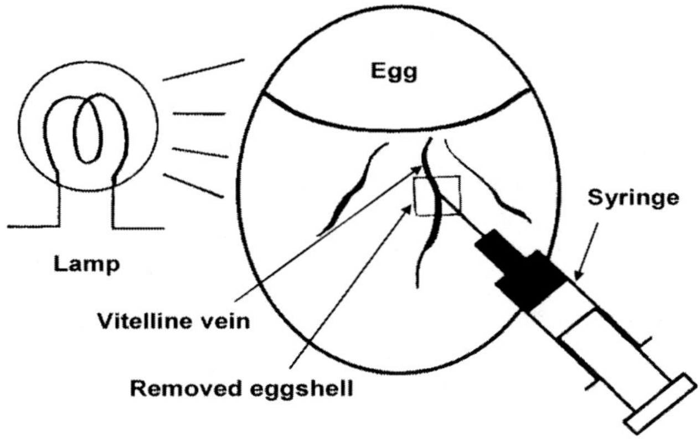

Figure 9.2. Chick embryo methodology (graphical abstract)

Collection of blood from the vitelline vein of fertile egg on the Day 17 of incubation.

Step 7. Inject STZ (100 mg/egg) into the albumen of each egg (n = 5 per group, negative control) on the Day 14 of incubation and collect blood on the Day 17 of incubation using the same methods. With the same methods, determine the levels of blood glucose and serum insulin.

Step 8. A test sample or a regular human insulin (4 U/egg, standard group) is injected into the air sac of STZ-treated eggs on the Day 17 day of incubation. After 5 min of insulin injection or 30 min of test sample injection, collect blood and measure blood glucose level in same methods.

Step 9. Perform suitable ANOVA statistics and compare the obtained results.

Part VI: Anti-Obesity Test

An excessive quantity of body fat is a complex medical disease called obesity. Numerous additional illnesses and health issues, such as heart disease, diabetes, high blood pressure, some malignancies, etc., are proven to be aggravated by it. Eating too much and moving too little have been found to be linked with obesity. However, genetic predisposition, high amounts of energy consumption (e.g., fat and sugar), low energy burning, low exercise and physical activity history are also associated with obesity. Assessment of physiological markers in animals is the basic principle of this study (Bays and Dujovne 2002; Müller et al. 2022). Examples of some popularly used models for anti-obesity tests of a wide variety of samples have been given below.

In Vitro Models

Pancreatic lipase (PL) inhibition assay

Porcine pancreatic lipase (PPL, type II) activity is estimated by using *p*-nitrophenyl butyrate (*p*-NPB) as a substrate in this study (Roh and Jung, 2012).

Step 1. Prepare 1 mg/mL PPL stock solution in 0.1 mM PPB (pH 6.0) and store it at -20 °C. The test material (at various concentrations) or Orlistat (at identical concentrations) is pre-incubated with PPL for 1 h in PPB at 30 °C before the PPL activity assay is conducted to assess the lipase inhibitory activity.

Step 2. Start the reaction by adding 0.1 μL NPB (adjust to a final volume of 100 μL).

Step 3. Measure the amount of p-nitrophenol produced in the reaction at 405 nm using a UV-Vis spectrophotometer after 300 sec of incubation at 30 °C. DMSO can be used as a negative control.

Step 4. Additionally, both with and without an inhibitor, the activity of the negative control is assessed. The following formula is used to determine the inhibitory activity:

$$\%\text{Inhibition} = 100 - ((B - b)/(A - a) \times 100)$$

where, A, a, B and b are the activity without inhibitor, negative control without inhibitor, activity with inhibitor, and negative control with inhibitor, respectively.

Cell Differentiation, Triglyceride and Glycerol Test in Adipocytes

Step 1. Collect preadipocytes (3T3-L1) and culture in DMEM supplemented with 10% (v/v) heat-inactivated FBS at 37 °C in 5% CO_2.

Step 2. To induce adipocyte differentiation, 48-h post-confluent 3T3-L1 (day 0) are stimulated for 48 h with an inducer (10 μg/mL insulin, 2.5 μM dexamethasone, and 0.5 mM 3-isobutyl-1-methylxanthine) including your test sample, and then maintained for 6 days (day 8) in DMEM supplemented with 10% FBS and 10 μg/mL insulin.

Step 3. Treat the cells with your sample in DMEM supplemented with 10% FBS for 2 days (day 10). Change the media and your test sample every 48 h until the end of the experiment at day 10.

Step 4. Utilize the MTT test to ascertain cell viability.

For this, a test sample is administered to cells grown in DMEM medium for 48 h at a specific final concentration, and then the cells are exposed to a 5 mg/mL MTT solution for 3 h.

The optical density (OD) at 570 nm is used to determine the formazane level after the cells have been dissolved in 0.04 N HCl (in isopropanol) (against OD at 630 nm). The PBS-washed cells are then fixed in 10% formalin for 0.5 h.

The cells are stained for at least 60 min at room temperature in a newly diluted Oil Red O solution (the Oil Red O stock solution used is 0.5% Oil Red O in isopropanol). This is done after two washes with distilled water.

Utilizing isopropanol to elute the dye still present in the cells, the amount was quantified by measuring the absorbance at 500 nm.

Step 5. TG levels in cells can be determined using a commercial TG test kit. Treat the cells for 6 days during adipocyte differentiation with your test sample at a specific dose in 6-well plates. After two PBS washes, the cells are scraped in 75 μL of a homogenizing solution (154 mM KCl, 1 mM EDTA, and 50 mM Tris, pH 7.4) and homogenized using a sonicator. To remove the fat layers, centrifuge the remaining cell lysate at 3000×g for 5 min at 25 °C. Check the supernatants for protein and TG levels. By utilizing BSA as a reference, normalize TG to the protein concentration using the Bradford test. Give your findings in mg of TG/mg of cellular protein.

Step 6. Glycerol discharged into the media can be used to quantify lipolysis. Treat differentiated 3T3-L1 cells with your test sample for 1 day to accomplish this. Following incubation, 50 μL of the medium is incubated at ambient temperature for 15 min with 200 μL of a free glycerol reagent. Measure the absorbance at 540 nm to determine the glycerol's amount (Roh and Jung 2012).

Lipoprotein lipase (LPL) Inhibitory Assay

According to Schotz et al. (1970):

Step 1. Dilute the activator (Apo C-II from human plasma to 1 μg/mL with 0.002 M Tris HCl, pH 8.0).

Step 2. Mix 0.6 mL of triolein with 24 mL of apo C-II, 3.6 mL of 1% BSA solution, 3.6 mL of 1% triton X-100, and 28.8 mL of 0.2 M Tris-HCl buffer to create a substrate (pH 8.0). For 180 sec, sonicate the mixture with ice.

Step 3. By dilution with 0.02 M Tris HCl (pH 8.0) to a concentration of 25 units/mL, prepare the enzyme LPL from bovine milk. Analyze the activities of LPL. This is done by mixing 0.5 mL of previously diluted LPL with 0.5 mL of your test sample, followed by pre-incubation at 4 °C for 30 min.

Step 4. Combine your test sample with the enzyme and add 1 mL of substrate emulsion to this combination. Hydrolysis is started by incubating the combination in a water bath at 37 °C. With the addition of 1 mL of 1 M NaCl, the process will be stopped. Only an enzyme and substrate mixture is present in control samples.

Step 5. Utilizing an auto titrator, titrate the freed free fatty acids (FFA) with 0.01 M NaOH until pH 9.4. The amount of base needed by the incubation mixture, which is equivalent to LPL activity, indicates the amount of freed FFA. A control sample has 100% of the enzyme activity. For each sample extract, the experiment is run three times, and the percent inhibition is calculated.

In Vivo Model

High-Fat Diet (HFD)-Induced Anti-Obesity Model in Mice

Step 1. In this study, we collect the required number and species of mice and maintain a suitable environment for them.

Step 2. Then administer an HFD (see **Table 9.1**) that contains 60% fat calories in order to quickly raise BW and cause obesity. Divide the adapted animals at random into the necessary number of groups (n), with weight differences between and within groups not exceeding 10% of the sample population's mean body weight.

Step 3. Divide all animals into normal and obese groups and then feed them with normal diets (ND) and HFD, respectively. The HFD groups can be divided into further groups and given treatments for a certain period (e.g., 64 days)-the HFD group receives HFD only, the HFD-treatment group receives HFD with a dose, and the HFD-standard group receives HFD with a suitable standard drug dose). Use water ad libitum and these diets throughout the experimental period.

Table 9.1. Composition of the typical experimental diets

Ingredients (g/kg)	**ND**	**HFD**	**HFD-0.25**	**HFD-0.5**
Casein	210.0	230.0	230.0	230.0
l-Cystine	3.0	3.5	3.5	3.5
Maltodextrin	50.0	160.0	160.0	160.0
Sucrose	325.0	90.0	90.0	90.0
Lard	20.0	310.0	310.0	310.0
Soybean oil	20.0	30.0	30.0	30.0
Cellulose	37.15	65.5	65.5	65.5
Corn starch	280.0	-	-	-
Mineral mix	35.0	48.0	48.0	48.0
CaH(PO4)2	2.0	3.4	3.4	3.4
Vitamin mix	15.0	21.0	21.0	21.0
Choline bitartrate	2.75	3.0	3.0	3.0
Blue food color	0.1	0.1	0.1	0.1
NAOs	-	-	2.5	5
Nutrition facts: % g (w/w) (% kcal)				
Protein	18.8 (20.1)	23.5 (18.4)	23.5 (18.4)	23.5 (18.4)
Carbohydrate	64.7 (69.8)	27.3 (21.3)	27.3 (21.3)	27.3 (21.3)
Fat	4.2 (10.2)	34.3 (60.3)	34.3 (60.3)	34.3 (60.3)
Kcal/g	3.6	5.1	5.1	5.1

Step 4. Collect blood from the inferior vena cava after 64 days and a 16-hour fast. Blood samples should be centrifuged to extract the serum into tubes, which should then be stored until testing. Measure the weight of the tissues (such as the liver, kidneys, and epididymis) and record it as a proportion of the body weight before the fast. Then, fix the tissues with 10% formalin and freeze them in liquid nitrogen.

Step 5. Use paraffin and 10% formalin to preserve the tissues of the liver and epididymis. Slice 4-μm standard slices, stain with hematoxylin and eosin, and then view with a 100x optical microscope. Based on the presence of macro-or micro-vesicular fat in >5% of the hepatocytes and an analysis of adipocyte size using the ImageJ tool, fatty liver is diagnosed.

Step 6. Utilize an auto-chemistry analyzer to measure the TG and TC levels in serum. Use an automated chemical analyzer and NEFA-HR reagents to evaluate the serum FFA. Analyze serum levels of adiponectin, leptin, and insulin using the ELISA method. Estimate the quantities of ALT, AST, and ALP as well.

Step 7. Obtain dried and powdered fecal waste from the experimental animals after 32 and 64 days. Fecal lipids can be extracted using a 2:1 mixture of chloroform and methanol, then dissolved in triton × 100 at 1%, and estimated using a kit approach. Utilize the tri-reagent to separate the total RNA from the animal's adipose tissue in accordance with the manufacturer's instructions, and then use a DNA synthesis kit to reverse-transcribe the RNA to produce cDNA. Use specified primers and 20 ng of cDNA for semi-quantitative PCR.

N.B. - This experiment can be continued for anti-diabetic effects of the test drug or controls as follows:

Step 8. OGTT can be done as follows at 64 days: Gavage feedings of 20% glucose solution (2 g glucose/kg, b.w.) are administered to 5-h-fasted animals (e.g., mice). A glucometer is used to measure blood glucose levels. At 0, 30, 60, 90, and 120 min, blood samples (3.5 μL) are drawn to measure the plasma glucose level (Nolan et al. 1997; Mopuri et al. 2015; Rasband and Image, 2016).

An anti-obesity study can also be performed by using S.C. administration of progesterone (depo-medroxyprogesterone acetate: DPMA) at a dose of 10 mg/kg induced obesity model. For this, administer 0.5 h after p.o. administration of your test sample for 4 weeks, except for the negative controls (Gundamaraju et al. 2012). Then follow the same procedure as mentioned above.

Part VII: Anti-Hemolytic Tests

Red blood cells are destroyed by hemolysis (RBCs). RBCs can live for up to 4 months on average. Our bodies automatically kill them after that. However, some illnesses and treatments may cause them to degrade more quickly than usual, which can cause hemoglobinemia, which can be a major factor in the pathogenesis of sepsis. Because this phenomenon has a suppressive effect on the innate immune system, it also raises the risk of infection. Certain types of hemolysis can lead to death. For example, malaria-associated hemolysis may cause death in adult patients. It has been speculated that conditions, pathogens, or causative agents producing oxidative stress and inflammation can damage RBCs and are potentially involved in hemolysis-related pathophysiology (Bhushan et al. 2021). This test can be performed by some popularly used models mentioned below.

Preparation of Rat Erythrocytes

Under general anesthesia, kill the animals, and draw blood from the heart into heparinized tubes. Isolate the erythrocytes and store them in Alsevier's solution at 4 °C until the test commences. Centrifuge the blood sample at 1500×*g* for 10 min at 4 °C. Separate the RBCs from the plasma and buffy coat before centrifuging the blood sample 3 times (at 3000×*g* for 300 sec) in 10 volumes of 10 mM PBS (pH 7.4). With each wash, gently remove the WBC buffy coatings and supernatant. For additional studies, keep the RBCs at 4°Cand use them within 6 h (Ebrahimzadeh et al. 2010).

CuOOH-Induced Hemolysis Assay

Step 1. Prepare a 1% RBC suspension in balanced phosphate buffered saline.

Step 2. 3.5 mL of aliquots should be incubated at 37 °C for 3.5 h while 50 μM CuOOH (dissolved in ethanol) is present. After that, check the cellular integrity turbidimetrically at 710 nm every 0.5 hours.

Step 3. Add CuOOH to the sample pre-incubated for 0.5 with 1% RBC suspension and read the absorbance similarly.

Step 4. Calculate %hemolysis setting as a 100% hemolysis (Ebrahimzadeh et al. 2010).

H_2O_2-Induced Hemolysis Assay (Model 1)

According to Yang et al. (2005):

Step 1. Take 5 mL of a healthy person's venous blood in EDTA vials, and centrifuge for 5 min at 1000×*g*.

Step 2. Before re-suspending the pellets in a saline solution (0.5%), remove the supernatant and wash the pellets 3 times with PBS (0.2 M, pH 7.4).

Step 3. Add 0.5 mL of the test sample to 1 mL of RBC suspension, and let it sit for 20 min at ambient temperature.

Step 4. To encourage oxidative breakdown of the membrane lipids, add 0.5 mL of H_2O_2 (0.82 M) solution (prepared in buffered saline) to the reaction mixture. The samples should be incubated for 180 min at 37 °C.

Step 5. The samples should be centrifuged at 1000×*g* for 10 min, and the absorbance of the supernatant should be measured at 540 nm.

Step 6. Analyze the relative hemolysis in relation to the H_2O_2 treatment (negative control), set at 100% hemolysis. Use 0.2 M PBS and 0.82 M H_2O_2 as a blank solution, and L-ascorbic acid as the standard (31.5-1000 μg/mL). Determine the inhibitory activity of the various groups, represent it as %inhibition of hemolysis, and duplicate each set of trials.

H_2O_2-Induced Hemolysis Assay (Model 2)

According to Ajila and Prasada (2008):

Step 1. Make a 4% RBC suspension in PBS (0.2 M). Add 1 g of your test sample to 1 mL of PBS, and then increase the volume of PBS to 5 mL.

Step 2. Incubate the mixture for 5 min at ambient temperature.

Step 3. After 4 h, 90% of the blood cells will have undergone hemolysis if you add 0.5 mL of H_2O_2 (0.82 M) solution diluted in PBS to cause oxidative breakdown of the membrane lipids. **Step 4**. Measure the absorbance at 540 nm, which corresponds to hemoglobin liberation, to assess the degree of hemolysis by centrifuging the reaction mixture at 1500×*g* for 10 min.

Part VIII: Thrombolytic Activity Analysis

Blood flow via the circulatory system is obstructed by thrombus formation inside blood channels, which can result in hypertension, heart attacks, anoxia, and other conditions. Thrombous formation occurs through several pathways in humans. A typical thrombolytic agent may act through one or more pathways. A popularly used *in vitro* clot lysis test model has been given below.

Clot Lysis Model

According to Prasad et al. (2007):

Step 1. Collect 5 mL of venous blood from the required number of healthy volunteers who are not currently using anti-coagulant therapy and disperse the blood in sterile pre-weighed (W_1) microcentrifuge tubes (0.5 mL/tube).

Step 2. Incubate the tubes at 37 °C for 45 min.

Step 3. Remove the serum carefully and take the second weight (W_2) of all tubes and determine the clot weight (W_2-W_1).

Step 4. Add a 100 μL test sample to each tube. As a standard, 100 μL of streptokinase (equivalent to 30,000 I.U.) can be used. For the control group, use only 100 μL of distilled water.

Step 5. Re-incubate the tubes at 37 °C for 90 min.

Step 6. Discard the lysed fluid from all tubes carefully and take the third weight (W_3) and calculate the clot weight after discarding the lysis and then %clot lysis using the below-mentioned equation:

%Clot lysis = (Weight of clot after treatment ÷ Weight of clot before treatment) × 100

$$\text{or } [(W_2 - W_1) - (W_2 - W_3) \div (W_2 - W_1)] \times 100$$

Part IX: Anti-Emetic Activity Study

The violent expulsion of stomach contents from the mouth is referred to as emesis (sometimes called vomiting). Motion sickness, the use of specific medicines, intestinal blockage, disease or dysfunction of the inner ear, head injury, and appendicitis are only a few of the many potential reasons. Medical science declares that our vomiting center is predominantly activated by three distinct mechanisms: (i) reflexive activation: by nervous impulses from the stomach, intestinal tract, and other portions of the body; (ii) stimulation: from the higher brain centers; and (iii) impulse generation: by the chemoreceptor trigger zone (Zhong et al. 2021). All these mechanisms can be targeted to develop the anti-emetic effect of your test sample. An example of one study model includes:

Chick (*In Vivo*) Model

According to Akita et al. (1998):

Step 1. Randomly divide chicks of 3-5 days of age into the required number in each group and keep each in a large plastic jar or glass beaker at ambient temperature for 10 min.

Step 2. Dissolve the test sample in 0.9% saline containing 5% DMSO and 1% tween 80 and administer it orally at 10 mL/kg body weight. Use 0.9% saline solution as a control. On the other hand, metoclopramide can be used as a standard drug (50 mg/kg, b.w., i.p.).

Step 3. $CuSO_4$ should be given orally at a dosage of 50 mg/kg body weight after 30 min, and the number of retches should be counted for 10 minutes. The latency and reduction in retches in the treatment group compared to the control group serves as an indicator of the antiemetic impact.

Step 4. Calculate the %inhibition using the below-mentioned equation:

$$\%\text{Inhibition of emesis} = ((A\text{-}B)/A) \times 100$$

where, A and B stand for retching frequency of control and test group, respectively.

Step 5. Calculate the %incidence of emesis (%IE) using the below-mentioned equation:

%IE = (Number of emetic chicks ÷ Total chicks in the group) × 100

Part X: Anti-Pyretic Activity Study

A person to have a fever when he or she has a measured temperature of 100.4 °F (38 °C) or greater, or feels warm to the touch, or gives a history of feeling feverish. The main symptoms of a fever include: elevated temperature (above 100.4 °F), chills, shivering, shaking, and body aches and headaches. It is not considered a disease. Fever is usually a sign that your body is trying to fight an illness or infection. Mostly, most pathogenic bacteria and viruses do well when your body is at your normal temperature. But if you have a fever, it is harder for them to survive. Fever also activates your body's immune system. High fevers that linger or worsen can cause significant health complications if left untreated, including febrile seizures, brain damage, and even death (Hellon and Townsend 1982; Kozak et al. 2000). An example of a widely used anti-pyretic test model includes:

Brewer's Yeast Induced Pyrexia (Mouse/Rat Model)

According to Abena et al. (2003):

Step 1. Take adequate fasted overnight with water *ad libitum* experimental animals (e.g., mice, rats) and record their initial rectal temperature using an Ellab thermometer.

Step 2. Administer 10 mL/kg body weight of a 20% aqueous suspension of Brewer's yeast to induce hyperpyrexia.

Step 3. After 18 h observe the rectal raised temperature of 0.3 - 0.5 °C for selecting qualified animals for this study.

Step 4. Treat the groups respectively with tests or controls. As a control, the vehicle can be used while, as a reference standard, an antipyretic drug such as paracetamol (150 mg/kg body weight orally) can be used.

Step 5. Record the rectal temperature at 1 h intervals for 4 h after treatment and compare the test group temperature with the control groups.

Yeast Induced Pyrexia (Chick Model)

According to Mousa et al. (2019) and Bashar QM & Albadrany (2022):

Step 1. Take adequate 4 - 5 h fasted broiler chicks 7 - 21 days old weighing between 48–125 g (n = 5/6) and record their initial rectal temperature using an Ellab thermometer.

Step 2. Administer 10 mL/kg body weight of a 15-20% aqueous suspension of Brewer's yeast (p.o.) or baker's yeast 0.135 g/kg (i.p.) to induce hyperpyrexia.

Step 3. After 12 h observe the rectal raised temperature of 0.3 - 0.5 °C for selecting qualified animals for this study.

Step 4. Treat the groups respectively with tests or controls. As a control, the vehicle can be used while, as a reference standard, an antipyretic drug such as paracetamol (150 mg/kg, p.o.) or ketorolac (20 mg/kg, i.m.) can be used.

Step 5. Record the rectal temperature at 0.5 h intervals for 2 h after treatment and compare the test group temperature with the control groups.

Part XI: Anti-Microbial Assays

Each year, infectious diseases cause more than 10 million fatalities. The term "infection" describes the invasion of tissues by pathogens (such as bacteria, fungi, and viruses), their growth, and the host tissues' response to the infectious agent and the toxins (such as exotoxins and endotoxins) they create. Transmissible or communicable diseases are other names for infectious diseases (Hutner et al. 1958). Our body can fight against pathogens using immune machinery through diverse mechanisms. Specifically, antibiotics, antivirals, antifungals, anti-protozoals, and anti-helminthics are used to treat infections. Diabetes, anxiety, lupus, shingles, psoriasis, schizophrenia, Lyme disease, HPV, herpes, pneumonia, fibromyalgia, scabies, chlamydia, endometriosis, strep throat, diverticulitis, and bronchitis are among the twenty significant disorders currently known to be caused by infection. It is to be noted that developing resistance to antibiotics is a common consequence. Therefore, searching for new antimicrobial agents from natural products and managing pathogens are two important objectives of antimicrobial studies.

Antimicrobial activity is the ability of a substance to act against microorganisms (e.g., bacteria, fungi, viruses, yeasts, and molds) by inhibiting or retarding the growth of microorganisms or their population. Some are *cidal* in nature and kill the microorganisms other than retarding or sustaining (*static*) the growth of microorganisms.

Factors Affecting Anti-Microbial Activity of Test Sample

1. Microorganisms:
   a. *Type:* Each microorganism is unique in its behavior, nutritional requirements, and sensitivity towards a particular anti-microbial agent. Therefore, the choice of sensitive microorganisms is an important issue.
   b. *Condition:* The microorganisms should be either vegetative cells or spores. In the case of vegetative organisms, we need to select the organisms from the log or exponential phase, while the spores should be activated by heat shock at a suitable temperature.
   c. *Density of the inoculum:* Another important factor for microbiological assay is that there is a quantitative relationship between the number of microorganisms and the amount of anti-microbial agents required to inhibit the growth or kill them. It may be 1-10 million per mL in the final medium.
2. Culture media:
   a. *Formulation and condition:* The selection of an appropriate culture medium rich in the adequate and right amount of nutrients is quite important, as each microorganism species is different from the others according to their nutritional requirements. Maintenance of an optimum pH in the culture medium is also important.
   b. *Thickness:* The thickness of the culture medium affects drug diffusion, growth of the microorganism and its population, and variation of nutrient amounts over the experimental period. The thickness of the agar medium should be between 3 and 5 mm.
3. Anti-microbial agents:
   a. *Dose/concentration*
   b. *Exposure time or period*
   c. *Susceptibility towards the microorganisms*
   d. *Excipient interference*
   e. *Nature and action mechanism(s)*

f. Potency: The test agent(s) under screening must have susceptibility towards the test microorganism(s). It must have adequate potency during the time of microbiological assay.

4. *Diffusion rate and time*: The test sample should be given adequate time for its diffusion; the diffusion rate should be optimized in the test medium.
5. *Incubation time and temperature*: Each organism requires an optimum time and temperature for its growth and multiplication.
6. *Aseptic process and environmental condition*: Sterilization process should be reliable along with the other microbiological lab supports.
7. *Standards selection*: Potent, appropriate, and susceptible reference standard(s) should be chosen.
8. *Method selection.*

Agar Disk-Diffusion (Simple) Method

Principle

One technique for measuring an antibiotic's capacity to prevent bacterial growth is the agar diffusion assay. Model-dependent analysis, which assumes that antibiotics permeate easily in the solid nutrient medium and sufficiently limit the growth or kill the injected microorganisms in the culture plate, is used to interpret the results of this assay. Zones of inhibition are calculated either linearly or circularly in mm. Table 9.2 presents the composition of the agar media.

Table 9.2. Composition of agar media

Ingredients	Grams/L
Peptone	5.0
Sodium chloride	5.0
HM peptone B#	1.5
Yeast extract	1.5
Agar	15.0
Final pH (at 25°C)	7.4 ± 0.2

Peptone - provides organic nitrogen, while Beef extract/Yeast extract - the water-soluble content of these contribute vitamins, carbohydrates, nitrogen, and salts.

Procedure

Preparation of Agar Media: In 1000 mL of distilled water, dissolve 28 g. To completely dissolve the medium, heat it until it boils. By autoclaving for 15 min at 121 °C and 15 lbs of pressure, sterilize. Cool to 45 to 50 °C.

Sub-culture preparation: A pure bacterial culture is standardized to turbidity, suspended in buffer, and uniformly swabbed on a culture plate.

Test plate preparation: Boiled required amount of powder medium until the agar is melted and sterilized in an autoclave for 15 minutes at 121°C. This allows it to cool at 55 to 60 °C in a water bath. Pure sterile culture medium in petri-dishes at an appropriate volume (3-5 mm thickness).

Microorganism inoculation, Placement of the disc and Incubation: Pre-determined volume of the inoculum is added to the medium. It is then mixed thoroughly and poured into the plates. For this, calculate the CFU of the organism by using a suitable colony counter, against which the susceptibility of the antimicrobial agent is to be determined.

Preparation of sample/standard paper disc: A specified amount (5 μL) of test/sample should be applied to a sterile paper disc.

Measurement of zone of inhibition: After solidification of the culture dish (at 4 °C for 10 min in a refrigerator), apply the paper disc containing the sample and/or standard towards the inoculated agar dishes. Then incubate for a specific time and temperature (for bacteria, 37 °C for 24 h; for fungi, 29 - 35 °C for 36 - 48 h). Then calculate the circular zones of inhibition (for simple technique) or linear zones of inhibition (for swab technique) in mm.

Latin Square (*agar well diffusion*) Method

Procedure

1. Assay plates of 30 × 30 cm size, glass plates with Al frames and lids are used. The plates are properly cleaned, dried and sterilized in a dry heat sterilizer.
2. To make 350 mL, mix 9.5 g of dried antibiotic medium with distilled water.
3. Boiled until the agar is melted and sterilized in an autoclave for 15 minutes at 121 °C.
4. This is allowed to cool at 55 - 60 °C in a water bath.
5. A pre-determined volume of the inoculum is added to the medium. It is then mixed thoroughly and poured into the plates.

6. The agar is allowed to settle in the plate for about 30 - 40 minutes and then transferred to a refrigerator at 4 °C for about an hour to harden the seeded medium.
7. After that, the plate is placed on a template made according to 2 × 2 or (8 × 8) designed as shown below:

T2	T1	S2	S1	T2	T1	S2	S1
S1	T2	T1	S2	S1	T2	T1	S2
S2	S1	T2	T1	S2	S1	T2	T1
T1	S2	S1	T2	T1	S2	S1	T2
T2	T1	S2	S1	T2	T1	S2	S1
S1	T2	T1	S2	S1	T2	T1	S2
S2	S1	T2	T1	S2	S1	T2	T1
T1	S2	S1	T2	T1	S2	S1	T2

Here, S1 = Low dose of standard; S2 = High dose of standard; T1 = Low dose of test sample; T2 = High dose of test sample.

1. S1, S2, T1 and T2 are placed in such a way that in a column or row, they do not appear more than two times.
2. 64 holes are punched in the plate with a sterile 8 mm cork borer, following the template design placed under the plate.
3. Thereafter, standards and samples of high and low-dose solutions are applied to their denoted places in the plate using a semi-automated micropipette which delivers the same amount of solution in each case.
4. Then the plates are put into a refrigerator for about 2 hours to diffuse the liquids. The plates are then kept in an incubator for 18–20 hours at 37 °C.
5. Then the sharp, clean, and round zones of inhibition of growth are obtained around the holes (if the treatments act against test organisms). The diameter of zones is carefully read by using a zone reader or Vernier scale.
6. The results are noted and the mean of the diameter of the inhibition zones (T1, T2, S1, and S2) is calculated.

Calculation

Dose difference (E) = $[\{(T2 + S2) \div 2\} - \{(T1 + S1) \div 2\}]$

Preparation difference (F) = $[\{(T2 + T1) \div 2\} - \{(S2 + S1) \div 2\}]$

Log ration of doses (I) = log2 or log4 = 0.301 or 0.602

Slope of the dose response line (b) = E ÷ I
Log potency ratio of T/S (M) = F ÷ I
Potency ratio of T/S = Antilog M
Sample potency = Potency ratio × Dilution factor

Turbidimetric or Serial Dilution (*broth dilution*) Method

The minimum inhibitory concentration (MIC) for your test sample against test microorganisms is determined using the nutrient broth method.

Principle

The tubes of broth medium containing a specified number of microorganisms require graded doses of antibiotics. After a suitable incubation, growth will occur in the tubes (turbidity formation of the colony), and if the antibiotic has susceptibility towards the organism, it will inhibit the growth of the organism inside the tubes.

Procedure

- Mix 25 g with 1000 mL of distilled or filtered water. If heat is required to entirely dissolve the medium, do so. By autoclaving for 15 min at 121 °C and 15 lbs of pressure, sterilize. Cool to 45 to 50 °C.
- Clean screw cap test tubes and sterilize (same as above) them along with the broth medium. Then mark the tubes for each dilution. Take 3 tubes for each concentration.
- Take one tube for medium (T_M), one for medium + inoculum (T_{MI}), one for medium + solvent (T_{MS}).
- Put 1 mL of sterile nutrient broth medium in all the marked tubes.
- Add the specified volume (1 mL of the antibiotic solution) and serially dilute until the final marked tube.
- Then inoculate with the specific microorganism (inoculums containing 10^6 CFU/mL of cells) of all the test marked tubes, and T_{MI}.
- For T_{MS} add only the solvent used for your test sample, while T_M contains only 1 mL of sterilized media.

- Incubate all the test tubes for 24 h at 37 °C (in the case of an anti-bacterial test, but for an anti-fungal test, do it at 29 - 35 °C for 36 to 48 h).

Calculation of MIC value: [(Lowest concentration of the test sample inhibits growth + Highest concentration of the test sample allows growth of microorganism) ÷ 2]

If-

a. all tubes remain clear: MIC is lower than the least concentration of the test sample.
b. all tubes are turbid: MIC is higher than the highest concentration of the test sample.
c. there are any variations in the T_{MI}, T_M and T_{MS} marked tubes: The test is invalid.

Challenge Test

Challenge testing is used for the assessment of growth, survival, or reduction of microorganisms when added to food products under well controlled conditions. Challenge testing is done by using a wide range of microorganisms such as pathogenic bacteria (e.g., *Listeria, Salmonella, Clostridium*), and spoilage bacteria, yeast, and molds. The challenge tests are performed on real food or in model systems mimicking food compositions. Most often, packaged products are carefully inoculated. Products may also be packaged (vacuum or MAP). Finally, the inoculated products are stored under well-defined temperature conditions and sampled at regular time intervals. When analyzing the samples, a number of methods are used to quantify the inoculum or in order to analyze the composition of the microbial background flora. *Examples* of some challenge tests:

- *Listeria monocytogenes* in cold smoked salmon
- *Clostridium botulinum* in sausage batter after heating
- *Debaromyces*, *Zygosaccharomyces*, *Penicillium* and *Aspergillus* in cold sauces
- *Lactobacillus*, *Debaromyces* and *Penicillium* in roe products.

In this case, nitrite, NaCl, pH-value, sorbate, benzoate, citric acid, lactate, bacteriophages, protective cultures, and so on values are tested.

E-Test (antimicrobial gradient method)

Previously it has been known as 'Epsilometer test'. It is a manual *in vitro* diagnostic device used by laboratories to determine the MIC and whether or not a specific strain of bacterium or fungus is susceptible to the action of a specific anti-microbial. This type of test is most commonly used in healthcare settings to help guide physicians in the treatment of patients by indicating what concentration of antibiotic would successfully treat an infection.

Principle

With a predetermined gradient of antibiotics covering a continuous range of concentrations, E-test is a "ready-to-use," inert, and non-porous plastic reagent strip that may be used to determine the exact MIC values of a diverse variety of antimicrobial drugs against various organism groups. The antimicrobial gradient is instantly released from the plastic carrier to the agar whenever the E-test is put to the surface of an agar plate inoculated with the test strain, forming a continuous and stable gradient below and close to the strip.

Based on the intrinsic growth features of the organism and the unique incubation conditions, test incubation and reading periods have been established. Consequently, the gradient's consistency must be maintained for many hours in order to produce results that are trustworthy and reproducible. The predetermined E-test gradient is stable for at least 18 - 24 h, which is long enough to encompass many species of fastidious and non-fastidious organisms' critical periods.

The antibiotic gradient on the E-test strip simply transfers to the agar matrix, leaving an impression of the gradient on the strip in the agar, when the strip is placed on an agar surface. Following incubation, the bacterial growth is apparent, and a symmetrical inhibition ellipse centered along the strip is observed. Where the elliptical edge touches the strip the MIC value is read from the scale in terms of μg/mL.

E-Test Medium

As long as the medium promotes healthy growth of the test organism and does not inhibit the antimicrobial agent's activity, the E-test (Figure 9.3: E-test strip) can indeed be utilized with a wide variety of AST agar media. The medium selected should, however, meet the fundamental specifications for a susceptibility test medium in order to maximize repeatability. It is advised to utilize the appropriate AST medium alongside E-test:

- Aerobes: Mueller Hinton agar (e.g., MHE, bioMérieux)
- Anaerobes: Brucella blood agar (with appropriate supplements)

Activity Identification

The MIC value can be determined at the point at which the margin of the inhibitory ellipse crosses the edge of the strip just after the necessary incubation period and only after an even lawn of growth is clearly apparent. If the culture seems mixed or if the growing lawn is too light or heavy, the plate shouldn't be read. Despite the possibility of varied growth and inhibition patterns, MIC test conclusions are typically unambiguous.

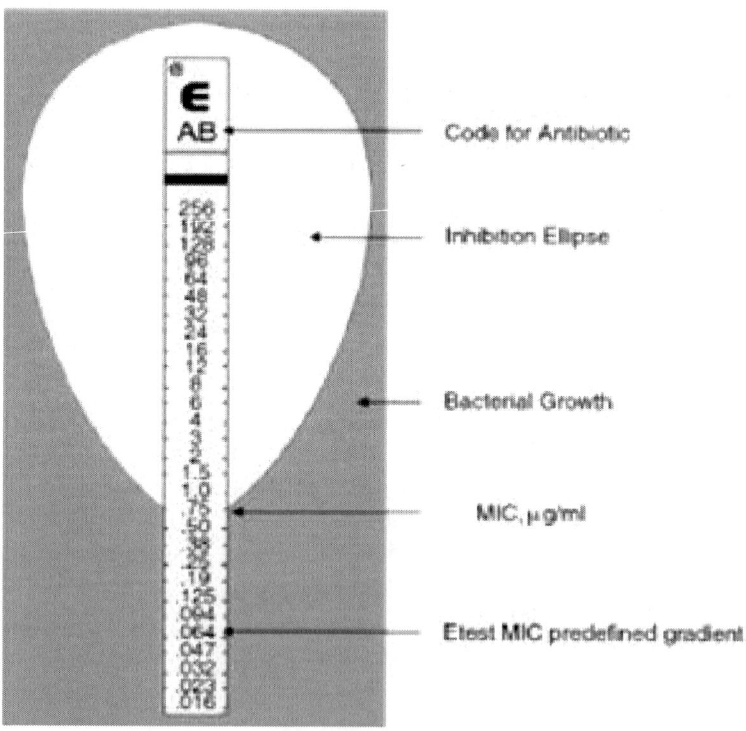

Figure 9.3. A typical E-test strip

Some Popularly Used Other Anti-Microbial Assays

Agar Plug Diffusion Method

Similar to the disk-diffusion approach, the agar plug diffusion method is frequently used to highlight the competition between microorganisms. Making an agar culture of the target strain using tight streaks on the plate surface requires using the strain's proper culture media. Microbial cells release chemicals that spread across the agar medium as they proliferate. Once the test microorganism has been incubated, an agar-plot or cylinder is sliced aseptically using a sterile cork borer and placed on the agar surface of another plate. The chemicals spread out into the agar media from the plug. The formation of the inhibition zone around the agar plug serves as a further indicator of the antibacterial activity of the chemicals released by the microbes.

Cross Streak Method

To quickly check for antagonism, bacteria are screened using the cross-streak method. A single streak in the middle of the agar plate seeds the target microbial strain. The microorganisms evaluated by a single-streak parallel to the center streak are seeded onto the plate after an incubation period based on the microbe. By measuring the size of the inhibitory zone after additional incubation, the antimicrobial interactions are examined.

Poisoned Food Method

The poisoned food approach is typically used to assess a substance's ability to fight mold. The extract or anti-fungal agent is added to the molten agar at the desired final concentration and thoroughly stirred. The medium is then added to the petridishes. An inoculation can be carried out using a mycelia disc between 2 and 5 mm in diameter that is deposited in the plate's center following an overnight pre-incubation. The diameters of fungal growth in the control and sample plates are measured after additional incubation under conditions appropriate for the tested fungus, and the anti-fungal effect is evaluated using the method below:

$$\%\text{anti-fungal effect} = [(Dc - Ds) \div Dc] \times 100$$

where, Dc and Ds are the diameter of growth in control and test agents, respectively. Comparing sporulation to control is also possible.

Direct Bioautography

One of the most widely used techniques for microbiological assay is this one. A microbiological suspension is poured or sprayed onto the prepared TLC plate. The bioautogram is therefore incubated for 2 days at 25 °C in a humid environment. Tetrazolium salts are widely employed for this purpose in order to visualize microbial development. The dehydrogenases in living cells convert these salts into the corresponding highly colored formazan. The best detection agent is p-iodonitrotetrazolium violet. The bioautogram is sprayed with these salts and then reincubated at either 25 °C for 24 h or 37 °C for 3 to 4 h. Agar has been added to Mueller Hinton Broth, which has been suggested to provide a medium with enough fluid to improve adhesion to the TLC plate and maintain the right humidity for growth of bacteria. Either fungi or bacteria may be used for direct bioautography.

Agar Overlay Bioassay

It is a combination of the agar diffusion and direct bioautography techniques and is also referred to as immersion bioautography. The seeded agar used to cover the TLC plate is molten. The plates might be kept at a low temperature for a few hours before incubation in order to facilitate the good diffusion of the tested chemicals into the agar medium. Tetrazolium dye can be used for staining once the test microorganism has been incubated under the proper conditions. Similar to direct bioautography, this technique can be used with any kind of microorganism.

Agar Dilution Method

The agar dilution method entails incorporating a variety of desirable anti-microbial agent concentrations into a molten agar medium using repeated two-fold dilutions as a regular practice, then inoculating a specific microbial inoculum onto the agar plate surface. The MIC endpoint is defined as the lowest concentration of anti-microbial agents that, under optimum incubation circumstances, totally stops growth.

Time-Kill Test (Time-Kill Curve)

The best technique for determining the bactericidal or fungicidal action is the time-kill test. It is an effective method for learning more about how the anti-microbial agent and the microbial strain interact dynamically. A time-dependent or concentration-dependent antibacterial action is revealed by the time-kill test.

ATP Bioluminescence Assay

The ability to quantify ATP, which is produced by bacteria or fungus, is the foundation of the ATP bioluminescence assay. All living cells use ATP as their chemical source of energy, hence it is always present in a cell in roughly the same quantity. The microbial population in a sample is therefore estimated using its quantification. When D-luciferin is exposed to ATP, luciferase converts it to oxyluciferin, which emits light. A luminometer measures the amount of light released and converts it into relative light units (RLUs), which can then be turned into RLUs per mole of ATP. As a result, there is a linear link between the measurement of luminescence and cell viability.

Microbiological Assay of Vitamin

It is a particular kind of biological test that uses microorganisms. A microbial assay is used to standardize several medicinal medicines that either prevent the growth of bacteria or are necessary for their growth.

Principle

Microorganisms require vitamin growth to flourish. The goal of this assay is to assess a test organism's capacity to use the chemicals under investigation under optimal nutritional conditions.

Assay for Vitamin B_{12}

The chosen test microorganism must be able to use cyanocobalamin. It is discovered that *Lactobacillus liechmanii* meets the parameters. It is a non-pathogenic, gram-negative bacillus. Its culture is simple, easily accessible and separated from dairy products like cheese. Either the titrimetric method or the turbidimetric method is used to conduct the assay.

Procedure

- Take clean test tubes and add serially diluted standard Vit B_{12}
- Add 5 mL of basal medium solution to each tube.
- Add water to make a final volume of 10 mL.
- Take the test solution in other test tubes.
- Treat these tubes similarly.
- Sterilize the tubes by autoclaving at 121 °C (15 lbs) for 15 min.

- Let the tubes cool to ambient temperature before adding a dose of prepared test-microorganism inoculum.
- Incubate the tubes for 64 - 72 h at 30 - 37 °C.
- Titrate each tube's contents with 0.05 N NaOH after incubation, using bromothymol blue as an indicator, until the color turns green, then record the reading.

Data Interpretation

- Calculate the titration values for each level of both the standard and test solutions on average.
- Plot a graph comparing the concentration of standard vitamin B_{12} solution to the average titration values (in mL) of 0.05 N NaOH. You will get a linear graph.

Terminology

- *Inoculum*: Inoculum is the term used to describe the substance that is introduced during an inoculation and contains microorganisms or similar things.
- *Inoculation*: Inoculation is the process of introducing a microbe or other substance into the body or a culture medium.
- *Incubation*: Incubation is the term used in microbiology to describe the process of exposing cultures of microorganisms to an environment (particularly temperature) that is conducive to their growth.
- *Microbial culture & sub-culture*: In microbiology, organisms isolated or from raw sources are led to grow in an artificially prepared medium that is assumed to contain a sufficient and required amount of nutrients. This is called microbial culture. On the other hand, the preparation of further culture from the primary culture is known as a sub-culture.
- *Strain*: A succession of cultures derived from an initial colony is called a strain.
- *Colony*: It is a microscopically visible growth of microorganisms in a culture medium.
- *Zone of inhibition*: In a microbiological assay, inhibition of the growth of microorganisms in a culture medium by an antibiotic substance appears as a clear zone, which is called a zone of

inhibition. The size of the zone of inhibition depends on the following *factors*:

- Intrinsic anti-microbial sensitivity of the test drug.
- Growth rate of the test microorganism.
- Concentration and diffusion rate of the test drug.
- Size of inoculum.
- Thickness of the culture medium.

- *Reference standard*: In a biological assay to compare the test sample's response we take a positive control treatment which is known as reference standard. The standard is thought to be pure, highly potent and active against the test microorganism.
- *MBC*: It is the minimum concentration or dose of a substance required to act against a bacterial strain.
- *MFC*: It is the minimum concentration or dose of a substance required to act against a fungal strain.
- *MIC*: The 'Minimal Inhibitory Concentration' (MIC) is the lowest concentration of an antibiotic that inhibits the growth of the particular no(s) organism(s) upon which it acts.
- *Dilution factor*: It is the ratio of the aliquot volume + diluent volume to the aliquot volume.

Q. What is the dilution factor if you add 0.1 mL aliquot of a specimen to 9.9 mL of diluent?

Solution:

V_f = Aliquot volume + Diluent volume
= 0.1 + 9.9 mL
= 10.0 mL

DF = $V_f \div V_i$
= $10.0 \div 0.1$
= 100 mL

IC_{50}: It means half the minimal inhibitory concentration of an antibiotic towards an organism.

EC_{50}: It means half the maximal effective concentration of an antibiotic towards an organism.

Anti-Viral Test

Anti-viral assay *(in vitro)* methods (Rumlová and Ruml, 2018) are mainly based on the –

- evaluating viral entry inhibitors
- screening viral capsid disassembly/uncoating inhibitors
- determining viral genome replication inhibitors
  - Polymerases
  - Methyltransferases
  - Helicases
  - Kinases
  - Integrase
- determining viral assembly inhibitors
- screening and evaluating viral maturation inhibitors

Typical anti-viral assays have been given below:

Cytopathic Effect Inhibition Assay (Model 1)

Step 1. Seed virus cells in 96-well culture plates and incubate for 24 h (check optimum temperature for your virus), replace the medium with 100 μL of standard medium like Dulbecco's Modified Eagle's Medium, containing the test sample, and 50 μL dilution of the test virus in quadruplicate.

Step 2. For 72 h, re-incubate the plates. The controls are made up of untreated non-infected (sample control), treated non-infected (virus titer), and untreated non-infected (cell control) cells.

Step 3. Determine the virus titers as 50% of the tissue culture infective dose per milliliter ($TCID_{50}$/mL). Calculate the test sample's anti-viral activity as the viral titer's logarithm reduction factor (log10) in comparison to untreated infected controls. Titer ($TCID_{50}$/mL) and inhibition percentage (IP) are appropriate units of measurement. Calculate IP according to the formula:

$$\%IP = (1 - T/C) \times 100$$

where, T and C are the antilog of the sample and control (without sample) treated viral titers, respectively. IP is positive when its value is ≥98% (Kohn et al. 2015).

MTT Assay (Model 2)

Step 1. Add 50 µL viral suspension (10^3 $TCID_{50}$) to the cells (e.g., vero) monolayer in 96-well plates. Then incubate at 4 °C for 1 h to promote cell attachment.

Step 2. Aspirate the media to remove any remaining viruses.

Step 3. PBS washes the cell monolayers before the test material is added in dilutions to the plates. Use uninfected cells as a control and infected cells without treatment. Run the experiment three times with the infected-untreated and uninfected-treated groups serving as controls.

Step 4. Use an inverted microscope to score the viral cytopathic effects (CPE) of the tests under light microscopy in contrast to the virus control and cell control. Incubate all plates at 37 °C in humidified 5% CO_2 (Xu et al. 2012).

N. B. – Anti-microbial activity studies have a broad sense in biological activity investigations. For example, *Porphyromonas gingivalis* and *Streptococcus mutans* are two major causative bacteria that are primarily responsible for periodontal inflammatory diseases and dental caries. If anyone wants to test whether his/her test sample possesses a dentoproteive effect or not, s/he can consider a simple anti-bacterial study against these bacteria. Similarly, microbes' responsible gastritis (*Helicobacter pylori*), diarrhea (*Escherichia coli*, *Shigella*, *Salmonella*, *Campylobacter*, *Yersinia* and *Clostridium* spp.), dysentery (*Shigella*, *Campylobacter*, *Salmonella*, or enterohemorrhagic *E. coli.*), typhoid (*Salmonella typhi*), paratyphoid (*Salmonella paratyphi*), hepatitis (*Hepatovirus* A, B, C, D, and E), gonorrhea (*Neisseria gonorrhoeae*), tetanus (*Clostridium tetani*), meningitis (meningococcal bacteria: several different types e.g., A, B, C, W, X, Y and Z. pneumococcal bacteria; *Haemophilus influenzae* type b), influenza (influenza viruses, RNA viruses of the *Orthomyxovirus* genus), pneumonia (*Streptococcus pneumoniae*, *Staphylococcus aureus*, Group A *Streptococcus*, *Klebsiella pneumoniae*, *Haemophilus influenzae*, *Moraxella catarrhalis*, anaerobes, and gram-negative organisms), botulism (*Clostridium botulinum*, *Clostridium butyricum* and *Clostridium baratii*), hand, foot, and mouth disease (viruses that belong to the *Enterovirus* family; Coxsackievirus A16), smallpox (*Variola virus*), respiratory distress syndrome (*Streptococcus* *pneumoniae*, *Haemophillus influenzae*, *Moraxella catarrhalis* and *Streptococcus pyogenes*, MERS, SARS), and so on can be target to investigate anti-microbial effect of your test sample aiming to see either it possesses such type biological effect or not.

Part XII: Anthelmintic Tests

Helminths, or parasitic worms, are one of the main global burdens. According to estimates, more than a billion people, mostly in developing nations, are infected with helminths that are spread through the soil. Helminth infection also poses a serious danger to global food security and is a major issue in cattle production globally. A few handfuls of synthetic anthelmintic medications are essentially the only means of controlling helminths (Jayawardene et al. 2021). The risks of parasites developing drug resistance (which is already common in some livestock production systems), the cost of medications for small-scale farmers in developing nations, and for some helminths, the lack of effectiveness of drugs currently available are the drawbacks of this reliance on chemotherapy. You can apply a number of anthelminthic test models to check your sample's anthelminthic properties. Some reliable and widely used methods include:

In Vitro Assay

Adult Motility Assay

According to Sharma et al. (1971):

Step 1. Collect the required number of adult parasites (e.g., *Haemonchus contortus*) parasites.

Step 2. As necessary, set up your test and controls. As a positive control, 0.25 mg/mL of albendazole can be used instead of the vehicle as the control group.

Step 3. Until the seventh hour following the treatments, check for worm death or paralysis at regular intervals. Take the immobile worms and soak them for 10 minutes in warm PBS. Number them (number of dead or motility).

Egg Hatch Inhibition Assay

According to Coles et al. (1992):

Step 1. Wash the eggs thrice with distilled water and adjust to a concentration of 100-200 eggs/mL using the McMaster technique.

Step 2. Centrifuge the suspension for 5 min at 1500×*g* and discard the supernatant.

Step 3. Pipette approx. 100 eggs in 200 μL of distilled water and keep into each well of a 48-well microtiter plate.

Step 4. Add 200 μL of your test sample or controls to each test well and adjust the final volume to 400 μL. Use 200 μL of albendazole (pure standard reference) at a concentration of 0.25 mg/mL as a positive control, and vehicle (200 μL) as a negative control.

Step 5. Conduct the experiment in duplicates. Incubate the plates at 37°Cfor 48 h.

Step 6. To prevent more hatching, add a drop of Lugol's iodine solution to each well. Then, using a dissecting microscope, tally the unhatched eggs and L1 larvae in each well to calculate the percentage of egg hatching inhibition.

$$\%\text{Inhibition} = 100\,[1 - P_{test}/P_{control}]$$

where, P stands for number of eggs hatched in EHIA.

In Vivo Assay

Larval Development Assay with Free-Living Stages

According to Várady et al. (1997):

Step 1. Collect two 8-week-old pigs and infect them with two doses of 5,000 third-stage larvae (L3) of *Oesophagostomum dentatum* by stomach tube, three weeks apart.

Step 2. Collect pig faeces and isolate the eggs of *O. dentatum* by sieving and saturating salt flotation.

Step 3. Keep your test sample or controls in 96-well plates together with 15% (v/v) of a larval feeding solution (1% yeast extract in Earle's balanced salt solution), antibiotics (300 U/mL penicillin, 300 μg/mL/streptomycin) and antimycotic (10 μg/mL, amphotericin B). Negative and positive controls consist of vehicles and 50 μg/mL of levamisole, respectively.

Step 4. Add 100 eggs to each well and incubate the plates at 25 °C in a humidified environment for a week.

Step 5. Kill the larvae by adding iodine and determine the number of L3 per well.

Larval Migration Assay

According to Williams et al. (2014):

Step 1. Collect third-stage larvae from the faeces of mono-infected donor pigs by standard copro-culture using the Baermann apparatus and store in water at 10 °C.

Step 2. On the day of the assay, L3 is rapidly exsheathed by the addition of 2% sodium hypochlorite (10 - 15% available Cl^-). Wash the L3 five times in sterile water.

Step 3. Suspend the larvae in RPMI 1640 media with HEPES containing L-glutamine (2 mM), 100 U/mL penicillin and 100 μg/mL streptomycin.

Step 4. Add 100 larvae in triplicate to each well of a 48-well plate containing medium with either your test sample or vehicle (negative control) or 50 μg/mL ivermectin (positive control).

Step 5. Incubate the larvae overnight at 37 °C in an atmosphere of 5% CO_2 before the addition of agar to a final concentration of 0.8%.

Step 6. By using a light microscope, count the number of larvae that can leave the setting agar after a four-hour migration period. However, as previously mentioned, you can pre-incubate your test sample using polyvinylpolypyrrolidone (PVPP) to specifically deplete CT during the course of an overnight incubation.

Larval Development Assay with Parasitic Stages

According to Stepek et al. (2005):

Step 1. Exsheath third-stage larvae as above, wash and seed approximately 100 larvae per well in 2 mL of culture medium (LB broth containing 10% heat-inactivated porcine serum, 200 U/mL penicillin, 200 μg/mL streptomycin and 1 μg/mL amphotericin B) in 24-well plates.

Step 2. Add your test sample at a concentration of 1 mg/mL. You can add 25 mM of diethylcarbamazine as a positive control in order to block the development of third-stage to fourth-stage larvae, whilst using vehicle or culture medium as a negative control.

Step 3. Incubate the larvae at 37 °C in an atmosphere of 5% CO_2 for 2 weeks, with the medium being replenished on days 5 and 10. Determine %L4 on day 14 in each well.

Motility Assay with Fourth-Stage Larvae

According to Stepek et al. (2005):

Step 1. Exsheath third-stage larvae as above, wash and then seed at a concentration of 1000 larvae/mL in tissue culture flasks containing complete LB broth culture medium.

Step 2. Incubate the larvae at 37 °C in an atmosphere of 5% CO_2 with medium changes every five days. Culture the larvae for 21 - 24 days to allow the development of large numbers of L4.

Step 3. Separate the L4 from L3 by repeated sedimentation, wash five times in warm sterile saline, and then suspend in the same medium as used for the L3 migration assay above.

Step 4. Add approximately 10 larvae to each well of a 48-well plate containing either a test sample or controls. Use ivermectin (50 μg/mL) as a positive control. Record the motility of the larvae daily for four days on a 0-5 scale, where 0 is no movement and 5 is vigorous movement.

Motility Assay with Adult Worms

According to Williams et al. (2014):

Step 1. Infect the donor pigs with *O. dentatum* larvae as described above.

Step 2. After 5 weeks of the second infective dose, kill the pigs by captive bolt pistol and exsanguination, and remove the large intestine.

Step 3. Pluck (manually) adult worms from the gut contents with forceps and rinse well with warm saline. The worms were washed repeatedly in the same sterile culture medium as used for the L3 migration assay.

Step 4. Seed 4 worms in each well of a 24-well plate containing either medium only, ivermectin (50 μg/mL) or hazelnut skin extract.

Step 5. Incubate the worms at 37 °C in an atmosphere of 5% CO_2 for 3 days and assess motility twice daily as described above.

Step 6. After 24 h, wash a subset of worms from the test or controls, fix them, and examine them by transmission electron microscopy as previously described.

N.B. - Parasitic attacks are one of the common consequences worldwide. To date, a number of parasitological methods have been introduced for testing a wide variety of test substances. Currently, we are using these models for the diagnosis of parasite attacks, for example, schistosomiasis. It is to be mentioned that, these methods are insensitive, particularly in areas of low endemicity, and labour-intensive. To overcome these issues, certain immunoassays based on detection of parasite antibodies have been introduced. These strategies have high sensitivity, economy, rapidity and ease of detection (Coulibaly et al. 2013).

Part XIII: Anti-Diarrheal Activity Tests

Loose, watery, and perhaps looser bowel motions are symptoms of diarrhea. It is a widespread issue everywhere. Diarrhea can occur on its own or in combination with other complaints such as nausea, vomiting, abdominal pain, or loss of weight. Although diarrhea often only lasts a few days, it can occasionally last longer. It is categorized as: watery, fatty (malabsorption), and inflammatory. Most people suffer due to watery diarrhea, which is further subdivided into osmotic, secretory, and functional types. This form also includes irritable bowel syndrome. Each year, diarrhea causes the deaths of thousands of people worldwide. Diarrhea is associated with many potential symptoms, and if left untreated, it can cause death (Schiller, 2000). Causative facts can be targeted for developing test protocols for assessing anti-diarrheal agents. Some widely used anti-diarrheal test models include:

Castor Oil-Induced Mouse Model

According to Abu Mohammed et al. (2013):

Step 1. Perform a pre-experimental screening in which you administer only 0.5 mL of castor oil to each animal (e.g., mice) to check their responses to this agent. Select only those animals which are found diarrheic in this pre-experimental action.

Step 2. Randomly divide these animals (n = required number in each group) after 24 h of fasting into control (vehicle), positive control (e.g., loperamide 3 mg/kg, p.o.) and test group(s).

Step 3. Orally administer 0.5 mL of castor oil for the induction of diarrhea in each animal 30 min after treatment and place each animal in a separate cage. Every hour, replace the floor lines with new translucent paper.

Step 4. Keep track of when diarrhea first appears (first diarrheal stool following castor oil administration) (onset of action) and how many feces were produced overall during the preceding 4 h (duration of action). Based on stool consistency, classify by using the following: 1 (normal), 2 (semi-solid), and 3 (watery) stools, respectively. Make a mean evacuation index calculation for each group.

Step 5. Utilizing the weight difference between the fresh and dry stool, determine the total amount of fluid present in the faces (dried for 24 hours at ambient temperature in a shaded area). Calculate each group's %reduction in diarrhea relative to the negative control group. The formula below is used to compute the %diarrhea inhibition:

$$\%ID = [(WFNC - WFT) \div WFNC] \times 100$$

$$\%ITFO = [(TFC - TFT) \div TFC] \times 100$$

where, ID, WFNC, WFT, ITFO, TFC, and TFT stand for inhibition of diarrhea, wet feces in the negative control group, wet feces in the test group, inhibition of total fecal output, total feces of control and total feces of treated, respectively. Figure 9.4 presents a general outline of the castor oil-induced diarrhea model.

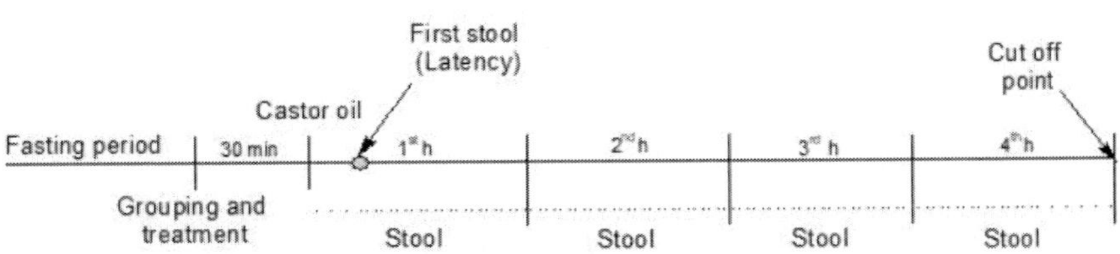

Figure 9.4. General outline of castor oil-induced diarrheal model.

Castor Oil Induced Chick Model

According to Sera et al. (2017):

Step 1. Collect 2-3 days old chicks (2-h fasted, only access to water *ad libitum*) and randomly divide the birds into Group I: Control, Group-II:

Positive control and Group-III: Test sample (if necessary other treatments/groups).

Step 2. Take their initial body weight and mark accordingly. Keep them separately or group wise.

Step 3. Give 1.0 mL castor oil orally to each chick after treating with test sample/controls.

Step 4. Observe for the first diarrheal stool (onset of action) and record diarrheal secretions in each hour up to 4 h. Also note the number of diarrheic birds in each treatment group. Calculate the incidence of diarrhea (ID) as follows:

$$\%ID = (\text{Number of diarrheic chicks} \div \text{Total chicks in the group}) \times 100$$

Step 5. Take final body weight (after 4th h of study). Calculate weight variation (WV) as follows:

$$\%WV = [(\text{Initial body weight} - \text{Final body weight}) \div \text{Initial body weight}] \times 100$$

Step 6. Sacrifice the chicks by jugular vein exsanguination. Collect and take the weight of the total viscera (liver, pancreas, and heart), the immune organs (thymus gland, and bursa of fabricius), and accessories (proventriculus and gizzard) by using an electronic balance. Then calculate the relative weight of each organ in relation to the live weight. Homogenize several portions of the small and large intestines of the chicks in a mortar. Then, mix 2 g of the sample with 10 mL of distilled water and vortex for 2 min. Adjust the pH 7-10. At the end of the experiment, draw 1 mL of blood from the jugular veins of five chicks per treatment and determine the hematocrits.

Castor Oil-Induced Enteropooling (Mouse Model)

According to Chitme et al. (2004):

Step 1. Use 18 h fasted animals (e.g., mice) with access only to water. Group the animals randomly as mentioned above.

Step 2. After giving each animal a 1 h oral dose of your test sample or the reference drug (loperamide 3 mg/kg), give them each 0.5 mL of castor oil.

Step 3. Laparotomy with a surgical blade is performed after cervical dislocation as the method of sacrifice for the animals. Lie down on both ends of the small intestine after cutting it from the pylorus and cecum.

Step 4. Determine the difference between the intestinal weights taken before and after the removal of bowel contents.

Step 5. By milking it into the calibrated cylinder for volume measurement, separate the intestinal content.

Step 6. Use the following formula to calculate the %change in weight and volume of the intestinal content compared to the negative control:

$$\%RWI = [(MW_{control} - MW_{test}) \div MW_{control}] \times 100$$

$$\%RVIC = [(MVIC_{control} - MVIC_{test}) \div MVIC_{control}] \times 100$$

where, %RWI, %RVIC, MW, and MVIC stand for %reduction in weight of intestinal content, %reduction in the volume of intestinal content, mean intestinal weight, and mean intestinal content volume respectively.

Magnesium Sulfate Induced Enteropooling

According to Sunilson et al. (2009):

Step 1. Use 18-h fasted animals (e.g., mice) with access only to water. Group the animals randomly as mentioned above.

Step 2. After giving each animal a 1-h oral dose of your test sample or the reference drug (loperamide 3 mg/kg), give them 0.5 mL of magnesium sulfate (10% w/v) orally.

Step 3. Sacrifice the animals after 30 min of magnesium sulfate therapy. Remove the small intestine after tying the ends with threads and taking weight.

Step 4. Collect the intestinal content into a graduated cylinder and measure its volume. Take empty intestinal weight and determine the difference between the full and empty intestine.

PGE_2-Induced Enteropooling

According to Robert et al. (1976):

Step 1. Divide overnight fasted animals (e.g., mice) into different groups (required number of animals in each group), such as Group I: 2% gum acacia (control); Group II (vehicle): 2% gum acacia + PGE_2 (0.5 mL of 100 μg/kg, i.p.); Group(s) for test sample and last group (standard): loperamide (3 mg/kg, p.o.).

Step 2. Induce diarrhea with 0.5 mL of a 100 μg/kg (i.p.) dose of PGE_2.

Step 3. Sacrifice the animals after 30 min and remove their small intestine.

Step 4. Measure the intestinal contents in a syringe after collecting them. Then, by comparing the results with those of the vehicle control, ascertain the %intestinal fluid inhibition.

Small Intestine Transit Model

According to Akah and Offiah (1992):

Step 1. Group 16 h fasted animals (e.g., mice, required number for each group) only accessed to water into Control: 2% gum acacia; Test group(s) and Standard (loperamide: 5 mg/kg, p.o.).

Step 2. Five minutes after the treatment, provide 0.5 mL of marker to the animals (3% charcoal solution in 2% gum acacia).

Step 3. After killing the animals (0.5 h later), determine how far the charcoal meal went from the pylorus and express it as %length of the intestine as a whole, from the pylorus to the caecum.

Gastrointestinal Motility Test (Charcoal Meal Model)

According to Akah et al. (1998):

Step 1. Randomly group animals fasted for 18 h with free access to water into different groups (control, positive control, and test).

Step 2. Administer 1 mL of 3% deactivated charcoal in normal saline after 1 h to each animal and wait for 1 h and dissect (after sacrifice).

Step 3. Measure the length of the small intestine after removing it from the pylorus to the caecum. Using the peristaltic index, calculate the intestinal charcoal transit as a percentage of the total length between the pylorus and the caecum and the distance traveled by charcoal (PI). Use atropine (100 mg/kg), a common spasmolytic, as a reference medication and a positive control. Using the following formula, determine %motility inhibition:

$$PI = (\text{Distance traveled}_{\text{charcoal}} \div \text{Total length}_{\text{small intestine}}) \times 100$$

$$\%\text{Motility inhibition} = [(PI_{\text{control}} - PI_{\text{test}}) \div PI_{\text{control}}] \times 100$$

Anti-Secretary Activity Study

According to Tadesse et al. (2014):

Step 1. Give the 1-day-fasted animals 20 μg/kg of misoprostol (e.g., mice). Animals will experience intestinal secretion as a result.

Step 2. Treat each group the same way as described in the castor oil-induced diarrhea procedure after 60 minutes.

Step 3. After 1 day, laparotomize the animals, sacrifice them by cervical dislocation, and then knot and remove the small intestine's pyloric and caecal ends.

Step 4. For each animal, calculate the fluid accumulation ratio (weight of the intestine/rest body weight of the animal) and express the anti-secretory activity as a %inhibition. By deducting the weight of the intestine before and after milking the excised intestine, you can also calculate the weight of the fluid content of the intestine.

In Vivo Antidiarrheal Index

To measure the *in vivo* antidiarrheal index (ADI), use the following formula (Than et al. 1989):

$$\text{ADI } (in\ vivo) = \sqrt[3]{Dfreq \times Gmeq \times Pfreq}$$

D_{freq} = [(Onset of diarrhea_{test} − Onset of $\text{diarrhea}_{control}$) ÷ Onset of $\text{diarrhea}_{control}$] × 100

where, D_{freq} is the delay in the onset of defecation or diarrhea, G_{meq} is the reduction in the travel time of the charcoal meal (as a percentage of the negative control) in the model of the gastrointestinal motility test, and P_{freq} is the reduction in the number of wet stools (as a percentage of the negative control) in the model of castor oil-induced diarrhea.

Shigella-Induced Diarrhea

According to Kamgang et al. (2005):

Step 1. Prepare the inoculum at 9×10^8 CFU/mL (McFarland 3 standard).

Step 2. Establish animal diarrhea caused by *Shigella flexneri* by looking for blood in the feces and WBCs in freshly prepared stools.

Step 3. Randomly distribute the animals into different groups of the required number of animals in each. To reduce the risk of reinfection from feces, put each animal in a cage with a bottom lined with a gauge that allows excrement to pass through.

Step 4. Treat the animals as Test group(s); Control (vehicle) and Standard (loperamide: 2.5 mg/kg) orally.

Step 5. Assess the fecal load of *Shigella* in stool by culturing on *Salmonella–Shigella* agar medium. Take a stool sample three days in a row before diarrhea is introduced and five days in a row after. To achieve this, suspend 0.5 g of feces in 4.5 mL of sterile isosaline, then dilute it in steps.

Step 6. To count the number of *Shigella* colonies per culture, 200 μL within each dilution. In this investigation, note the variance in animal weight and the frequency of feces.

Step 7. The total number of proteins and blood cells should be determined after all the animals have been sacrificed and their blood, hearts, and livers have been collected. Use standardized kits to measure the amounts of creatinine and serum TG.

Magnesium Sulfate-Induced Diarrhea Model

According to Doherty (1981):

Step 1. Randomly divide 12 h fasted animals (e.g., mice) into different groups containing required number of animals in each such as Control: vehicle (10 mL/kg, p.o.); Standard (loperamide: 10 mg/kg, p.o.) and Test group(s).

Step 2. After 60 min of therapy, administer $MgSO_4$ (2 g/kg, p.o.) to each animal.

Step 3. Place each animal in a cage with white filter paper on top, and for 4 h, count the quantity of wet feces.

Step 4. Express the antidiarrheal activity as percent inhibition (%) of defecation and percent inhibition (%) of diarrhea similarly as the castor oil method.

Gastrointestinal Motility Test (Barium Sulfate Milk Model)

According to Afroz et al. (2006):

Step 1. Randomly divide 12 h fasted animals (e.g., mice) into different groups containing required number of animals in each such as Control: vehicle (10 mL/kg, p.o.); Standard (loperamide: 10 mg/kg, p.o.) and Test group(s).

Step 2. Treat each mouse with 15% $BaSO_4$ milk after 30 min of treatment and sacrifice the animals.

Step 3. Calculate the $BaSO_4$ milk's travel distance and convert it to %small intestine's overall length. By using the following equation, calculate the proportion of GI motility inhibition in comparison to the control group:

$$\%\text{Inhibition intestinal length} = [(\text{Test sample} - \text{Control})/\text{Control}] \times 100$$

Part XIV: Anti-Cancer Activity Test

Trillions of cells are arranged into tissues and organs in our body. Each cell's nucleus contains genes that control when it divides, grows, works, and dies. Normally, our cells carry out these directives, and we maintain our health. However, a gene can be modified when our DNA is altered or damaged. Since the DNA instructions in genetic mutations get confused, they are unable to function properly. Because of this, cells that ought to be resting may instead divide and proliferate uncontrollably, which can result in cancer. Although a number of strategies have been introduced as effective treatment modalities, cancer remains the most feared disease in the world. Cancer is a complex disease in the sense of its diverse occurrence pathways, treatment scopes, and associated interactions with other pathophysiological conditions and so on. Cancer can result in different ways. Each pathway has its own mechanisms. To date, a number of anti-cancer drugs have been introduced that act through diverse pathways on cancer cells (Mans et al. 2000; Willoughby et al. 2013). Thus, evaluation methods of anti-cancer agents are usually unlimited. Some frequently used anti-cancer methods are given below.

Cell Viability Model

According to Lombardi et al. (2017):

Step 1. Prepare your test sample at different specified concentrations in a suitable vehicle and store in −20 °C until use.

Step 2. Collect and grow target cancer cells in a suitable medium.

Step 3. Treat the cells in a 24 - 96 well plate with various doses of your test sample (if you use DMSO, its final concentration in the treatment should not exceed 0.25%).

Step 4. To wash the cells with PBS, aspirate the media.

Step 6. Add MTT solution (0.5 mg/mL) to each well, and then incubate the plate for the prescribed amount of time and at the specified temperature (for example, 37 °C in the dark).

Step 7. Replace 200 mL of the MTT solution with DMSO (if you use it for dissolving your test sample).

Step 8. Use a plate reader to measure the optical density at 490 nm after shaking the plate at 150×*g* for 300 sec. Triplicate the experiment and calculate the data by plotting a graph.

Additionally, you can examine the *morphology of cells* by putting them on 24-well plates, dosing them for 1 day with your vehicle or test material (at IC_{50} concentration), and then taking pictures using a phase contrast microscope.

For a *clonogenic* study, cells can be grown to an approximate ~80% confluency and then treated for 1 day with a certain dose of a vehicle or test substance. After 24 hours, trypsinize the cells, seed roughly 10×10^3 cells per well on a 6-well plate, and allow them to develop for 2 weeks. After giving the cells a PBS wash, culture the cells in 0.5% crystal violet solution, which contains 3.7% formaldehyde, for 0.5 h. The plates should then be dried at room temperature after being washed with running tap water. Utilize Gel Doc XR + to capture the image and calculate the cell density (Bio-Rad) (Banerjee et al. 2016).

When a consistent scratch or wound is produced in each well with a 10 μL pipette tip, cells can be seeded in 6-well plates and allowed to develop to 80-90% confluency for the purpose of studying *wound healing*. Images of the cells are captured using an inverted microscope after the cells have been treated for 1-2 days with various doses of your test sample or vehicle after being cleaned with sterile PBS to eliminate any debris. To collect data, conduct each experiment at least three times (Bolla et al. 2019).

Potato Disc (Anti-Tumor) Bioassay

According to McLaughlin et al. (1998) and Karakaş et al. (2012):

Step 1. Preparation of *Agrobacterium tumefaciens* (48 h before assay): Add 0.5 g sucrose, 0.8 g nutrient broth, and 0.1 g yeast extract to 100 mL of distilled water. Take the contents and sterilize them in an autoclave for 12 min. Cool the medium and add 1 loop of *Agrobacterium tumefaciens* aseptically. Shake the mixture for 48 h below 30 °C by using a shaker.

Step 2. Prepare 1.5% agar in distilled water and sterilize by autoclaving all the required items for 15 min.

Step 3. Pour 20 mL of sterilized agar solution per petri dish and allow it to cool. Dissolve 4 mg of test material in 1 mL of DMSO. Use 1 mL of DMSO as a blank.

Step 4. Preparation of inoculum: Mix 1.5 mL of water with 2.0 mL of the 48-h bacterial culture (1×10^9 CFU) and 0.5 mL of your sample. As a control, replace the sample with 0.5 mL of DMSO.

Step 5. Wash the potatoes (*Solanum tuberosum*) with running tap water and soak in bleach (10% commercial). Place the tubers on sterile paper towels and cut along either side, revealing the largest surface area available. Immerse the trimmed tubers in 20% commercial bleach for 15 min. Cut cylinders (10 mm in diameter) from the center of the potato tissue (skin portion was eliminated) using a cork borer on sterile paper towels and place them in sterile distilled water with lactic acid (pH 4.0). Rinse the cylinders twice more using sterile distilled water with lactic acid. Cut each cylinder into 0.5-cm disks after excluding the 1-cm end pieces.

Step 6. Place 5 potato discs per Petri dish using aseptic technique by gently pushing the discs into the agar.

Step 7. Prepare at least 3 Petri dishes per sample and control. As a positive control, you can use camptothecin (a tumor suppressant). Add 1 drop (0.05 mL) of bacterial suspension per disc.

Step 8. Seal the edge of each Petri dish with parafilm strips to prevent moisture loss during the incubation period in the dark at 27 °C.

Step 9. After the incubation period, stain the disks with Lugol's reagent (I_2KI; 5% I_2 + 10% KI in distilled water). Count the tumors on each disk after 12 to 21 days. (**N.B.** - Lugol's reagent stains the starch in potato tissue dark blue to dark brown in color, but the tumors do not take up the stain and appear creamy to orange.)

Step 10. Calculate %inhibition of crown gall tumors as follows:

$$\%\text{Inhibition} = [100 - (\text{Tumor}_{\text{sample}} \div \text{Tumor}_{\text{control}})] \times 100$$

DMBA-Induced Breast Cancer Test

According to Alencar et al. (2019):

Rodent Model

Step 1. Divide the animals like mice or rats randomly into the following groups:

1. Control group (vehicle, p.o.)
2. 2,4-Dimethoxybenzaldehyde (DMBA) group: 6 mg/kg, p.o., for 7 weeks
3. Test drug group with recommended dose, p.o., once per week
4. Standard drug group: Cyclophosphamide 25 mg/kg, intra peritoneal (i.p.), once per 7 days.

Step 2. Dilute DMBA in natural vegetable oil and apply 0.2 mL weekly by gavage. Observing the tumor generation in 7 weeks' duration by physical palpation and measuring with a digital caliper to measure the length 'C' along with the lagura L to determine the tumor volume by using the following equation:

$$4/3 \times \pi \times (C/2) \times (L/2)\ 2.37.$$

Step 3. After treatment, resect both mammary lines and subject all animals to macro and microscopic evaluations of primary neoplasms.

Step 4. Breast necropsies and resections are intended for macroscopic examination (paying particular focus to determining the dimensions and variations in the cutting surface of the pieces), fixation in 10% buffered formalin, and automatic histological processing for inclusion in paraffin and slide preparation.

Step 5. Histo*pathological and immunohistochemical assessment*: All animals are administered pentobarbital sodium (150 mg/kg, i.p.) and lidocaine (10 mg/kg, i.p.) to cause their death after 7 weeks of observation. This is followed by a mastectomy of the paraffin-embedded mammary glands, sectioning of the sagittal plane into cuts of 7 mm thickness, and mounting on gelatin-coated blades. Sections go through a series of ethanol treatments to be dewaxed and rehydrated. Slides should be treated for 20 min each with 1 N sodium borate buffer and 1 N sodium acetate, followed by a PBS wash. Sections are treated with serum, incubated with anti-BrdU monoclonal antibodies (1:500 solution for 2 h, 1:200 solution for 1 h, and then stained with avidin-biotin complex and 3,30-diaminobenzidine). Entellan is used to cover the slides. Additionally stained with hematoxylin and eosin, all tissue sections are then examined using a 400x optical microscope. The Nottingham System (modified Scarff-Bloom-Richardson (SBR)), which assesses the degree of tube development, degree of nuclear pleomorphism, and mitotic index, provides the basis for histological grading. Each variable is given a score between 1 and 3, and the total of the partial values determines the "final histological grade." After performing a light microscopy inspection of the entire cutting area, spontaneous necrosis is evaluated.

N.B. - Some other chemical-induced cancer models are also available in experimental animals. For example –

N-ethyl-N-nitrosourea (ENU) Induced Brain Tumor Test
According to Laskera et al. (1992):

Rodent Model

Step 1. *Brain tumor induction*: Collect the pregnant test animals (e.g., rats). Within 24 h of birth, 16 new-born rats are given a single subcutaneous injection of 0.1 mM/kg (12 mg/kg) ENU in 20 μL of saline. Fifteen newborn control rats are given injections of 20 μL of saline within 24 h of birth. After weaning, these animals are grouped as follows: 6 males and 10 females in the ENU group, and 10 males and 5 females in the control group. The rats are identified by ear punching as young adults. They are housed 3 per cage under standard conditions, with a standard diet and water *ad libitum*. Measure their body weight every 4 weeks. Sacrifice the rats when moribund to prevent autolysis.

Step 2. *Plasma NMR determinations*: Beginning at age 6 months, draw 1 mL of blood from each animal by orbital bleeding into microcentrifuge tubes containing 0. 1 mL of 15% EDTA solution. Centrifuge the blood sample at 3000×*g* for 15 min, isolate the plasma, and store it at 5 °C until MRS analysis. Use a Fourier NMR Spectrometer for this analysis. Within 3 weeks of blood collection, add 0.1 mL of D_2O to 0.5 mL of plasma and determine the spectra at 22 ± 1 °C.

Step 3. *Histopathological analysis*: Prepare and analyze the brain sections as mentioned in various sections.

Part XV: Spasmolytic Activity Tests

A spasm is an uncontrollable, convulsive, or abrupt muscle contraction. Irritable bowel syndrome (IBS) is a functional gastrointestinal condition with symptoms including diarrhea, constipation, stomach pain, and different cramps. Its etiology is currently unknown. The first type of compound is anti-muscarinic or anticholinergic. These medications can occasionally have negative side effects, including urine retention, dry mouth, irritation, headache, nausea, vomiting, and constipation, which are sometimes linked to anti-muscarinic and calcium blocker medications depending on the situation (Stern and Bayes de Luna 2009; Lanza et al. 2011). The following models can be used to test your test drug's spasmolytic effects:

Isolated Tissue Model

According to Kandsi et al. (2021):

Step 1. After being anesthetized, collect about 2 cm of jejunum fragments from the animals (e.g., rabbits, guinea-pigs) and maintain them in the oxygenated normal Krebs–Henseleit buffer (KHB) solution (in mM): NaCl, 118; KCl, 4.7; $CaCl_2$, 2.5; $MgSO_4$, 1.2; $NaHCO_3$, 25; KH_2PO_4, 1.2; and glucose, 10. The KHB solution should be maintained at a temperature of 37 °C and a pH of 7.4 with continual oxygenation for 1 h to have the same physiological conditions as the animal. Mount each piece of jejunum in an isolated organ tank. Change the physiological fluid every 15 min to balance the organ before adding the test sample or controls. Record the effects of each dose/treatment for at least 7 to 8 min.

Step 2. Test myorelaxant activity by applying your test sample against controls at different concentrations in an isolated organ chamber.

Step 3. Test for an antispasmodic effect using pre-contracted jejunal smooth muscle through the application of carbachol 10^{-6} M. Then add your test sample or controls. Calculate the IC_{50} of your test and standard drug.

Ach-Induced Contraction Model

According to Devi et al. (2011):

Step 1. To the previously prepared rabbit ileum, add increasing doses of ACh (range: 10^{-7} to 10^{-2} M) into the bath and record the change in the strength of contractions. Prepare a dose-response curve.

Step 2. Wash the preparation several times, and when the spontaneous contraction re-establishes, add your test drug's doses or atropine (reference drug) at 0.01 to 1 μM, respectively, into the bath, 5 minutes prior to the addition of ACh (10^{-3} M).

Step 3. Calculate the response as %inhibition of the maximal force of contraction induced by the optimal dose of ACh. Compared the concentration-response curve with the control curve obtained without the test materials.

Kcl-Induced Contraction Model

It determines the calcium channel blocking activity of your test sample or controls (Ghayur and Gilani, 2005).

Step 1. Use high K^+ (80 mM) to induce a maximum sustained contraction.

Step 2. Add your test drug's doses or controls. Verapamil (0.01 to 3 μM) can be used as a reference drug. It is due to its potent calcium channel blocker.

Step 3. Express the responses as %inhibition of the KCl-induced contraction and plot the concentration-response curves.

Nitric Oxide Pathway Model

In order to disrupt the NO pathway, add L-NAME at 1 μM into the tissue bath, incubate for 0.5 h, and allow the ileum to contract spontaneously. Add your test materials or controls. Calculate concentration-response curves of the %inhibition of the contraction induced by the test materials in the presence of N-(gamma)-nitro-L-arginine methyl ester (L-NAME). Then plot and compare with the concentration-response curve obtained in the absence of L-NAME (Estrada-Soto et al. 2007).

Calcium Antagonistic Activity Test Model

According to Estrada-Soto et al. (2007):

Step 1. To confirm the Ca^{2+} blocking activity of the test substances, allow the tissues to stabilize in normal Tyrode's solution.

Step 2. Subsequently, replace it with Ca^{2+}-free Tyrode's solution containing EDTA (0.1 mM). Keep the ileal strips in this solution for 0.5 h.

Step 3. Replace the solution with K^+-rich and Ca^{2+}-free Tyrode's solution with the following composition (mM): KCl (50), NaCl (91.04), $MgCl_2$ (1.05), $NaHCO_3$ (11.9), NaH_2PO_4 (0.42), glucose (5.5) and EDTA (0.1).

Step 4. Incubate the mixture for 0.5 h at ambient temperature. Add $CaCl_2$ in increasing doses (range: 0.03 to 30.0 mM) to prepare a concentration-response curve for calcium.

Step 5. Repeat the process for your test sample and standard drug, verapamil (1 μM).

Rat Ilium Model

According to Sadraei et al. (2014):

Step 1. Kill the required number of adult male Wistar rats and collect longitudinal strips of them and place them in oxygenated Tyrode's solution.

Step 2. Suspend each strip between parallel platinum electrodes in a 50 mL organ bath (in Tyrode's solution at 37 °C and gassed with oxygen) under 1 g weight tension.

Step 3. Monitor the ileum tension with an isotonic transducer and display on a pen recorder device.

Step 4. Perform electrical field stimulation using rectangular pulses produced by a stimulator.

Step 5. Stimulate the tissues with a maximum of 6 volts using 1 s trains of stimuli at 50 Hz.

Step 6. Add ACh (0.5 μM) and 5-HT (2 μM) into the bath with contact time of 20 s. Perform stimulation once every 10 or 15 min as appropriate.

Step 7. Measure contraction to your test sample or controls relative to the tissue baseline and express as %initial response prior to addition of your test sample.

Step 8. Calculate IC_{50} values by plotting a full concentration-response curve for each tissue.

Part XVI: Evaluation of Biological Effects on Specific Organs

Numerous external and internal factors affect your body each day. Some agents are specific for some organs due to the toxicity of these agents. For example, digitalis glycosides exert toxic effects on the heart. Effects on your organs range from mild irritation to severe changes, such as irreversible damage, hypersensitivity, and even cancer. Certain drugs can alter or prevent organ damage. Therefore, the effects of a substance on body organs can be evaluated by using suitable test protocols. Examples of some widely used assay methods include:

Neuroprotective Activity Tests

Pain can be induced in experimental animals in a variety of ways; these include:

- *Mechanical stimuli*: dynamic (triggered by brushing), punctate (triggered by touch), and static (triggered by pressure).
- *Heat stimuli*: evoke sensations of warmth, hotness, or pain.
- *Cold stimuli*: decreases in temperature (usually starting at 32°C).

GABA Enzyme Inhibition Assay (In Vitro)

Briefly, the reaction mixture contains potassium pyrophosphate buffer (150 mM, pH 8.0), α-ketoglutarate (228.5 mM), GABA (873 mM), and GABAse (1,5-1,7 units/mg). The test substance is added to the reaction mixture and pre-incubated for 30 minutes at 37 °C. Then followed by addition of NADP+ (26.1 mM) and re-incubation for 30 and 60 min at 37 °C and monitoring absorbance changes at 337 - 340 nm due to the reduction of NADP+. Water and vigabatrin are used as negative and positive controls, respectively (Jakoby 1962).

Anti-Nociceptive Activity Study

Hot-Plate Model

According to Eddy and Leimbach (1953) and Coelho et al. (2005):

Step 1. Randomly distribute the required number of animals into the required number of groups.

Step 2. Administer treatments to the respective groups.

Step 3. Keep the hot plate's temperature at 55 ± 1 °C. For the study, a baseline latency is recorded before treatment. Nociception is the term used to describe acute responses, including jumping, forepaw licking, and paw(s) withdrawal. The latency durations are measured at intervals of 15, 30, 45 and 60 following the administration of conventional drugs (such as morphine or diclofenac) or test samples to animals (such as mice). In order to prevent tissue damage, you should only heat the animals for 15-20 sec at a time for this. Using naloxone (i.p.) 15 min prior to the injection of a standard or test sample in mice, the procedure is repeated in order to assess the participation of opioid receptors. The maximum reaction time is fixed at 45 sec to prevent any injury to the tissues of the paws. If the reading exceeds 45 sec, it would be considered as maximum analgesia. Use the following formula to determine the percentage of the maximum impact (%MPE):

$$\%MPE = (Latency_{Postdrug} - Latency_{Predrug}) \div (Cutoff\ period - Latency_{Predrug}) \times 100$$

where, MPE stands for maximum protective effect.

Analgesic Test in Chick Model

According to Mousa (2019):

Step 1. Take adequate 4-5 h fasted broiler chicks 7 - 21 days old weighing between 48 - 125 g (n = 5/6) and group as per your need.

Step 2. Induce voltage (volt) by electrostimulation for each chick and record before and after 30 min of your treatment. As a standard you can use ketorolac injection (20 mg/kg, i.m.).

Step 3. Determine the percentage of analgesia in each group.

Tail Immersion Model
According to Janssen et al. (1963):

Step 1. Randomly distribute the required number of animals into the required number of groups.

Step 2. Administer treatments to the respective groups.

Step 3. 52 ± 1 °C should be the water bath's consistent temperature. The study used animals (such as mice) that exerted tail deflection from heated water within 1.5 to 3.5 sec.

Step 4. Using "Chux," animals are gently immobilized for 25 to 30 sec while a 1 to 2-cm portion of their tails are immersed in warm water. Animals' violent flick responses are considered the culmination of nociception. To prevent harm to animals, a 20-second cutoff time is maintained. Following administration of a vehicle, a standard (such as morphine), or a test sample, the latency time at 30, 45, 60, 90, and 120 min is noted. Prior to administration, one obtains a pre-treatment latency. The identical test is run as stated in the hot plate test with naloxone (i.p.) administered beforehand, and %MPE is computed from the delay periods. The test group's values are contrasted with those of the control groups.

Acetic Acid-Induced Writhing Model
According to Vogel (2007):

Step 1. Randomly distribute the required number of animals into the required number of groups.

Step 2. Administer treatments to the respective groups.

Step 3. 0.7-1% acetic acid (10 mL/kg, i.p.) is administered to cause writhing 0.5 h after the administration of the controls or your test sample and 15 min of the recommended course of treatment (such as diclofenac sodium). The number of animals (such as mice) writhing during the following 10 min is counted after the animals are kept in the box for 5 min. Abdominal contraction, stretching or bending of the torso, trunk, and/or pelvis, followed by limb extension, are the characteristics of writhing. Latency (first writhing time after the administration of acetic acid) and total number of writhings (in 10 min, observation time) are determined for this purpose. The values of the test group are compared with the control groups.

Formalin-Induced Licking Model

According to Coelho et al. (2005):

Step 1. Randomly distribute the required number of animals into the required number of groups.

Step 2. Administer treatments to the respective groups.

Step 3. Animals (such as mice) used in this study are given injections of formalin to cause discomfort in the sub-plantar area of the right hind paw. 20 μL of a 1.35% formalin solution (or 0.5% formaldehyde) prepared in normal saline is injected into each animal. 0.5 h after the administration of the controls or test sample, formalin is administered. The typical medication is administered 15 min prior to the formalin injection (e.g., sodium diclofenac, morphine). Animals' right hind paw licking is timed from 0 to 5 min for the early phase (neurogenic phase) and from 15 - 25 min for the late phase (inflammatory phase). Licking is thought to be a sign of nociception. Analyze the data with the control groups and establish the latency and overall number of paw licks for the test sample group.

Glutamate-Induced Paw Licking and Edema Model

According to Rodrigues et al. (2012):

Step 1. Randomly distribute the required number of animals into the required number of groups.

Step 2. Administer treatments to the respective groups.

Step 3. In this study, the animals (such as mice) are given the standard medicine (such as diclofenac sodium), the test sample, or the control (a vehicle). At this point, digital slide calipers are used to measure the thickness of each animal's right hind paw. Each animal receives 1 μL/1 μM of glutamate in the sub-plantar region of the right hind paw, 30 min after the injection of the controls or your test sample and 15 min following conventional medication treatment. The preparation's pH is set at 7.4 to prevent irritation. The mice are kept in observation chambers after the glutamate challenge. Following a 15-minute counting period, each animal's paw thickness is once more measured. The degree of edema (Δ) in mm is calculated by subtracting the measurement of paw diameter prior to glutamate injection from the paw diameter following glutamate challenge.

Hargreaves Model

When a radiant or infrared heat stimulus is applied, this model measures the heat thresholds that develop in the hind paws of animals (such as mice and rats). It is typically done in a glass enclosure with a heated bottom to reduce errors brought on by heat sink effects. A radiant or infrared heat source is placed and directed at the plantar surface of the rear paw. The withdrawal latency is measured as the amount of time it takes for the subject to stop responding to the heat stimulus; depending on the model of the apparatus, this measurement may be made manually by the subject or automatically by the subject. In order to detect heat allodynia and hypoalgesia in naive animals, the intensity of the light source should be adjusted to generate withdrawal latencies of 10 - 12 sec, with a predetermined cutoff period to minimize tissue injury. Each animal can act as its own internal control in unilateral pain models thanks to this apparatus's ability to measure ipsilateral and contralateral heat thresholds. Additionally, it makes it possible to measure the heat thresholds of free-moving animals, which lowers the likelihood of stress-related reactions. However, you need to acclimate your animals to the equipment to reduce ambulation so that withdrawal latencies can be precisely calculated (often for 5 - 30 min) (Hargreaves et al. 1988).

Thermal Probe Model

The heat thresholds of animals are likewise quantified by this model (e.g., mice and rats). A mouse enclosure that allows access to a 2 mm thermal probe on the hind paw can be used to conduct this test. The hand-held device's handle is rotated to start heating at a rate of 2.5 °C/sec from room temperature to 60 °C, which is terminated automatically upon paw withdrawal, operator removal of the probe from the paw, or upon reaching a predefined cut-out (typically 60 °C). The temperature at which paw withdrawal took place is automatically recorded, making it possible to record the temperature without having to wait for an investigator to manually note it (Deuis and Vetter, 2016).

Cold Plate Model

This model examines how experimental animals behave in response to cold temperatures that are both harmful and harmless (e.g., mice, rats). Similar to the hot plate test, the cold plate test can be used to measure a variety of endpoints. The reaction to a particular temperature (usually between -5 and 15 °C) can be measured *first*. Here, the mouse is set down on the plate once it has cooled to the proper temperature, and the length of time it takes for the animal to exhibit nociceptive activity like shaking, jumping, or licking is noted as the response time. *Second*, at a particular temperature, the number of flinches during a predetermined time can be counted. *Third*, the threshold for the cold reaction can be calculated using the unpleasant response to a cooling ramp. It is to be noted that certain animal strains tend to prevent weight bearing on the affected paw or adjust their posture to minimize contact with the chilly surface rather than flinching or licking. Therefore, all observations should be tailored to the particular model animal (Allchorne et al. 2005).

Acetone Evaporation Model

This model evaluates evaporative cooling-induced unpleasant behaviors and is often regarded as a gauge of cold allodynia. Acetone is dabbed or sprayed on the plantar surface of the hind paw during the test, which cools the skin to safe temperatures of 15 - 21 °C, albeit the exact temperature varies depending on the room temperature, the skin's temperature, and the dose of acetone used. In contrast to the tail flick assay, exposure of the hind paw to acetone did not cause paw withdrawal in mildly sedated animals. Instead, ethyl chloride administration results in skin temperatures of around 5°Cor less, which is widely regarded as an unpleasant cold stimulus. Acetone can be difficult to apply consistently since it has a lower surface tension than water (25.2 mN/m *vs* 72.8 mN/m), which makes it difficult to create consistent droplets with a pipette or syringe. Some labs choose to utilize a spray instead. Sensitivity to cold is measured by counting or timing nocifensive reactions or by rating the intensity of the reaction (e.g., 0 (no response); 1 (brisk withdrawal or flick of the paw); 2 (repeated flicking of the paw); 3 (repeated flicking of the hind paw and licking of the paw)). As a control, water that has been heated to 30 °C and administered similarly is typically utilized. Video recordings that are played back in slow motion may be necessary in order to appropriately examine the response to acetone since the nocifensive response can sometimes be too quick for a researcher to quantify in real time (Carlton et al. 1994).

Cold Plantar Assay Model

The animal is housed in this model in an enclosure with a spotless glass floor. A cut off syringe filled with dry ice (for temperatures between 5 and 12 °C) or wet ice (for temperatures between 17 and °C) is used to administer a cold stimulation to the glass beneath the paw. When the glass is chilled, the hind paws are exposed in one direction to the cooled surface, whose temperature can be measured by sticking a thermocouple probe to the glass or skin. Cold allodynia and hyperalgesia are measured by the latency to paw withdrawal. The paw being tested must remain in contact with the glass in order to accomplish efficient temperature transfer, even if application of the ice pellet to the glass produces a cooling ramp that is roughly connected to estimations of the paw withdrawal temperature. Nevertheless, acclimatized animals are capable of regular measures, though guarding or an altered weight distribution may cause mistakes (Bernner et al. 2012).

Temperature Preference Model

Animals' preferences for different temperatures are measured using this as a substitute for a thermal aversion test (e.g., rodents). The animal can select between two nearby regions that are kept at various temperatures in their most basic form. The two-temperature choice assay, commonly known as the thermal place preference test, can be employed to measure a person's aversion to or preference for cold or heat. A test plate at a specified temperature, typically between 5 and 55 °C, is put next to a reference plate at a neutral temperature, typically between 25 and 30 °C. The amount of time an animal spends on the test plate in comparison to the reference plate is measured over a predetermined period and compared to the time spent on the control plate in order to determine temperature sensitivity. This model is widely utilized in the investigation of the function of thermosensitive transient receptor potential (TRP) channels, such as TRPA1, TRPM8, TRPM3, TRPV3, and TRPV4, in thermal nociception (Wibbenmeyer et al. 2011).

Non-Stimulus Evoked Nociception Model

Most of the time, the underlying or impulsive pain arises without a clear provocation. Animals' impulsive pain can be measured by the use of mechanized behavioral psychology, gait analysis, weight bearing, and burrowing assays (Wibbenmeyer et al. 2011).

Grimace Scales

Animal facial expressions, such as those of mice and rats, can be used to rate the subjective degree of pain. Five facial characteristics—orbital tightening, nose bulge, cheek bulge, ear position, and whisker position—are evaluated using the rodent grimace scale. Orbital tightness is the tightening or squeezing of the eyes and a narrowing of the orbital region. While cheek bulge refers to the rounded extension of the cheek muscle in contrast to its usual look, nose bulge refers to the bulge visible on the nose's bridge. An abnormal ear posture is one in which the ears are moved back and apart from their normal position (they may feature vertical ridges). Lastly, the term "whisker alteration" describes a shift in whisker location (may be backward, forward, or clumped together). These expressions are scored on a scale of 0 to 2, with 0 being normal, 1 being moderately changed, and 2 being substantially changed features. The severity of these expressions changes with the level of felt "pain" (Langford et al. 2010).

Burrowing Models

Rodents' spontaneous and self-driven behavior of burrowing can be utilized to assess whether their nociception is stimulus- or non-stimulus-evoked. A long tube is used to create a burrow that is filled with a suitable substrate (such as food pellets, sand, or marbles), and the other end is locked and elevated by screws to prevent non-burrowing behaviors from shifting the substrate inside. For a predetermined period of time, the burrows are placed in the rodent's cage, and the amount of material moved is weighed and recorded.

Weight Bearing and Gait Analysis Model

Rodents' gait and weight bearing can be used as a substitute for measuring nociception and are often regarded as indicators of non-evoked or stimulus-independent "pain." It can be argued that ambulation itself provides a nociceptive mechanical stimulus to the affected limb(s), and thus it may be a measure of stimulus-evoked nociceptive behavior, particularly in dynamic weight-bearing tests or gait analysis tests. Weight bearing is typically thought of as a measure of non-stimulus evoked nociception. Static weight bearing or incapacitance assays, which commonly include putting the animal in an elevated holder and forcing the positioning of the hind paws on two different pressure sensors, evaluate the weight distribution over the hind paws. Uneven weight distribution between the ipsilateral and contralateral paws has been seen in a variety of models, such as osteoarthritis caused by monosodium iodoacetate (MIA), pain brought on by bone cancer, inflammation brought on by carrageenan, and sciatic nerve crush injury. These results are interpreted as a natural adjustment to the level of nociception felt.

The CatWalk XT (Noldus) and GaitLab (ViewPoint Behavior Technology) are two commercial automated gait analysis systems that use internally reflected light to illuminate paw prints as an animal walks across an elevated glass floor. Other systems include DigiGait (Mouse Specifics Inc.) and GaitScan/TreadScan (CleverSys), which use video recordings and automated software to analyze the paw prints of animals walking on a transparent belt treadmill or clear floor.

Automated Behavioral Analysis Model

More and more, non-stimulus-induced pain in rats is being studied utilizing automated methods that analyze the activities of uncontrolled animals. Aspects of behavior such as locomotion (such as stillness, walking, trotting, and running), distance traveled, velocity, grooming, posture, eating and drinking, and foraging are all examined. It is possible to draw conclusions about various "pain" states, and particularly about spontaneous nociception, by comparing the frequencies of behaviors in animal models of pain in comparison to control states. The fact that no "pain-specific" actions are recorded raises the possibility of medication or phenotypic effects interfering and masking nociception or anti-nociception. With this technique, operator subjectivity is removed and animal stress is decreased because the animal is not aware of the researcher and does not need to be restrained or trained. Automated video analysis, vibration sensors, photobeams, and combinations of these can be used to undertake automated behavioral analysis in a dedicated apparatus (Behavioral Spectrometer, Behavioral Instruments) or in a home cage (HomeCageScan, CleverSys; PhenoTyper, Noldus). The Behavioral Spectrometer (Behavioral Instruments) is a specially designed instrument that consists of an enclosed box (about 30 x 30 x 30 cm) with a fish-eye lens mounted on the ceiling, an accelerometer, and a line of photobeams mounted on the wall. 23 different sorts of behaviors, such as ambulation (such as stillness, walking, trotting, and sprinting), grooming and rearing behaviors, as well as distance traveled and average velocity, may all be captured in real time by the spectrometer. The Behavioral Spectrometer has been proven accurate in a mouse model of inflammation of the hind paw caused by carrageenan, where there is a clear increase in grooming frequency and a decrease in ambulation. The HomeCageScan (CleverSys) classifies 38 pre-defined actions of mice in a home cage using automated video analysis. These behaviors include walking, rearing, smelling, stretching, jumping, burrowing, foraging, sleeping, eating, drinking, hanging, and grooming, as well as the distance traveled. It has been proven effective in mouse models of pain after laparotomy and vasectomy.

Memory-Enhancing Capacity Test

Rodent Model

Animals are sorted into the necessary number of groups, each containing the necessary number of animals (such as mice or rats), at random. Before beginning the behavioral evaluations, the animals receive the test drug or controls for a period of 4 weeks. Galantamine at 3 mg/kg can be utilized as a standard drug. On the first day of the behavioral test, animal locomotion is evaluated in an open field. Step-down passive avoidance tests are evaluated on days 15 to 16 and 28, respectively, while Morris water maze tests are conducted from days 2 to 8 and 23 to 25. The mice are then promptly beheaded, and the brain tissues are quickly dissected on ice to check for the presence of MDA. Figure 9.5 shows a general outline of a typical memory-enhancing study in rodents.

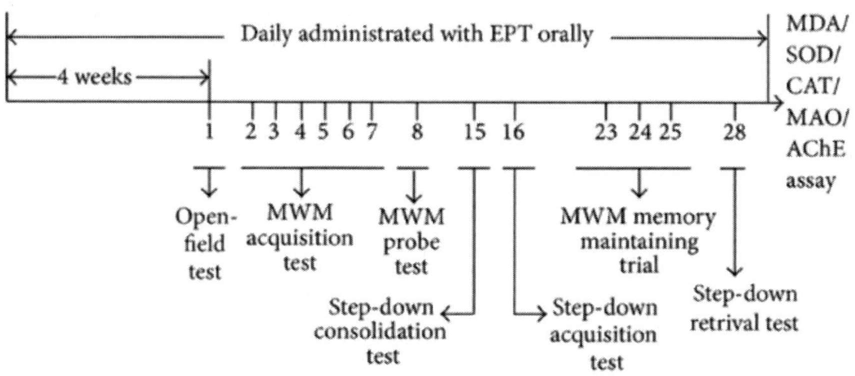

Figure 9.5. General outline of a typical memory-enhancing study in rodents.

Open-Field Test

Follow the previously discussed protocol.

Morris Water Maze Test

It is a circular swimming pool (diameter: height = 100 × 40 cm) with continual cues placed outside the maze to help animals navigate it. To make the water opaque and keep animals from seeing the submerged platform, black ink is added to the water. Throughout the experiment, the water's temperature is maintained between 24 and 26 °C. The only way out of the water is a 6 × 15 cm invisible platform that is positioned 1.5 cm below the water's surface. Through the use of a computerized tracking and picture analysis system, the pool is separated into four quadrants. The maze's two main axes cross perpendicularly to one another to form an imagined "+." One of the four cardinal points-north (N), south (S), west (W), and east (E)-is marked at the end of each line (E).

Steps

1. The spatial reference memory is tested using the Morris water maze, which consists of an acquisition phase and a probe trial, from days 2 to 8 of behavioral testing. On days 23 through 25, the animals' capacity for memory is examined.
2. Animals are introduced to the environment in the pool-containing platform during the acquisition phase so they can get used to it before training.
3. Animals are then put through two trials per day for six days to train them to locate the submerged platform, which is placed in the middle of the pool's southeast quadrant and stays there for the duration of the experiment. Four trials over two days of training make up a session. The mouse is placed on the learning platform for 15 sec prior to each trial, after which it is gently released into the pool with its back to the wall. For each session, one of four release points (NE, SE, SW, and NW) is randomly chosen. Animals have up to 60 sec to locate the platform. If the animal is gently led to the platform and remains there for 10 seconds after being lost for 60 sec, its escape latency is recorded as 60 sec. If an animal locates the platform in less than 60 sec, it is permitted to stay there for 10 sec before being put into a cage until the next attempt. The animals are brought back to their cages for rest after finishing their daily training. To assess the mice's capacity for learning and memory, data on escape rate, escape delay, and swimming speed are gathered.
4. The spatial probe trials are put to the test on Day 8 of the behavioral evaluation. Each animal is lowered into the water on the opposite side of the SE quadrant when the platform has been removed. For 120 sec, they are free to swim. Spatial memory is measured by keeping track of the crossing numbers over the platform's location, swimming time, and swimming distance spent in the target quadrant.

5. Testing for memory retention is conducted two weeks following Morris water maze trials. Mice are launched in the opposite quadrant; neither the platform nor the starting location are fixed. For three days, this training is done twice each day. For the purpose of assessing an animal's capacity for memory retention, escape latency is defined as the average of two trials per day.

Step-Down Test

To assess how EPT affects the learning and memory abilities of aged mice, step-down passive avoidance tests are conducted in a chamber. The chamber's floor is made of copper rods, and one of the corners has a rubber platform that is highly insulated. At the start of training, the animals are placed in the chamber for a three-minute adaptation period. Animals are placed on the floor after adaptation, and they immediately receive a minor electrical shock lasting five minutes (25 V). Animals instinctively jump back onto the platform in order to avoid the shock. It is measured by how long it takes to step down on the grid with all four paws. Within 4 min, the time spent in the safe zone (on the platform) and the error zone (on the grid) are both recorded. Three phases of the tests-acquisition, consolidation, and retrieval are run on days 15, 16, and 28 of the experiment, respectively.

Preparation of brain tissue samples and biochemical analysis: After behavioral measurements, all the animals are sacrificed by decapitation; the brain tissues are quickly removed, washed with cold saline solution, followed by 50 mM Tris-HCl buffer (pH 7.4), and weighed. Then, it is placed into a glass bottle, labeled, and stored in a deep freezer (-25 °C) until processing (maximum 10 h). The tissues are homogenized in four volumes of ice-cold Tris-HCl buffer using a glass Teflon homogenizer for 2 min at 5000×*g* after cutting them into small pieces. The homogenate is then centrifuged at 1000×*g* for 10 min to remove the debris. The clear upper supernatant fluid is extracted with an equal volume of ethanol and centrifuged at 17000×*g* for 30 min; the clear upper ethanol layer is taken and used for biochemical assay. All the preparations are performed at 4°C, and then MDA, SOD, CAT, and AChE are estimated using commercial kits according to the manufacturer's protocols or as mentioned above (antioxidant test section).

MAO Can Be Determined as Below

The activity of MAO is based on the production of benzyl aldehyde from the reaction and its specific substrate, aniline hydrochloride. Briefly, the protein concentrations are determined by the Lowry method using bovine serum albumin as a standard. The homogenate is then incubated (37 °C, 30 min) in reaction buffer containing aniline hydrochloride. The absorbance of the reaction product is measured at 242 nm. One unit (U) of MAO activity is defined as the amount that increases the absorbance by 0.01 at 37 °C. Therefore, MAO activity is expressed as U/mg protein (Li et al. 2014).

Anti-Alzheimer's Disease Activity Test

According to Oyeleke et al. (2022):

Rodent Model

Step 1. Collect and randomly divide required number of animals (e.g., rats or mice) into required groups.

Step 2. *Surgery and induction of Alzheimer's disease*: Develop Alzheimer's disease through a single bilateral intra-cerebroventricular (ICV) injection of the previously obtained Aβ 1–42 aggregates. Use Paxinos and Watson atlas to get the appropriate coordinate and the following stereotaxic coordinates: anteroposterior: -0.8 mm from bregma, medial/lateral: +/-1.4 mm and dorsal/ventral: - 4.0 mm are employed to inject substances into the lateral ventricles through a stainless steel cannula using a Hamilton microsyringe. Aβ 1-42 (4 μg/μL/site) is injected into experimental rats while sham rats are injected with the same volume of isosaline (1 μL/site).

Step 3. House the animals after surgery individually and give the free access to food and water. Apply an antibiotic cream daily and allow them 7 days to recover from surgery. Monitor the general condition of the animals such as body weight, food and water intake daily after surgery.

Step 4. *Behavioral assessment*: Subject the animals to some behavioral tests such as Y-maze and Novel object recognition (NOR) test for spatial memory on Days 19 and 20 of administration respectively. Assess short-term memory by spontaneous alternation behavior in the Y-maze task using a standard rats' Y-maze.

Step 5. *Animal sacrifice, excision of brain tissues and sample preparation for biochemical and histological analysis*: After 1 day of completion of treatment, sacrifice the animals by cervical dislocation and collect blood through cardiac puncture. Excise brain tissues using appropriate forceps. For biochemical assays, sagitally divide the cerebrum into two at the corpus callosum and isolate the hippocampus on ice surface.

The hippocampi tissues should be immediately homogenized (10% w/v) in 100 mM PBS (pH 7.4) and fix some whole brain tissues in 10% formal saline for the histological procedure.

Step 6. *Biochemical assays*: Assess for MDA, GPx, released inorganic phosphate (Pi), AChE activity, glutamate and Aβ1-42 by using suitable methods.

Step 7. *Histological analysis*: Prepare the hippocampus specimens and perform histopathological analysis as mentioned above.

Anti-Convulsant Activity Tests

Strychnine-Induced Seizure Model

According to Obese et al. (2021):

Step 1. Randomly distribute the required number of animals (e.g., mice) into the required number of groups.

Step 2. Induce seizure by injecting strychnine nitrate at a dose of 0.5 mg/kg (i.p.) 1 h after administration of your test sample or 0.5 h after the reference drug (e.g., diazepam at 0.1 - 1.0 mg/kg, i.p.).

Step 3. Record the frequency, duration, and latency of myoclonic jerks in all groups in comparison to a control group receiving the vehicle. These parameters can be observed by using a video recording system.

Pilocarpine-Induced Status Epilepticus Model

According to Obese et al. (2021):

Step 1. Randomly distribute the required number of animals (e.g., mice) into the required number of groups.

Step 2. Administer your test sample 1 h before seizure induction while 0.5 h for standard drug (e.g., diazepam at 0.1 - 1.0 mg/kg, i.p.) or vehicle (control at 10 mL/kg, p.o.).

Step 3. Administer pilocarpine (300 mg/kg, i.p.) to induce seizures in animals.

Step 4. Administer *N*-butyl-bromide hyoscine (1 mg/kg, i.p.) 0.5 h prior to induction to counter the peripheral autonomic effects produced by pilocarpine. Then place the animals separately into the transparent Plexiglas testing chamber and record the latency and duration of clonic tonic seizures through video recordings and tracking systems.

Isoniazid-Induced Seizure Model

According to Obese et al. (2021):

Step 1. Randomly distribute the required number of animals (e.g., mice) into the required number of groups.

Step 2. Adapt the animals in the chamber for 60 min prior receiving your test sample, standard drug (e.g., diazepam: 0.1 - 1 mg/kg i.p.), or control (vehicle: 10 mL/kg, i.p.).

Step 3. Induce seizures with isoniazid (INH) (300 mg/kg, p.o.) 0.5 or 1 h after the above-mentioned treatments and record the seizure parameters as mentioned before.

Picrotoxin-Induced Seizure Model

According to Obese et al. (2021):

Step 1. Randomly distribute the required number of animals (e.g., mice) into the required number of groups.

Step 2. Administer picrotoxin (3 mg/kg, i.p.) 0.5 h (standard) and 1 h (test drug) after the treatments.

Step 3. Record the latency of tonic convulsions, latency to myoclonic jerks, and also the frequency and duration of tonic convulsions similarly.

Evaluation of Gabaergic System Involvement

According to Obese et al. (2021):

Step 1. Randomly distribute the required number of animals (e.g., mice) into the required number of groups.

Step 2. For this, use a selective benzodiazepine receptor antagonist (e.g., flumazenil; 2 mg/kg) and an agonist (e.g., diazepam; 0.3 mg/kg, i.p.).

Step 3. Treat the animals with your test drug at a specified dose 0.5 h prior to the administration of picrotoxin (3 mg/kg, i.p.).

Step 4. Treat with the antagonist (e.g., flumazenil: 2 mg/kg, i.p.) 5 min before the administration of your test and agonist group, and 65 min or 35 min before the injection of picrotoxin (3 mg/kg, i.p.), respectively.

Step 5. Record the latency to the frequency and duration of clonic convulsions as mentioned above.

Anti-Epileptic Activity Tests

6 Hz Seizure Model

According to Viswanatha et al. (2016):

Step 1. Randomly distribute the required number of animals (e.g., mice) into the required number of groups.

Step 2. Treat the animals with your test drug for 3 days. On Day-3, 1 h after the last dose, apply tetracaine ophthalmic solution (0.5% tetracaine hydrochloride), wet the corneal electrodes 30 min later with saline, and give electrical stimulation for 3 sec (200 μs-duration, 32-mA mono polar rectangular pulses at 6 Hz) to all animals, using a constant current device (e.g., ECT Unit 5780). Use vehicle as control and treat similarly.

Step 3. After the seizures, resume the animals' normal exploratory behavior. Define the end point as protection against seizures. Consider the animals that gain their normal exploratory behavior within 10 seconds of stimulation as protected.

%protection = 100 – [(Number of animal show seizures ÷ Total number of animal use) × 100]

Maximal Electroshock (MES)-Induced Convulsions Model

According to Viswanatha et al. (2016):

Step 1. Randomly distribute the required number of animals (e.g., mice) into the required number of groups.

Step 2. Treat the animals with vehicle, your test drug or reference drug (e.g., phenytoin: 25 mg/kg) orally for 3 days.

Step 3. On the 3rd day, exactly 1 h after the assigned treatment, apply tetracaine ophthalmic solution (0.5% tetracaine hydrochloride) to their cornea.

Step 4. Apply immediately an electrical stimulation (150 mA, 0.2 s) through corneal electrodes using Electro convulsiometer to produce generalized tonic-clonic seizures in all the groups of animals.

Step 5. Observe all animals individually in an open-top plastic cage for 0.5 h. Observe and record the parameters: duration of hind limb flexion, hind limb extensor, stupor, and death/survival; and calculate %protection using the survival rate as mentioned above.

Pentylenetetrazole (PTZ)-Induced Convulsions Model

According to Viswanatha et al. (2016):

Step 1. Randomly distribute the required number of animals (e.g., mice) into the required number of groups.

Step 2. Treat the animals with your control, test drug, or reference drug (e.g., diazepam: 3 mg/kg) orally for 3 days.

Step 3. On the 3rd day, after 1 h, treat the animals with PTZ (80 mg/kg) intraperitoneally and observe them individually in a plastic cage for 0.5 h.

Step 4. Count the survivors later, up to 1 day. During the individual observation, record the parameters: onset of clonus, onset of tonic convulsions, and death/survival and express %protection as mentioned above.

Lithium-Pilocarpine-Induced Seizures

According to Patel et al. (1988):

In this case, the animals (e.g., mice, rats) receive lithium sulphate (3 meq/kg, i.p.), 24 h before pilocarpine (30 mg/kg, i.p.). The animals also receive your test sample, standard drug (e.g., diazepam: 2 mg/kg, i.p.) or vehicle, 30 min before receiving pilocarpine. Evaluate the severity of convulsions until the maximum effect is produced, using the following scoring system: 0 (no response); 1 (fictive scratching); 2 (tremors); 3 (head nodding); 4 (forelimb clonus); 5 (rearing, falling and clonus).

Brain GABA Level Detection

According to Viswanatha et al. (2016):

Step 1. Randomly distribute the required number of animals (e.g., male mice) into the required number of groups.

Step 2. Treat the animals with vehicle, your test drug or reference drug (e.g., diazepam: 3 mg/kg) orally for 1 and 3 days in two different experimental sets.

Step 3. Sacrifice the 1st experimental set of animals on day 1, 1 h after the dosing. Sacrifice the 2nd set of animals on day 3, 1 h after the assigned treatment.

Step 4. Collect the brain and freeze, and subsequently, separate the cerebellum and whole brain using a microtome blade.

Step 5. Take the weight of these tissues and transfer them to 10 mL of ice-cold 0.1 M perchloric acid containing 15 μg/mL of valine (internal standard).

Step 6. Homogenized the contents under ice-cold conditions and centrifuge at 5000×*g* for 10 min at 4°C.

Step 7. Collected the supernatant and subjected it to brain GABA level estimation. For this, add 100 μL supernatant or the standard GABA to a micro-tube containing 100 μL of 0.1 M potassium carbonate solution. It will induce a dansylation reaction. Vortex the mixtures thoroughly and centrifuge at 10000×*g* for 10 min. Transfer 100 μL supernatant from each into a Pyrex tube containing 100 μL of 0.1 M sodium hydrogen carbonate solution. Add 400 μL of working dansyl chloride solution (1.25 mg/mL anhydrous acetone). Vortex the tubes for 30 sec and incubate at 90°Cin benchtop oven for 0.5 h. Avoid capping the tubes to allow most of the solvent to evaporate.

Step 8. Then collect the tubes and allow them to cool at an ambient temperature. Transfer the contents to 1.5 mL microtubes and subject them to high-performance liquid chromatography (HPLC) analysis. Express the brain GABA level as ng/g of tissue in comparison to a pre-prepared standard calibration curve.

Actophotometer Study

According to Viswanatha et al. (2016):

Step 1. Randomly distribute the required number of animals (e.g., mice) into the required number of groups.

Step 2. Treat Gr-I with the vehicle (control: 10 mL/kg, p.o.), while Gr-II with reference drug (e.g., diazepam: 4 mg/kg, i.p.) and Gr-III with your test drug (at a specified dose via recommended route).

Step 3. Observe the activity of animals after 0.5 or 1 h of treatments by placing them in the actophotometer for 5 min in a square (30 cm) closed arena fitted with infrared light-sensitive photocells. Calculate %reduction of locomotor activity using the following formula.

%Reduced locomotor activity = 100 – [(Photocell counts after treatment ÷ Photocell counts before treatment) × 100]

Depression Behavior Models

Forced Swimming Test

It contains a glass container with a height-diameter of 25 × 12 cm, filled up to 8 cm with water at 25 °C. Conduct the experiment for all groups between 9:00 AM and 4:00 PM under similar conditions (Porsolt et al. 1977; Porsolt et al. 1979).

Step 1. Place the animal (e.g., mouse) gently into the water from 20 cm above. Consider the discontinuation of the movement of the animal's limbs immobility for 5/6 min. The first 1-2 min are taken as the adjustment time to the conditions of the animals and their immobility during this time is not recorded.

Step 2. Record the immobility for the next 4 min. Compare your test group data with the controls.

Head Dip Test

It consists of a wooden hole-board apparatus measuring 20 × 40 cm with 16 evenly spaced holes (each of diameter 3 cm). The apparatus elevates to a height of 25 cm. Thirty minutes after treatment, place the animal (e.g., mouse) individually on the center of the board and count the number of heads dipping and the latency until the first entry using a tally counter during a 5-minute trial period (Somani et al. 2010).

Light-Dark Box Test

It is an open-topped rectangular box (46 × 27 × 30 cm high) divided into a small (18 × 27 cm) area and a large (27 × 27 cm) area with an opening door (7.5 × 7.5 cm) located at the center of the partition at floor level. One compartment is painted black and has a dark environment, whereas the large compartment is painted white and brightly illuminated by a 60-W (400 lx) light source. The light is placed in the center of the white compartment. The time spent in the illuminated and dark compartments, as well as the number of transitions in each space and the latency of the first crossing from one compartment to the other, is recorded for 5 minutes. The environment during the test is dark (Shahed-Al-Mahmud and Lina, 2017).

Anti-Compulsive Model

Marble-Burying Test

In this study, each animal (e.g., mouse) is individually placed in a plastic cage (21 × 38 × 14 cm) containing 5-cm thick sawdust bedding. Keep 20 small glass marbles (diameter 10 - 12 mm) on the bedding, evenly spaced in four rows (Figure 9.6).

Count the number of unburied marbles after 10-30 min of an animal's exposure. A marble covered at least two-thirds of its size by saw dust is considered "buried" (Njung'e and Handley 1991).

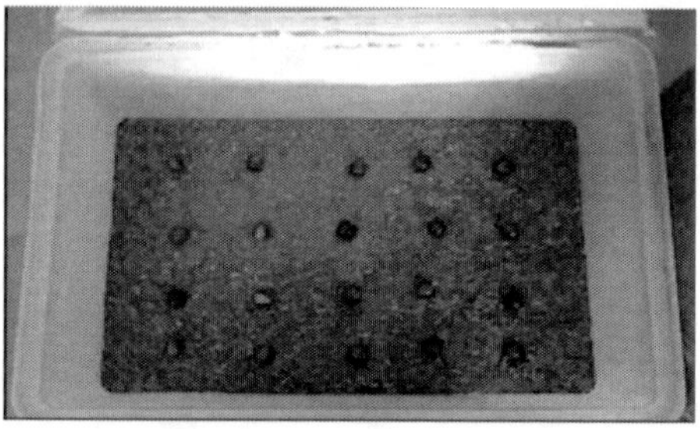

Figure 9.6. A marble burying field.

Motor Coordination Model

Rota-Rod Test

It is an automated, electrically-operated biological research apparatus. It is used to evaluate the activity of drugs interfering with motor coordination. The instrument (a horizontal rotating device) is set at a rate of 17 revolutions per minute (rpm) (Samson et al. 2011).

Step 1. To select the testing animals (e.g., mice or rats), place them individually on the horizontal rod. Among them, select those that are able to remain on the rod longer than 3 min for the study.

Step 2. Group the animals and treat them as required.

Step 3. Place the animals individually on the rotating rod at least for 3 minutes. Measure the performance time and count the total number of falls within 3 minutes.

Cage Crossing Movement Test

In this study, a box is specifically designed to have a rectangular shape. Briefly, transparent perpex cages (26 × 26 × 26 cm) with sawdust covered floors are used to monitor the activity in a familiar environment. After random distribution and treatments, place animals (e.g., mice, rats) singly in these cages to get them familiarized with the environment, and count the number of cage crossings for 10 min (Najam and Anser 2011).

Stationary Rod Test

For this, allow the animals to balance on a stationary rod after training. Note the time during which each animal maintains balance and then falls from the stationary rod (Najam and Anser 2011).

Inclined Plane Test

The plain consists of two rectangular boards connected at one end by a hinge. One board is the base, and the other is a movable inclined plane. Allow the animals to move on the plane and record the movement (Najam and Anser 2011).

Other Popularly Used Neruopharmacological Test Models

Open-Field Test

This test is run to determine the impact of the test sample on mouse movement. Choose a remote, quiet, and poorly lighted spot for this. The open field apparatus has an overall size of 50 × 50 × 50 cm^3. The open field's floor is divided into rows of squares, with the colors of each square alternately black and white (Gipta et al. 1971).

Step 1. Randomly distribute the required number of animals into the required number of groups.

Step 2. Administer treatments to the respective groups.

Step 3. Each animal (e.g., mice) is positioned in the field's center following treatment with the vehicle, the drug diazepam (2 mg/kg, i.p.), or the test agent. Then, for 180 sec at 0, 30, 60, 90, and 120 min, the number of squares crossed is counted. Using the following formula, where "MST" stands for mean squares traveled, and "% inhibition" is calculated:

$$\%\text{Inhibition} = (\text{MST}_{\text{Control}} - \text{MST}_{\text{Test}}) \div \text{MST}_{\text{Control}} \times 100$$

Step 4. Similarly, also count the number of grooming (e.g., licking, scratching, and nibbling) and rearing (maintaining physiological stasis, comfort, and appearance through maintenance behavior) of each animal.

However, *'Rearing test'* can be performed individually. For this, take a 1000 mL glass beaker lined with white paper on its bottom to evaluate this exploratory behavior. Count the upward movements of the animals in the beaker for 20 minutes (Turner 1965).

Hole Cross Test

According to Takagi et al. (1971):

Step 1. Randomly distribute the required number of animals into the required number of groups.

Step 2. Administer treatments to the respective groups.

Step 3. The experiment is carried out by using a cross box with holes that measures 30 × 20 × 14 cm^3. The box is split into 2 compartments by a fixed divider in the middle. To allow animals (such as mice) to slip through the barrier easily, there is a 3 cm opening. Animals are administered a vehicle, diazepam, or test sample and are then immediately placed next to the wall of one compartment with their backs to the hole. Then, for a period of three minutes at 0, 30, 60, 90, and 120 min, the number of movements from one compartment to another via the opening is counted. The number of motions is used to compute %inhibition.

Sodium Thiopental-Induced Sleeping Time Test

According to Ferrini et al. (1974):

Step 1. Randomly distribute the required number of animals into the required number of groups.

Step 2. Administer treatments to the respective groups.

Step 3. Each animal is given sodium thiopental (40 mg/kg, i.p.) to put them to sleep 0.5 h after receiving the treatments before being placed in an observation chamber.

Step 4. Once the righting reflex has been lost, record the latent period and the amount of time that has passed while sleeping between the loss and recovery of the reflex.

Diazepam-Induced Sleeping Time Test

According to Rakotonirina et al. (2001):

Step 1. Randomly divide the animals (e.g., mice or rats) into test and control groups, having 5-6 animals in each.

Step 2. The control group receives the vehicle (10 mL/kg, p.o.). Test groups receive test samples (different doses, p.o.). Other groups receive flumazenil (1 mg/kg, p.o.) only and flumazenil with your test sample (one effective dose or all). Administer flumazenil 15 min before the administration of your test sample in the latter group.

Step 3. Administer diazepam (3 mg/kg, p.o.) 30 min after administration of all the above-mentioned treatments.

Step 4. Measure the time between the loss of the straightening reflex and the regain of this reflex as the sleep time.

N.B. – 7-8 days old chicks can be used for this purpose. You can apply both sodium thiopental and diazepam models in chicks (Warnick et al. 2009).

Elevated Plus Maze (EPM) Test

This test is used to determine whether test samples have any calming effects. Two open arms (50 × 10 cm) and two enclosed arms (50 × 10 × 40 cm) make up the maze. The arms are placed in such a way that each type is opposed to the other and is lifted to a height of 50 cm above the floor. The experiment was conducted in a silent, remote location (Pellow et al. 1985).

Step 1. 0.5 h before the experiment, the control or test sample is administered.

Step 2. Each animal (such as a mouse) should be placed separately in the maze's center, facing a closed arm. Four paw entries into an arm are considered arm entries.

Step 3. Count the following metrics during the course of a 5-min observation period: (a) the number of entries; and (b) the time spent in closed and open arms. Each animal's proportion of time with an open arm is computed as follows:

$$\%\text{Time spent in open arm} = \text{Time}_{\text{Open arm}} \div (\text{Time}_{\text{Open arm}} + \text{Time}_{\text{Closed arm}}) \times 100$$

$$\%\text{Time spent in closed arm} = \text{Time}_{\text{Closed arm}} \div (\text{Time}_{\text{Open arm}} + \text{Time}_{\text{Closed arm}}) \times 100$$

%Open arm entries = (Number of entries$_{\text{Open arm}}$ ÷ Total number of entries) × 100

Elevated Zero Maze (EZM) Test

It is a modification of the formerly described EPM model of anxiety test in animals (e.g., mice, rats). The apparatus consists of an elevated (50 cm above the floor) circular platform (6 cm in width and 40 cm in inner diameter) that is equally divided into four quadrants. Two quadrants on opposite sides of the platform are enclosed by 12 cm high walls, while the other two quadrants are open and bordered by a 0.6 cm high lip. As a result, any ambiguity in the interpretation of the time spent in the traditional design's central square (elevated plus maze) is removed, allowing for uninterrupted exploration.

Place each animal at the center of the open arm (facing toward the closed chamber) after dividing the animals and giving respective treatments. Record the times spent in both the open and closed arms of the maze. Thoroughly clean the maze between tests with a tissue paper moistened with 70% ethanol (Yahaya et al. 2014).

Y-Maze Model

According to Heo et al. (2009):

This model is used to measure immediate spatial working or short-term memory in experimental animals (e.g., mice, rats). It consists of a three-arm horizontal maze (40 cm long and 5 cm wide with walls 10 cm high) in which the three arms are symmetrically separated at 120°.

After dividing the animals and giving respective treatments, place the animals initially within one arm (A), and the arm entry sequence (e.g., ABC CAB, where letters indicate arm codes) and record the number of arm entries manually for each animal over a 5/6-min period. Clean the maze arms with 70% ethanol between tasks to remove residual odors. Determine the alternation of successive entries into the three arms of overlapping triplet sets in which three different arms are entered. An actual alternation is defined as entries into all three arms consecutively (i.e., ABC, CAB, or BCA but not BAB). An entry is defined as placing all four paws within the boundaries of the arm. Determine the percentage alternation for each animal as the ratio of actual to possible alternations (defined as the total number of arm entries minus 2), multiplied by 100, as shown by the following equation:

$\%$Alternation = (Number of alternations $\div$ Total arm entries-2) $\times$ 100

Swing Test

According to Islam et al. (2014):

Step 1. Randomly distribute the required number of animals into the required number of groups.

Step 2. Administer treatments to the respective groups.

Step 3. After 30 min, place each animal (e.g., mouse) immediately in the center of the swing box and observe the spontaneous movement of the animal from one side to another for 5 min.

Step 4. After each test, clean the floor of the swing box with 70% ethanol and dry. Compared the average number of swings of the test group with the control groups. Vehicles and diazepam can be used as control and positive control, respectively.

Amphetamine-Induced Stereotyped Behavior Study

According to Ayoka et al. (2006):

Step 1. Prior to the experiment, give the animals (such as mice) a maximum of 0.5 h to become acclimated to the observation cage. An unbiased observer scores amphetamine-induced stereotypy every 5 min for 0.5 h. Stereotypy scoring: 0 (normal behavior), 1 (intermittent sniffing), 2 (constant sniffing), 3 (constant sniffing with intermittent licking and/or false biting), 4 (constant or false licking), 5 (constant licking), 6 (constant biting and moving around), 7 (constant biting and restricted to a small area in the cage) and 8 (rearing).

Step 2. Group the animals into the necessary groups, with the necessary number of animals in each group. They are placed individually in the cage and given either the control sample (10 mL/kg, i.p.) or the test sample (various doses). 0.5 h following the administration of your test drug, inject amphetamine (1 mg/kg, i.p.). Note the stereotypical actions.

Haloperidol-Induced Catalepsy Test

According to Ferre et al. (1990):

Step 1. After grouping, administer control (vehicle: 10 mL/kg, i.p.) or test sample (specified doses, i.p.) to the experimental animals (e.g., mice, n = required number in each group).

Step 2. Treat the animals with haloperidol (1 mg/kg, i.p.) after 0.5 h and then use the Bar test to determine how long the animals were in catalepsy (a medical issue characterized by a state or seizure with a lack of sensibility and awareness coupled with stiffness of the body).

Step 3. The animal's forepaws are placed on a horizontal bar that is 3 cm off the ground, and the time it takes to remove them is measured as the length of the catalepsy. In every experiment, the treatment of the animals is concealed from the spectator. The animals are returned to their home cages after each experiment.

Metoclopramide-Induced Catalepsy Test

According to Muruganandam et al. (2000):

In this study, metoclopramide (20 mg/kg, i.p.) is administered to animals (e.g., mice, n = required number in each group) pre-treated with control (vehicle: 10 mL/kg, i.p.) or test sample (specified doses, i.p.) and measures the duration of catalepsy as in the above-mentioned study.

Foot Shock-Induced Aggression Test

According to Kastur (2006):

Step 1. Pairs of animals (such as mice) are subjected to a series of impulses delivered through an electronic stimulator to a grid floor for three minutes in order to provoke foot shock-induced aggression (FSIA) behavior. Divide the animals into the necessary number of groups, with the necessary number of animals in each group, for this.

Step 2. Give the test sample (specified dosages, i.p.), haloperidol (1 mg/kg, i.p.) as a reference, and vehicle (10 mL/kg, i.p.) 0.5 h before the experiment.

Step 3. Count the number of fights and latency of each pair of animals to observe aggressive behavior.

Acetylcholinesterase Enzyme Inhibitory Test

According to Falé et al. (2009):

Step 1. Mix 90 μL (50 mM/L) Tris-HCl buffer (pH 8.30) with 7.5 μL of acetylcholinesterase solution containing 0.26 U/mL in a microwell plate. Incubate the mixture for 15 min.

Step 2. Add 22.5 μL of AHCI (0.023 mg/mL) and 142 μL of 3 mM/L 5,5′-dithiobis(2-nitrobenzoic acid) to the mixture.

Step 3. When the reaction has reached equilibrium, check the absorbance at 405 nm. When water is used as the test sample in the control reaction, it is deemed to have 100% activity.

$$\%IP = 100 - (A_1/A_0) \times 100$$

where, A_1 and A_0 are the absorbance of the test sample and vehicle, respectively. IP is the %inhibition. Tests are run in triplicate, and an enzyme solution-free blank is utilized in place of the real thing. As examined materials are dissolved in this organic solvent, methanol, a blank is run using the standards.

GABAergic Activity Assay

According to Jakoby (1962):

Step 1. Mix PPB (150 mM, pH 8.0) with α-ketoglutarate (228.5 mM), GABA (873 mM) and GABAse (1.5-1.7 units/mg).

Step 2. Add the test sample to the reaction mixture and conduct a 0.5-h pre-incubation at 37 °C.

Step 3. Add $NADP^+$ (26.1 mM) to the reaction mixture. Then incubate (0.5-1 h at 37 °C). By monitoring the variations in absorbance at 340 nm brought on by the lowering of $NADP^+$, GABA-T activity was monitored. With the use of a microplate spectrophotometer, the absorbance is calculated. Utilize vigabatrin, a GABA-T inhibitor, as the positive control.

Use water as the negative control instead of the inhibitor.

Anti-Dopaminergic Activity Assay

According to Goyal (2003):

Step 1. Adult male animals (e.g., rats) can be sacrificed by cervical dislocation, with the vas deferens removed and the body kept in Krebs-Henseleit solution.

Step 2. On the Sherrigton rotating drum, note the concentration-related contraction response (CRC) to dopamine (10-160 μg/mL) (INCO, Ambala, India).

Step 3. In the context of the test sample, the repeat concentration-related contraction response to dopamine (0.5 mL of the specified concentration). Keep the dopamine's contact time with the tissue at 1 min.

Traction Model (Muscular Relaxant Test)

An iron rod of 1 m is used in this test. Animals (e.g., mice) are trained to make them able to walk on an iron rod. After 30 - 40 min of your test sample or control administration, subject the animals to the plat form of the rod and note an increase or decrease in time for 10 min.

You can use chlorpromazine (10 mg/kg, i.p.) as a reference drug for this purpose. You should place the forepaws of each animal on a small twisted wire rigidly supported above a bench top. A normal animal grasps the wire with its forepaws and, when it is allowed to hang free, it places at least one hind foot on the wire within 5 seconds. Consider the inability to place at least one hind foot to be a traction failure (Turner 1965; Rudzik et al. 1973).

Passive Avoidance Response (PAR) Model

According to Dilts and Berry (1967):

PAR is used to evaluate the learning and memory capacity of animals after receiving treatments. In this case, you should train the animals (e.g., rodents) to avoid punishment (normally an electric shock) by curbing a normal behavior (such as exploratory behavior). At specified intervals after training, test the animals again for retention of such learning. The study chamber consists of the following length×diameter×height: 34 × 34 × 20 cm. It also contains a metal floor that has an electric shock capacity of 20 mV whenever any animal gets in contact. A shock-free zone (SFZ) is provided in the center of the chamber by placing an inverted Petri dish.

After randomly distributing and treating, each animal is initially placed on the SFZ and observes the following parameters for a specified time:

- Latency of step down (how long the animal stayed in SFZ).

- Error of step down (number of attempts made by the animal to go to the shock zone).
- Time spent (total) in the shock zone.

Moreover, you can perform the Lim test (evaluation of loss of spontaneous movements, muscular tone, and righting reflex). Use the Varimex test to see the locomotor activity of the animals after receiving your test and control groups (Tyler et al. 1979). Additionally, a laser light projection test can be done to check the anti-depression, sedative/hypnotic, and anxiolytic behaviors of your test sample in mice or rats.

Cardio-Protective and Cardiological Activity Studies

Our lives are now threatened on a global scale by cardiovascular disorders. It now accounts for 17.1 million fatalities annually. It's anticipated that there will be over 30 million deaths from cardiac illnesses in 2030. To date, many important natural products have been introduced for cardiovascular diseases. Some are still in use, even after knowing the fact that these compounds have potential side effects on the heart. At present, medicinal scientists use some methods to investigate the cardiological effects of test samples. Some popularly used methods include:

Rat Model

According to Tesfaye et al. (2021):

Step 1. Collect the required number of rats and randomly distribute them into different specified groups (required animals in each group).

Step 2. Select the test doses and prepare your test sample in a suitable vehicle.

Step 3. Treat the animals for a specified time and then give them a suitable cardiotoxic drug (e.g., cyclophosphamide 200 mg/kg, i.p.). For activity comparison, you should take a positive control (e.g., EN 10 mg/kg, daily p.o. for the same specified time, then treat with cardiotoxic drug similarly), a negative control (treat only with the vehicle similarly but except for the infliction of cardiac injury), and a normal control (vehicle with cardiotoxic drug similarly). Treat the animals with test sample/controls based on each day's measured weight.

Step 4. After the specified time, collect blood from the retro-orbital plexus of the animals into heparinized tubes post-ketamine 100 mg/kg (i.p.) treatment. Centrifuge blood samples at 3500×*g* for 15 min to get the plasma. Collect the clear supernatant and estimate different cardiac biomarkers such as troponin I, AST, ALT, and lipid (e.g., cholesterol and triglycerides) profiles.

Step 5. Dislocate the animals' cervical spines to sacrifice them. Cut a transabdominal incision into the thoracic cavity that is visible after the diaphragm. Following cartilage connection to the ribs, the thorax is sliced open on both sides, exposing the heart, which should be gently elevated in the fingertips to prevent contusion injury. Place the heart into a beaker with a standard saline 0.9% solution as soon as the heart has been removed for washing purposes. After cleaning, dry the heart by placing it on a piece of filter paper, then weigh it to determine the relative weight of the heart in relation to the body. Place the heart in a container with 10% formalin (fixation) and place it in the freezer (- 80 °C) until you are ready to conduct another experiment.

Step 6. An automatic processing device can be used to take a sample of heart tissue, dehydrate it in various concentrations of ethanol (such as 40, 70, 80, 95, and 100%), and then clear it with xylene. Additionally, use an automated tissue processing machine to clear xylene with paraffin wax. Block the tissues in the coronal plane after embedding them in paraffin wax. Utilizing a microtome, tissue sections of 4 - 5 μm in thickness were created, which were then stained with hematoxylin and eosin dye to reveal histological alterations.

Isoproterenol-Induced Myocardial Infarction Model

According to Zafar et al. (2015):

Step 1. Prepare your test drug and animals (e.g., rats) similarly as mentioned in the previous study. You can follow the below-mentioned grouping for this purpose.

- Group I (normal control): receive isosaline for 7 days.
- Group II (toxic control): receive a toxic substance at a specified dose for a specified posttreatment period of 2 consecutive days.
- Group III (standard): receive standard drug at a specified dose for 7 days and subject to toxicant posttreatment period for 2 days.

- Group IV (test sample): receive a single or two consecutive doses for 7 days and be subject to a toxicant posttreatment period for 2 days.
- Group V (test sample + standard): you will receive a high dose of your test sample and standard drug for 7 days and be subject to a toxicant posttreatment period for 2 days.

Step 2. Animals are anesthetized with ketamine (70 mg/kg, i.p.) and xylazine (10 mg/kg, i.p.) 2 days after receiving their initial toxicant dosage, and blood is then removed through retro-orbital puncture.

Step 3. Centrifuge sera to separate it for biomarker estimates and lipid profile analysis. To record an ECG, use Pb (II). Animals are put to death by CO_2 asphyxiation. Half of the hearts are used to prepare a homogenate to calculate antioxidant levels, and the other half are embedded in formalin (10%) for histological analysis.

Step 4. Evaluate the following parameters to see the cardiological effects of your test sample in comparison to the control groups: LDH, CK-MB, CK-NAC, ALT, AST, TC, TG, SOD, and CAT, etc.

Ischemia-Reperfusion Injury (Modified Langendorff Setup) Model

According to Zafar et al. (2015):

Step 1. Prepare your test drug and animals (e.g., rats) similarly as mentioned in the previous study. You can follow the below-mentioned grouping for this purpose.

- Group I (normal control): receive physiological saline for 7 days, subject to IRI posttreatment.
- Group II (standard drug): receive standard drug at a specified dose for 7 days and subject to IRI posttreatment.
- Group III (test sample): receive a single or two consecutive doses for 7 days and subject to IRI posttreatment.
- Group IV (test sample + standard): receive a high dose of your test sample and standard drug for 7 days and be subject to IRI posttreatment.

Step 2. Anesthetize the animals similarly, remove their hearts quickly and mount them on an updated Langendorff apparatus through the aorta.

0.5 h before inducing anesthesia, heparinize the animals with 100 IU of heparin. Using a controlled perfusion pump, begin retrograde perfusion at a flow rate of 5.5 mL/min with modified Krebs-Henseleit (KH) buffer solution (pH 7.4) bubbled with carbogen (95% O_2 + 5% CO_2).

Step 3. During routine recordings, include a 10 min equilibration and a 15 min perfusion period. With the aid of a force-displacement transducer, determine the contractile force. Block the flow of KH solution and carbogen supply after 15 min of reperfusion to cause a 15-min period of global no-flow ischemia after the initial pre-ischemic perfusion. Calculate the post-ischemic period and recovery (%) by measuring the heart rate and stress that formed during the pre-ischemic period. Calculate the diagnostic marker enzymes in perfusate collected during the post-ischemic period. Take the heart out, weigh the individual, and prepare the heart tissue homogenate (HTH) or do a histological analysis. Record the answers on graph paper using a force transducer attached to a physiograph that has been previously calibrated and has a resting tension of 2 g. Set the transducer's highest sensitivity, or 0.1 mV, and the paper speed to a minimum of 0.05 mm/sec.

Step 4. Evaluate different cardiological parameters as mentioned above.

Step 5. Anesthetize the animals using a mixture of ketamine (70 mg/kg, i.p.) and xylazine (10 mg/kg, i.p.) at the conclusion of the procedure. For recording, use a digital physiograph. Assess heart rate, QRS, QT, PR, and RR intervals by attaching leads to each of the four limbs in the dermal layer.

Step 6. Perform histopathological analysis of the hearts as mentioned above.

Rabbit Model

According to Zafar et al. (2015):

Step 1. Collect male albino rabbits (avg. b.w., 1 - 1.5 kg) for this study. Manage them in a standard environment and randomly divide them into different groups with a specified number of rabbits in each.

Step 2. Prepare your test sample. You can follow the following grouping technique:

- Group I (normal control): give only standard diet.
- Group II (toxic control group): give toxicant (e.g., salbutamol at 60 mg/kg) for 2 successive days to induce oxidative stress/myocardial cell necrosis.

- Group III (test group): receive your test sample in a single or two successive doses once daily for 3 weeks.
- Group IV (preventive group): receive pretreated test sample once daily for 3 weeks and then treat with toxicant orally.
- Group V (curative groups): treat the animals with a toxicant for two days to induce cardiotoxicity. Then treat them with a test sample once daily for 5 days.
- Group VI (standard: curative group): treat the animals orally with toxicants for 2 days to induce cardiotoxicity. Then treat with a standard drug (e.g., norvasc, capoten) once daily for five days.

Step 3. Collect blood samples from the jugular veins of animals. Separate the serum and analyze cardiac biomarkers. Also, separate the cardiac tissues after surgery and wash with isosaline. Homogenize the heart tissues in 10% ice cold PBS (pH 7.0). Centrifuge the mixture and use the supernatant to analyze SOD, CAT, and GPx levels.

Anti-Hypertensive Test

In Vitro Assay

ACE and HLL Treatment Assay

According to Mao et al. (2015):

Step 1. Mix 50 μL of test solution with 200 μL of PBS (100 mM, pH 8.3) containing 0.2 M NaCl and 6.5 mM hippuryl-histidyl-leucine (HHL).

Step 2. Add 100 μL ACE solutions (0.1 U/mL) to start the reaction and incubate the mixture at 37 °C for 0.5 h.

Step 3. Add 50 μL of 1 M HCl for stopping the reaction. This will cleave the Gly-His bond of HHL and produce a Bz-Gly (hippuric acid) bond. Then extract it with 1.5 mL of ethyl acetate.

Step 4. Collect the ethyl acetate supernatant after centrifuging at 1200×*g* for 15 min. Remove the solvent by heat evaporation in a water bath. Dissolve the product in 3 mL of distilled water and measure the absorbance at 228 nm using a spectrophotometer. To calculate the inhibition activity, use the following equation:

$$\%Inhibition = [(A_a - A_b) \div (A_a - A_c)] \times 100$$

where, A_a is the absorbance with ACE and HHL without the sample (positive control, no inhibition, and maximum activity); A_b is the absorbance with ACE, HHL, and the sample or standard; and A_c is the absorbance with HHL without ACE and the sample (control).

Ex Vivo Assay

Aorta Ring Tie Model

According to Mao et al. (2015):

Step 1. Tie 4-5 mm-diameter rings of isolated thoracic aorta to stainless steel hooks.

Step 2. Immerse into organ baths containing 10 mL Krebs solution at 37°C.

Step 3. Oxygenate (with O_2:CO_2 at 95:5.2 g weight) all tissues for the creation of basal tension and record the changes in basal tension.

Step 4. Maximize the contraction of each prepared aorta by administering KCl (120 mM) and keeping a record.

Step 5. Pre-incubate the tissues with your test sample. Express the relaxation as a %change from the KCl contracted levels.

In Vivo Studies

Model 1 *(Salt-Induced Hypertension Model)*

According to Mao et al. (2015):

Step 1. Divide the normotensive animals (e.g., rats) into different groups with the required number of animals in each group.

Step 2. Gr-I receives vehicle and serves as normotensive group. Gr-II receives an 18% NaCl salt solution at a 10 mL/kg dose per day for 4 weeks (10.00 to 11.00 AM). Gr-III group receives saline and captopril at 10 mg/kg per day for 4 weeks. The last group (Gr-IV) receives a salt solution with your test sample per day for 4 weeks. Give all the treatments orally.

Step 3. Measure SBP/DBP as mentioned below by using a tail cuff machine.

Model 2 (BP, ACE and Renin Assay Model)
According to Junh et al. (2018):

Step 1. Collect the required number of male animals (e.g., rats) and randomly divide them into 3 groups: Gr-I for vehicle; Gr-II for captopril 100 (reference drug); and Gr-III for your test drug. Give the treatment daily for 4 weeks.

Step 2. Measure systolic and diastolic blood pressures using invasive and non-invasive methods before and after your test drug administration.

Step 3. Measure SBP/DBP once weekly using a computerized tail-cuff plethysmograph (non-invasive approach).

Step 4. Measure SBP/DBP at the end of the 4th week using MP36 (invasive approach) after carotid artery cannulation with PE20 tubes. Take 6 measurements and calculate the mean value for each animal.

Step 5. Anesthetize the animals with pentobarbital sodium. Then collect blood samples in a vacutainer tube containing clot activator from the inferior vena cava. Maintain the samples at an ambient temperature for 15 to 20 min and centrifuge at 3000×*g* for 10 min for serum collection. Use the aliquot and analyze the concentration of Angiotensin I-Converting Enzyme (ACE) and renin using ELISA kits. Express the value in ng/mL.

Hepatoprotective Activity Tests

Table 9.3. Merits and demerits of toxicity study strategies

Model	Examples	Merits	Demerits
In vitro	Fresh or primary hepatocyte culture	Rapid and economic	Complexity in result interpretation
	Cell lines (immortalized)	Small sample size	Do not allow biotransformation processes
		Larger control variables; reproducible	
		Possible to analyze diverse samples in the same test	
Ex vivo	Precise liver cuts	Resemble the *in vivo* environment	Low oxygenation rates in the internal cells
	Isolated perfused liver	Requires a few animals	Low cut viability (1-10 dias)
		Human tissue model can be developed	Significant differences in size and function between human and murine tissue

In vivo	Murine model	Widely used	Requires large number of animals
		Greater correlation with the humans	Exist species variations
		Allow to see biochemical and histological changes	Larger sample size
			Expensive and time-consuming

Different Strategies

One of the major consequences worldwide is diseases in our hepatic system. Medicinal scientists are in a continuous search for new molecules, especially from natural origins, to counteract and prevent hepatic problems. According to the WHO, liver disease results in 2.4 million deaths each year. The liver is a key organ. As a result, if there is a problem with it, it may affect other parts of our body. We know that the liver regulates many important functions in our body, including the metabolism of food materials and drugs or chemicals, the secretion of metabolites and wastages, the storage of nutrients and drug molecules, and detoxifying toxins that are harmful to us. Thus, damage to our liver will affect all these biochemical processes.

Unfortunately, our lives face a vast amount of toxins each day. It receives these toxins from the portal vein through the blood supply after intestinal functioning (e.g., absorption and secretion). We do check both, i.e., effects of toxins on the liver as well as hepatoprotective effects of drugs and chemicals, by using a number of non-clinical and preclinical (*in vitro*, *ex vivo,* and *in vivo*) strategies utilizing experimental animals or their derivatives (e.g., cells, tissues). Natural products, especially plants or their extracts or isolated compounds, are also evaluated for their toxicity or protective properties by using these models. Table 9.3 presents the merits and demerits of toxicity study strategies.

In Vitro Strategies

Hepatoprotective effects of drugs or chemicals or natural products are checked by using fresh hepatocytes, primary hepatocytes (cultures) and immortalized cell lines. You can draw a possible mechanism of action for a drug candidate by using these test systems. This gives a potential window for preliminary screening of a wide variety of test substances as well as establishing molecular interactions at a cellular level. It is due to fresh or primary hepatocytes retaining and maintaining normal liver functions that it is possible to maintain them over a time period. There are a number of cultural media available for this purpose. Additionally, it is also possible to evaluate some essential parameters such as protection capacity, transaminase activity, cell morphology and multiplication, macromolecular synthesis profile, oxygen consumption rate and extent, etc.

Ex Vivo Strategies

You can use precision cut liver slices for this purpose. In a suitable culture medium it is able to maintain cumulative hepatic characteristics like a whole *in vivo* organ. It is more precise for the study of liver morphology upon the treatments. As it retains functionally active metabolizing enzyme systems and biliary canaliculus supply it can be also used to study drug metabolism profile, liver functioning, biliary functions, hemodynamic parameters, and interaction between real organ function and *in vitro* and *ex vivo* test modalities using hepatocytes. In short, this model can give an *in vivo* outlook in a laboratory environment. Livers from pork, rats, mice and rabbits are frequently used for this purpose.

In Vivo Strategies

Currently, medicinal scientists are frequently using *in vivo* models. A number of experimental animals, such as pigs, rats, mice, and rabbits, are commonly used for this purpose. It is because these models provide a greater extent of relevance to human liver functions. By using these *in vivo* models, you can investigate the effects of many substances on the human liver. Therefore, these models are capable of sharing data directly with the clinical programs of a drug candidate. For this purpose, you can determine the magnitude of liver damage and/or protection, hepatic biomarkers along with the histopathological profile after giving a treatment to your laboratory animals. Ethanol, CCl_4, thioacetamide, acetaminophen, tert-butyl hydroperoxide, D-galactosamine, etc. are frequently used hepatoxicants in laboratory animals for this approach. All these substances cause characteristic hepatic damage in laboratory animals. Transaminases or aminotransferases, phosphatases, transpeptidase-glutamine, bilirubin, total proteins, lactato deshydrogenase, hepatic antioxidants, and other hepatic function biomarkers can all be tested.

Examples of some widely used methods include:

Cell Viability Assay (In Vitro)

According to González et al. (2017):

Step 1. Collect the necessary cells (such as HepG2), maintain and grow them under the prescribed conditions (added DMEMA at 37 °C in a humidified 5% CO_2 atmosphere, for example). Depending on the result, trypsinize the cells at 80-90% confluence and maintain 30,000 cells per well in a 96-well microplate, 1×10^6 cells per well in 6 plates, or 5×10^7 cells per well in a single dish. You should use these cells after attachment.

Step 2. You can perform CCl_4-induced toxicity in these cells. For all this, incubate the cells in the medium or treat them for 1, 1.5, 2, or 180 min with the toxic agent (20, 30, or 40 mM CCl_4 in 0.05% DMSO).

Step 3. You can also perform APAP-induced toxicity on these cells. For this, treat the cells with the toxic agent (2, 4, or 8 mM APAP) or incubate with medium only for 12, 24, 48, or 72 h.

Step 4. The cytotoxic effect can be measured in these cells by exposing your test sample for 12 h to a specified concentration in supplemented culture medium (e.g., DMEMA). Use cells in freshly prepared medium only as a negative control.

Step 5. The normal control cells should be incubated with DMEMA in DMSO (0.05% v/v) for 12 h. Toxic group: Incubate cells with DMEMA in DMSO (0.05% v/v) for 12 h, followed by 1.5 h of treatment with DMEMA in 40 mM CCl_4. Similar action should be taken for the other toxic agent and your test sample. Triplicate the experiment.

Step 6. Only live cells have mitochondrial succinate dehydrogenase, which transforms the medium into a purple formazan derivative when a conversion to MTT takes place. After removing the media and giving the cells MTT (0.5 mg/mL) for 120 min, the formazan crystals should be dissolved in 200 μL of DMSO per well.

Step 7. Measure the absorbance at 570 nm. Viability is defined as the percentage difference between the absorbance of treated and control cells. Calculate the IC_{50} values using regression analysis.

Step 8. Measure AST, ALT, LDH, TAOxC, GSH, SOD, and MDA levels with automatic instruments. In order to do this, withdraw the supernatant from the wells and take an instantaneous enzyme activity reading. Summarize the findings in IU/L.

CCL_4-Induced Hepatoxic Mouse Model

According to Meharie et al. (2020):

Step 1. Randomly divide 3-4 h fasted (only free accessed to water) laboratory animals (e.g., mice) into negative control, positive control, toxicant control, and test sample group(s) consisting of specified number of animals in each group.

Step 2. Treat the negative control with the vehicles used for reconstitution of your test drug 1 mL/kg orally for 6 days. CCl_4 (50% dissolved in liquid paraffin in 1:1, 2 mL/kg, i.p.) is administered to the positive control on day 4 in addition to the reference drug silymarin (100 mg/kg) for 6 days. On day 4, toxicant controls receive CCl_4 (2 mL/kg, i.p.) and then the vehicle. For 6 days, deliver your test sample in the same manner (with varied doses as needed). On day 4, administer CCl_4 (2 mL/kg i.p.) to all test groups.

Step 3. On day 7, take b.w. of the animals before sacrificing them while lightly sedated with ether. Centrifuge the blood sample at 3000×*g* for 10 min after heparinizing it with a heart puncture. Measure the amounts of albumin, total protein, total bilirubin, and liver indicators like ALT, AST, and ALP after collecting clear serum. Each mouse's liver should be removed, weighed, and checked for microscopic and gross pathology.

Step 4. Use the below-mentioned formula to determine the hepatoprotectivity of your test sample as %protection:

$$\%\text{Protection} = [(a - b) \div (a - c)] \times 100$$

where, **a**, **b** and **c** are the mean values of the markers observed in hepatotoxin, toxin plus your test sample, and the vehicle group, respectively.

Step 5. Perform histopathological analysis of the liver tissue mentioned in many of the models above.

N.B. - This study can also be conducted by using rats and chicks. Treatment days and doses of standard and CCl_4 can be varied from model to model (Nipanikar et al. 2017; Tokofai et al. 2021).

Paracetamol-Induced Hepatotoxicity (Mouse Model)

According to Kiran et al. (2012):

Step 1. After acclimation, randomly distribute your test animals (e.g., rats) into various groups (required number of animals per group) and orally treat them for a week.

Step 2. Group I acts as a normal control group and receives 1% Na-CMC (sodium carboxymethyl cellulose) at 1 mL/kg, while Group II acts as paracetamol control group and receives paracetamol (1 g/kg). Group III receives silymarin (50 mg/kg) plus paracetamol, and Group IV receives your test sample plus paracetamol. However, you can use different doses for your test sample.

Step 3. Collect blood samples from each animal's retro-orbital plexus 1 day after the last treatment, let them clot for 60 min at ambient temperature, and then separate the serum by centrifuging at 2500×*g* for 15 min at 30 °C. Serum should be collected, and it should be examined for a number of biochemical factors, including SGOT/AST, SGPT/ALT, ALP, TB total protein (TP), serum transaminase activity, serum bilirubin, and others.

Step 4. Perform histopathological analysis of the liver tissue mentioned in many of the models above.

N.B. - This study can also be conducted by using rats. Treatment days and doses of standard and paracetamol can be varied from model to model. Additionally, you can measure MDA, GSH, SOD, CAT, etc. levels in the liver tissue of the animals (Hanafy et al. 2016).

Lead-Induced Hepatotoxicity Test in Chick Model

According to Kodama et al. (1986), Sadasivudu et al. (1977) and Kumar et al. (2011):

Step 1. Collect one-day aged male chicks for this study and randomly group into normal control, negative control, positive control and test sample, respectively taking 5-6 birds in each group. Provide standard feed and water *ad libitum* throughout the experiment. Diet can be maintained with the daily treatment with/without the controls and test sample. Except the normal control keep other groups' birds on lead for 6 and 4 weeks, respectively.

Step 2. Draw blood samples from the wing vein at the end of 4th and 6th weeks for the assay of ALT. After 6th week, sacrifice the birds and collect the livers. Prepare liver sample as follows: cut liver into small pieces in cold conditions by using pre-cooled petri dishes and blot free of blood and tissue fluid. Take weight and cross-chop the pieces with surgical scalpel into fine slices, chill in ice-cold 0.25 M sucrose and then blot on a filter paper. The tissues are minced and homogenized in 10 mM Tris-HCl buffer (pH 7.4) at a concentration of 10% w/v with 25 strokes of tight Teflon homogenizer at a speed of 2500×*g*. The prolonged homogenization under hypotonic condition disrupts the ventricular structure of cells so as to release soluble proteins and leave membrane and non-vascular matter in sediment form. Centrifuge the homogenates at 10,000×*g* at 4 °C for 20 min. Re-centrifuge the supernatant for 1 h at 100,000×*g* at 4 °C using high-speed cooling centrifuge. Re-suspend the sediment in Tris-HCl buffer (pH 7.4) to get the final concentration of 10% and use for the assay of membrane-bound enzymes.

Step 3. Determine total ATPase and Mg^{2+}ATPase activities as follows:

2 mL of the assay mixture for the total ATPase contains 320 μM of Tris-HC1 buffer (pH 7.4), 10 μM of $MgC1_2$, 300 μM of NaCI, 40 μM of KC1, and 6 μM of ATP. In the assay mixture for Mg^{2+}-ATPase, sodium and potassium chlorides are replaced with equal volumes of distilled water. The 5% homogenate is pre-incubated at 37 °C for 20 min, and 0.1 mL of this is added to the assay mixture to initiate the reaction. After 20 min of incubation at 37 °C the reaction is terminated with 0.5 mL of 22.5% trichloroacetic acid and centrifuged. Inorganic phosphate (Pi) is estimated in a 1.0-mL portion of the supernatant. The activity of Na^+K^+ATPase is calculated as the difference between total and Mg^{2+}- ATPases, express as/ μM of Pi liberated per g wet weight of tissue per h.

Ca^{2+}ATPase activity can be determined as follows:

1 mL of reaction medium is quickly mixed with 1 mL of ice-chilled 0.6 M perchloric acid (PCA) and centrifuge at 1,700×*g* for 1 min. An aliquot of the supernatant, usually 1 mL, is incubated in a water-bath at 25 °C for 35 min after mixing with an equal volume of the Malachite Green reagent, and the absorbance is measured at 650 nm in a Hitachi 100-50 or a Gilford 503 spectrophotometer with cuvettes of 1 cm light path. The incubation period is kept constant for all samples and standards. To do so, the Malachite Green reagent is added to the supernatant at regular intervals and the absorbance is measured accordingly. In addition, a water-bath is placed by the side of a spectrophotometer so that the absorbance can be measured immediately after incubation.

Step 4. For CYP assay, remove the livers rapidly, take weight and perfuse with ice-cold 1.15% KCl solution containing 0.05 M EDTA. Homogenize each of the perfused livers with two volumes of ice-cold 0.25 M sucrose in the homogenizer. Centrifuge the homogenate at 10,000×*g* for 0.5 h in a refrigerated centrifuge. Collect the microsomes as above and wash the pellets once with 1.15% KCl solution containing 0.05 mM EDTA, re-suspend in PBS (pH 7.4) and use this suspension for microsomal enzyme assays.

Step 5. Estimate total protein by using Lowry method. For this, treat the microsomal suspension in PBS (1.0 mg protein/mL) with a few grains of sodium dithionate and taken in the reference and sample cuvettes and record the baseline from 400 to 510 nm. Transfer the contents of the sample cuvette into a tube and bubble gently with CO for 1 min. Then, transfer the contents back to the sample cuvette and record the difference in spectrum from 400 to 510 nm again. Use the difference in absorbance between 450 and 490 nm for the calculation of CYP_{450} content using the extinction coefficient difference ($\Delta E_{450\text{-}490}$ nm of 91 cm/mM).

Some Other Parameter Analysis

According to Sadasivudu et al. (1977):

Glutamine Synthetase

For this 5% homogenate (0.2 mL) is added to 0.9 mL of the assay mixture consisting of 50 µM of imidazole-HC1 buffer (pH 7.2), 20 µM of 2-mercaptoethanol, 50 µM of sodium glutamate, 100 µM of hydroxylamine, 20 µM of $MgC1_2$, and 10 µM of ATP. In the controls, glutamate is omitted. Incubations are carried out for 15 min at 37 °C and 1.5 mL of ferric chloride solution (0.37 M $FeC1_3$, 0.67 N HCI, and 0.27 M trichloroacetic acid) is added to stop the reaction. The optical density of the supernatant is measured at 535 nm, and the enzyme activity is expressed as µM of y-glutamyl hydroxamate formed/per g wet weight of tissue per h.

Aspartate and Alanine Aminotransferases

For this 5% homogenate (0.1 mL) is added to 1 mL of the substrate mixture consisting of 150 µM of PBS (pH 7.45), 200 µM of aspartate or alanine, and 20 µM of α-ketoglutarate. At the end of 15 min of incubation at 37°C 0.05 mL of aniline citrate (equal volumes of aniline and 100% citric acid are mixed freshly) is added, followed by 1 mL of 2,4-dinitrophenylhydrazine (0.02% in 0.1 N HC1). The color is developed with 10 mL of 0.4 N NaOH and is measured at 520 min. Controls receives the homogenate after the addition of aniline citrate. Enzyme activity is expressed as µM of pyruvate per g wet weight per h.

Glutamate Dehydrogenase

The assay mixture (2.5 mL) consists of 80 μM of triethanolamine buffer (pH 8.0), 13 μM of EDTA, 1 μM of NADH, 20 μM of α-ketoglutarate, and 120 μM of ammonium chloride. The reaction mixture is incubated for 5 min with 0.2 mL of 1% homogenate in the absence of α-ketoglutarate, and the reaction is started by the addition of α-ketoglutarate. Change in the absorbance is measured at 366 nm for 15 min at 3-min intervals. The enzyme activity is calculated using the molar extinction coefficient of 3.3 $cm^2/\mu M$, and express as μM of NADH oxidized per g wet weight of tissue per h.

Tyrosine Aminotransferase

The reaction mixture (1.8 mL) contains 160 μM of triethanolamine buffer (pH 7.5), 12 μM of tyrosine, 2 μM of a-ketoglutarate, 0.2 μM of pyridoxal-5-phosphate, 2 μM of EDTA, 2 μM of dithiothreotol, and 0.2 mL of 1% homogenate. The assay mixture is incubated at 37 °C for 15 min, and 0.2 mL of 10 N KOH is added to terminate the reaction. Controls receives the KOH prior to the addition of the homogenate. After 0.5 h at 37 °C the optical density is measured at 331 nm, and the enzyme activity is calculated using the extinction coefficient of 19,900 M^{-1}. The enzyme activity is expressed as μM of *p*-hydroxyphenylpyruvate formed per g wet weight of tissue per rain.

Ammonia

After separation of the brain, different regions are excised quickly and dropped into 10% trichloroacetic acid (TCA). The tissues are homogenized in ice-cold 10% TCA to get a 1% (w/v) homogenate. After centrifugation of the mixture, ammonia content is determined in 1.0 mL of the supernatant with Nessler's reagent.

Amino Acid

Immediately after decapitation, the tissues are dropped into ice-cold 80% alcohol. The tissues are weighed and homogenize in 5 mL of 80% alcohol and centrifuge at 8000×*g* at 0 °C for 20 min. The clear supernatant is evaporated to dryness at 70 - 80 °C and the residue is dissolved in 200 μl of distilled water. The amino acid content is determined by paper chromatography using butanol-acetic acid-water (65:15:25, vol.); solvent and ninhydrin (0.25% in acetone with 1% pyridine) is used to locate the amino acids. The amino acids are eluted with 3 mL of 75% alcohol (with 0.005% $CuSO_4$), and the color is measured at 515 nm. The amino acid content is expressed as μM of amino acid per g wet weight of tissue.

For *ribonucleic acid* (RNA) assay you can use 1.0 mL of the 5% homogenate by using Schneider (1957) model and for ***protein*** analysis you can follow Biuret method as described by Varley (1969).

Renal (Kidney) Protective Activity Tests

Kidneys filter extra water and waste out of blood and make urine. Many factors, including smoking, obesity, hypertension, diabetes mellitus, older age, underweight (birth), and genetic defects, can lead to renal disease. Risks include things like exposure to heavy metals, drinking too much alcohol, smoking, and taking analgesics. Additional risk factors include acute renal injury, circulatory system disease history, hyperlipidemia, metabolic syndrome, hepatitis C virus, HIV infection, and malignancy. Initial screening of kidney disease includes serum creatinine level estimation and urinalysis in patients. Additionally, some medications can cause nephrotoxicity in people, which is now known to be a major cause of kidney illness like acute renal injury and chronic kidney disease. It seems certain drugs can not only treat but also induce kidney diseases. Therefore, evaluation of the effects of drugs or drug-like substances on the kidney is also important. Some widely used methods for this purpose include:

Ischemia-Reperfusion (I/R) Induced Kidney Injury Model

According to Torres-Gonzálezb et al. (2018):

Step 1. Use vascular clamps to occlude the renal pedicle for 45 min to create ischemia, then remove the clamps and permit reperfusion to occur for 15 h to cause kidney damage. Give the animals (like rats) unlimited food and water access throughout this time. The surgical method for the control and your test groups involved a laparotomy with no obstruction. Control and sample should be given for 7 days.

Step 2. To anesthetize your laboratory animals, use xylazine: ketamin at 10:100 mg/kg (i.p.).

Step 3. After the surgery, take blood samples from each animal. To separate the serum, centrifuge at 3500×*g* for 15 min. Then, check the levels of pro-inflammatory cytokines (such as IL-6, IL-1β, and TNF-α), alanine aminotransferase (ALT), and kidney function indicators. As soon as samples of kidney tissue are taken, one portion of it should be fixed in 10%

formaldehyde for histopathological analysis, and the remaining tissue should be frozen at 80°Cagain for determination of MDA and SOD levels.

Step 4. Spectrophotometry is used to measure blood urea nitrogen (BUN), creatinine level, and ALT activity in accordance with the commercial kit supplier's guidelines.

Step 5. From the above fixed kidney sample, use only a representative sample (taken from both kidneys) from each animal in your test sample or control groups. Process and fix in paraffin. Using a microtome, slice the paraffin blocks into 4 μm-thick sections. Then, deparaffinize, hydrate, and color with hematoxylin and eosin. The sections should be examined microscopically to determine the presence of semiquantitative signs of cellular damage, including tubular necrosis and eosinophilic casts. The following scoring systems can be used to evaluate renal histopathology: 0 (no damage or intact), 1 (mild damage), 2 (moderate damage, damage <25%), 3 (severe damage, damage 25–50%) and 4 (severe damage, >50% damage).

Gentamicin-Induced Nephrotoxicity Model

According to Kumar et al. (2013):

Step 1. Distribute experimental animals randomly into three groups, containing the required number of animals in each. Treat Group I animals with a vehicle for 8 days and mark them as a control group. Treat Group II animals receive gentamicin at 80 mg/kg (i.p.) for 8 days to induce nephrotoxicity. Group III animals receive a test sample and 80 mg/kg of gentamicin intraperitoneally for 8 days. From the 9th to the 18th day of the study, the administrator administered test samples to the animals.

Step 2. Place the animals' individually in metabolic cages over a period of 24 hours and collect their urine. At the end of the experiment, i.e., 24 h after the last dose, anesthetize the animals with chloroform. Collect blood samples by cardiac puncture in plain plastic tubes, leave them to stand for 1 hour, and centrifuge (900×*g* for 15 min) to separate serum. Store the serum at -5°C until analysis.

Step 3. Analyze the serum creatinine, urea, and total protein using commercial diagnostic kits. Also, measure the body weight and relative kidney weight of the animals. And perform histopathological analysis as mentioned above.

Part XVII: Miscellaneous Activity Studies

Hair Growth Promoting Activity Test

Hair is an important constituent of mammals' bodies. Skin is the source of hair. The skin functions as a physical barrier, a thermal insulator, and a sweat and sebum dispersal organ. While unwelcome, rapid hair loss that affects both sexes has clinical repercussions and is typically linked to diffuse scalp hair thinning. Any therapy that promotes hair regrowth or prevents additional thinning may lessen the psychosocial effects of ongoing hair loss. Drugs that alter the quantity and appearance of scalp hair are in high demand. The only synthetic medications that are currently on the market that have received FDA approval are minoxidil and finasteride. The related negative effects and unpredictable success of current treatments for androgenic alopecia, however, place restrictions on their use. Numerous pharmacological products and hair transplants are being marketed for the treatment of alopecia and to increase scalp hair development. Some of these include vitamins (such as vitamin D3) and amino acids, although their effectiveness is still debatable, and transplant success is unpredictable and costly. However, natural solutions have become increasingly popular in the hair care sector. Almost a thousand different plant extracts have been tested for their ability to promote hair growth, and some of them have great potential. You can check the hair growth-promoting effect of your test sample by using the following models.

Rodent Model

According to Begum et al. (2015) and Bhinge et al. (2022):

Step 1. Randomly divide animals (e.g., mice or rats) into the required number of groups with the required number of animals in each.

Step 2. Shave (with an area of $4 \times 3 = 12$ cm^2) of their dorsal portion. You can use minoxidil 1% suspension as a standard drug, while vehicle as a negative control. Continue these treatments for 28 days.

Step 3. Observe for any irritating effects on the shaved region and skin lesions such as itchy eyes, skin rashes, inflammation, stuffy nose etc. Clean the shaven dorsal region of the selected animals properly with surgical spirit. Then apply your test drug or controls to the shaved region over 1 cm^2 and monitor the animals for 2 days for any skin lesions.

Step 4. Visually observe the hair growth using two parameters: hair growth initiation (the less period in days to begin detectable hair growth) and hair growth completion period (the less period in days taken to fully cover the shaved skin area with new hair).

Step 5. Pull 20 hairs from the early denude region of the selected animal on Days 20, 25, and 30 of study. Measure the hair lengths and express them in cm, and represent them as the mean length ± S.D. (standard deviation) of plucked 20 hairs.

Step 6. Euthanize the animals on Day 28 with a suitable anesthetic agent. Excise their skin and set them on a frame consisting of a metal coin with a radius of 0.9 cm. Calculate the difference in weight as a hair weight after weighing skin with and without hair.

Step 7. Collect the dorsal skin biopsies of the animals from each group and fix them in buffered formalin (10% neutral) solution. Perform the histopathological analysis as mentioned above. Measure the size and number of hair follicles (manually counted by a blinded viewer at a fixed size area from the dermis and subcutis layer).

Testosterone Model

According to Patel et al. (2015):

Step 1. Prepare a 1% testosterone solution in arachis oil. Use a vehicle for your test drug and standard (finasteride) solution (2%).

Strep 2. Follow the below-mentioned grouping for this test:

- Group I: Testosterone (S.C.) + Vehicle (Topically)
- Group II: Testosterone (S.C.) + Finasteride (2%) (Topically)
- Group III: Testosterone (S.C.) + Test drug (Topically)

Step 3. Administer 0.1 mL of testosterone to all animals (e.g., rats) in all groups. Carry out this study for 20 days.

Step 4. Observe hair growth activity differences in different groups visually.

Step 5. Using an ocular micrometer, determine the cyclic phase of hair follicles anagen and telogen, as well as the number of hair follicles, and calculate the A/T ratio (anagen/telogen). For this, select animals from each group erratically and sacrifice them on day 21. In skin biopsy, keep the balding site of each group of animals and samples of skin in PBS formalin for paraffin sectioning. Perform histopathology as mentioned above.

Reproductive Capacity Test

Certain agents can have bad impacts on the reproductive systems of humans and other animals. It reduces spermatogenesis, oogenesis, and the development of gonads. However, bad impacts on the reproductive system also include toxicological damage to parts and impairment of biochemical activities associated with this system. You can check the toxic/protective effects of your test sample on this system by using a number of models. One popularly used model has been shown below.

Rodent Model

According to Allan et al. (2009):

Step 1. Randomly divide male animals (e.g., mice or rats) into groups with the required number of animals in each.

Step 2. Give the treatments by oral gavage once daily for a period of 65 days prior to mating and 21 days during mating.

Step 3. Observe mortality and clinical signs every day and record the events.

Step 4. Record their BW at the beginning of the experiment and thereafter 2 times a week till they are sacrificed. Also record their feed consumption 1 day before the initiation of treatment and thereafter weekly during the premating period of 65 days.

Step 5. Perform the sperm count by using one of the epididymides of each animal. Incise the cauda epididymis and homogenize in a homogenizer glass vial containing 30 mL of 0.01% (w/v) Triton X-100 in 0.9% NaCl for approximately 15 to 20 min. Rinse the homogenate probe with distilled water and collect it. Adjust the final volume of the homogenate up to 50 mL using distilled water. Sonicate the mixture for 15 to 20 min. Add 0.5 mL of 1% eosin Y stain solution to it. Count the sperm using a hemocytometer.

Step 6. Collect the sperm from the vas deferens and observe under a microscope to determine the percentage of motile sperm. Immediately after sacrifice, isolate one vas deferens and excise it from the testis. Cut the vas deferens into small pieces and place in a petri dish containing 3 to 5 mL of PBS maintained at 35 – 37 °C. Transfer the sperm suspension to a test tube placed in a water bath at 35 – 37 °C and incubate for 5 to 10 min. transfer 10 μL of the suspension to a microscope slide with concave chambers kept on a slide warmer maintained at 35 - 37 °C and roof with a coverslip for evaluation of sperm motility.

Step 7. Collect blood samples at the time of sacrifice under CO_2 anesthesia, from the orbital sinus of all animals. Analyze serum levels of testosterone using the ELISA method.

Step 8. After 65 days of the treatment period, mate each male animal in the control and treated groups (1:1) with an untreated female. Cohabitate the females with the males till the vaginal smear examination confirms the presence of spermatozoa. The females that show positive vaginal smears are considered successfully mated and designate that day as Day 0 of gestation. Sacrifice the females on Day 15 of gestation and examine their uteruses for confirmation of pregnancies.

Step 9. Sacrifice the males at the end of the experiment. Remove their testes and epididymides, examine macroscopically, preserve in 10% neutral buffered formalin, and process for histopathological examination.

Wound Healing Capacity Test

Everyone may face a problem in their lifetime. A wound can be defined as a loss or breaking of cellular, anatomical, and/or functional connections of living tissues that results in a breach, contravention, or interruption of tissue integrity. Wounds could be injuries, cuts and bites, diabetic, gastric, or duodenal ulcers. Therefore, it affects public health worldwide with significant resource expenses. The majority of currently available wound healing drugs are expensive and exert many adverse biological effects, including allergy and drug resistance. Therefore, we should search for alternative treatment approaches for wound healing. You can calculate the wound healing capacity of your test sample by using the following models:

Rodent Model

Step 1. *Dermal toxicity test*: Before determining the wound healing capacity of your test sample, perform an acute dermal toxicity study. For this, take 2 groups of animals with 3 animals (e.g., mice) in each. Acclimatize them for 5 days. Then, shave around 10% of the body surface area from the dorsal area of the trunks of each animal 1 day prior to the test procedure. First, give a testing dose of 2000 mg/kg (limit dose: 10% sample ointment) and normal ointment base (control group). Then cover it with gauze and a non-occlusive bandage soon after and let it rest for 1 day. After 1 day, the entire materials and residual test substances are removed with care, and the test site of each animal is washed with distilled water. Observe the animals for the development of any adverse skin reaction for 1 day. Then, take 4 additional, two from each group, and give the dose, cover and wash following the same procedure, and similarly observe for 1 day for any skin reaction such as edema and erythema with close follow-up for 24 h after washing and then daily for 2 weeks.

Step 2. *Preparation of extract and control ointments*: At first, prepare a normal ointment following the below-mentioned general formula provided by the British Pharmacopoeia.

Ingredients	Master formula (g)	Reduced formula (g)
Wool fat	50	5
Hard paraffin	50	5
Cecostearyl alcohol	50	5
White soft paraffin	850	85
Total	1000	100

Now you can use this base as a vehicle and prepare your test sample at the required dose, such as 5, 10, or 15%.

Step 3. *Excision wound model*: Anesthetize animals by using suitable anesthetic agents, for example, ketamine (80 mg/kg) plus diazepam (5 mg/kg, i.p.). Make a wound by using the excision process under sterile conditions by utilizing a full-thickness circular excision wound measuring 314 mm^2 and 2 mm in depth in the shaved dorsal thoracic region. Then apply test ointment, control, or standard drug topically daily on the wounded surface of the animals. Consider the wounding day to be Day 0.

Step 4. *Linear incision wound model*: In this case, make a 3 cm long longitudinal paravertebral incision into their dorsal fur region and suture 1 cm apart using a surgical thread (no. 000) and curved needle (no. 11). To achieve better wound closure, the thread is tightened continuously on both wound edges. After 1 day of wound creation (Day 1), apply your topical test sample or controls daily for 9 days. Remove the sutures on Day 8 and measure the tensile strength on Day 10 using the continuous water flow technique.

Step 5. *Burn wound model*: After anesthetizing, shaving, and decontamination with 70% alcohol, a burn wound is created on four groups of animals (e.g., mice) through hot molten wax. For this, hot molten wax at 80°Cis poured into a cylinder with a 300 mm^2 circular opening and placed on the shaven skin of each animal until it solidifies (normally takes 10–12 min). Remove the cylinder. Then place the animals in individual cages and start treatments. Observe wound conditions every 2 days.

Step 6. *Infected wound model*: Prepare full-thickness circular excision wounds sized about 300 mm^2 aseptically as mentioned above. After achieving complete hemostasis by blotting the wound with a cotton swab soaked in normal saline, inoculate with a standard strain of *Staphylococcus aureus* (fresh culture) suspension (1×10^6 CFU/mL). Place the animals' singly in separate cages and treat them similarly from Day 2. Observe and measure the wound similarly. Every 24 h, check for the presence or absence of phlogistic characteristics such as infiltration, edema/localized swelling, abscess, lesion, and exudates.

Step 7. *Observation of period of epithelialization*: Observe the number of days required for the falling scar without any residue from the raw wound.

Step 8. *Measurement of wound contraction*: Assess the wound closure rate by tracing the wound on Days 2, 4, 6, 8, 10, 12, 14, and 16 using transparent paper and a permanent marker. In the case of the infected wound model, measurement of wound contraction continues till Day 18. Record wound areas by using a 1 mm^2 scale of graph paper. Use the following equation for measuring wound closure.

$$\%\text{Wound closure} = [(\text{Wound area}_{\text{Day } 0} - \text{Wound area}_{\text{Day } n}) \div \text{Wound area}_{\text{Day } n}] \times 100$$

Step 9. *Measurement of tensile strength*: Tensile strength is the force required to open the healing skin. For this, they fixed shelves with a table and 2 Allis forceps; one is fixed to the opposite side of the shelf, and the other is tied with rope attached to the empty IV bag on which the weights are placed. On Day 10, after wounding, anesthetize each mouse using diethyl ether to secure the animal to the table. The two forceps are firmly applied 1 cm away from the healed tissue on the incised part of the skin along the line facing each other. Allow water to flow into the bag from tap water through the IV line. A gradual increase in weight is transmitted to the wound site, pulling apart the wound edges. As soon as wound gaping appears, water flow is stopped, and the volume of water collected in the container is determined and noted as an indirect measure of breaking strength in grams. Measure %tensile strength by using the following equation.

$$\%\text{Tensile strength} = [(TS_{test} - TS_{control}) \div TS_{control}] \times 100$$

$$\%\text{Tensile strength of normal ointment} = [(TS_{\text{normal ointment}} - TS_{\text{left untreated group}}) \div TS_{\text{left untreated group}}] \times 100$$

Step 10. *Histopathological investigation*: At the end of the experiment, the animals were given 320 mg/kg of ketamine plus 20 mg/kg of diazepam (four times the anesthetic dose) intraperitoneally. Collect the cross-sectional full-thickness skin specimens. Fix the samples in 10% buffered formalin, process them, block them with paraffin, section them into 3-5 m sections, and stain them with hematoxylin and eosin. Make microscopic examinations as mentioned above (OECD 2017; Demilew et al. 2018; Tessema and Molla 2021; Abeje et al. 2022).

Insect Repellent Test

Insect Introduction Model

According to Mondal et al. (2012):

Step 1. *Preparation of test sample*: Prepare your test sample using a serial dilution technique at a series of concentrations using as $\mu g/cm^2$ unit. Organic solvents that readily evaporate can be used for this purpose.

Step 2. *Dose application*: Use half filter paper discs (Whatman any grade, diameter 9 cm) and separately apply onto each of the half-discs and allow to dry out in the air for 10 min. Then attach these discs lengthwise, edge-to-edge, to a control half-disc with adhesive tape and place them in petri dishes.

Step 3. *Introduction of insects*: Keep 10 adult insects in the middle of each of the filter-paper circles.

Step 4. *Observation*: Count the insects that settle on the non-treated/control half of the filter paper discs after 1 h and then at hourly intervals for 5 h. Use a suitable insect repellent as a standard drug.

Step 5. *Calculation*: Convert the average of the counts %repellency using the formula:

$$\%\text{Repellency} = 2 \times (C - 50)$$

where, C is the percentage of insects on the untreated half of the disc. Express positive values as repellency and negative values as attractant activity.

Mosquito Repellent Tests

Human-Bait Model 1

According to Idris et al. (2014):

Step 1. Collect a suitable mosquito species, such as *Anopheles gambiae*.

Step 2. Select 5 adult volunteers for this study. Spray test samples or controls on the exposed body surface ($3 \times 10 = 30$ cm^2 on each forearm) for up to 8 h over 2 weeks.

Step 3. Expose them to *An. gambiae* at night in a large room at room temperature. Constitute your test sample with an evaporable solvent such as ethanol. Triplicate the procedure. Or

Step 4. Each volunteer put the test forearm in a mosquito cage ($80 \times 40 \times 40$ cm^3), containing 50 female mosquitoes (3 - 5 days old), for the first 3 min of every 30 min exposure. However, before the start of each exposure, the bare hand, used as the control area of each volunteer, is exposed for up to 30 sec. If at least two mosquitoes land on the bare hand, continue the repellency test. This was done to ensure that the mosquitoes were host-seeking. The number of mosquitoes probing the treated area of each volunteer is noted for 30 min. Calculate %repellency as follows:

$$\%\text{Repellency} = [(C - T) \div C] \times 100$$

where, C is the number of mosquitoes that landed on the control and T is the number of mosquitoes that landed on the treated volunteers.

Human-Bait Model 2

According to WHO (2009):

Step 1. Collect 3-day-old blood-starved 100 female *Anopheles stephensi* mosquitoes and keep them in a net cage ($45 \times 30 \times 45$ cm^3).

Step 2. Select the required number of volunteers who have no contact with lotions, perfumes, oils, or perfumed soaps on the day of the assay.

Step 3. The arms of a volunteer, only 25 cm^2 dorsal side of the skin on each arm is exposed, and they cover the remaining area with rubber gloves.

Step 4. Prepare the samples similarly and topically apply the test sample or controls separately to the exposed area of the forearm.

Step 5. Perform the test with *An. stephensi* during the night. Triplicate the procedure. The volunteers conduct their test of each concentration by inserting the treated and control arms into the cages at the same time for one full minute every 5 min. The mosquitoes that land on the hand are recorded and then shaken off before they imbibe any blood. Calculate %repellency as follows:

$$\%\text{Repellency} = [(\text{Ta} - \text{Tb}) \div \text{Ta}] \times 100$$

where, Ta is the number of mosquitoes in the control group and Tb is the number of mosquitoes in the treated group.

Adulticidal Activity Test

Mosquito-Exposure Model

According to WHO (1981):

Step 1. Collect 5-6-day-old sugar-fed adult female mosquitoes for this study.

Step 2. Impregnate test samples or controls on filter papers (140 × 120 mm). Left to dry the papers at room temperature to evaporate off the solvent (e.g., ethanol) overnight.

Step 3. Impregnated papers were prepared fresh prior to testing. The bioassay system (kit) consists of two cylindrical plastic tubes, both measuring 125×44 mm. One tube serves to expose the mosquitoes to the test sample, and another tube is used to hold the mosquitoes before and after the exposure periods. The impregnated papers are rolled and placed in the exposure tube.

Step 4. Close each tube at one end with a 16-mesh size wire screen. Sucrose-fed and blood-starved mosquitoes (20) are released into the tube, and the mortality effects of the test sample are observed every 10 min for a 3 h exposure period.

Step 5. At the end of the 1, 2, and 3 h exposure periods, the mosquitoes are placed in the holding tube. Cotton pads soaked in 10% sugar solution with vitamin B complex are placed in the tube during the holding period of 24 h. Mortality of the mosquitoes is recorded after 24 h. The above procedure is carried out in triplicate for each test sample concentration.

Anti-Vitiligo Activity Test

An autoimmune cutaneous disease of pigmentation known as vitiligo causes distinct white patches to appear on the skin and mucous membranes. Melanocytes are destroyed, and the mechanism for making melanin is blocked. Melanocytes from the skin of vitiligo patients respond to exogenous oxidative stress more quickly than normal melanocytes do, with higher amounts of reactive oxygen species and more endoplasmic reticulum stress. There is currently no effective treatment for this agonizing condition. The following method can be used to test your sample for anti-vitiligo effects.

Rodent Model

According to Abuduaini et al. (2021):

Step 1. *Preparation of blood and skin samples*: Sera are separated from blood samples by centrifugation, and they are then chilled to -70 °C for storage. After being mixed and homogenized for 60 min at 4 °C in an oscillator, skin tissue samples are centrifuged for 15 min at 4 °C to separate the supernatant.

Step 2. *Animal preparation*: Animals should be divided into the necessary groups at random, 50/50 between male and female. The normal control group had their dorsal skin hairs removed, and they were rubbed with distilled water for 50 days, while the other groups were rubbed with hydroquinone or H_2O_2 (5%) for 50 days while receiving test samples orally for 30 days beginning on day 21. 12 h after the last dose is administered, sacrifice the animals and harvest their blood and skin tissue.

Step 3. *Measurement of melanin-containing hair follicles*: By using traditional histology investigation, the melanin-containing hair follicles are seen. A section of skin is cut, fixed with 10% neutral-buffered formalin, and then embedded in paraffin. On sections of about 5 mm, hematoxylin and eosin staining are carried out; fifty hair follicles are viewed under a light microscope (100×), and the number of hair follicles that contain melanin is counted.

Step 4. *Biochemical analysis*: Using commercial kits, identify the presence of acetylcholinesterase (AChE), monoamine oxidase (MAO), and malondialdehyde (MDA) in skin tissue. Using a microplate reader, the absorbance of AChE, MAO, and MDA are measured at 520, 242, and 532 nm, respectively.

Step 5. *Measurement of IL-6, IFN-γ, TYR, cAMP, and β-EP*: Determine the concentrations of cytokines, namely, interferon-gamma (IFN-γ), interleukin- (IL-) 6, tyrosinase (TYR), cyclic adenosine monophosphate (cAMP), and β-endorphin (β-EP) quantitatively in collected serum and tissue samples by enzyme-linked immunosorbent assay.

Step 6. *Histopathological analysis*: Prepare skin sections and stain by hematoxylin and eosin (H&E), or L-DOPA and examine under a light microscope.

Step 7. *Immunohistochemistry analysis*: Determine the expression of TYR, TRP-1 (tyrosinase-related protein 1), and TRP-2 (tyrosinase-related protein 2) in the shaved areas of the skin by staining with monoclonal antibodies for tyrosinase, TRP-1, and TRP-2, and the protein expression is determined using Image-Pro Plus 6.0.

Cell Line Assay Model

According to Abuduaini et al. (2021):

Step 1. Collect murine B16 melanoma cells and culture in HG-DMEM and supplemented with 10% FBS, 100 μg/mL streptomycin, and 100 U/mL penicillin, in a humidified incubator with 5% CO_2 at 37 °C and sub-culture every 2 days to maintain logarithmic growth.

Step 2. *Cell viability assay*: Perform this assay like the anti-cancer test.

Step 3. *Melanin content determination*: Seed B16 cells in a 6-well plate at a density of 1.8×10^5 cells/well. After 24 h of incubation, treat the cells for 48 h with your test sample or controls. Wash the cells twice with PBS (PH 7.4), lysed in 100 μL RIPA buffer for 40 min at 4 °C, and centrifuge at 12,000×*g* for 20 min at 4 °C. Measure the protein content of the supernatants using the BCA assay, and mix the pellets with 190 μL of 1 M NaOH (with 10% DMSO) for 2 h at 60 °C. Detect the melanin content at 405 nm by a multiplate reader and correct for the concentrations of proteins.

Step 4. *Tyrosinase activity assay*: Seed B16 cells in a 6-well plate at a density of 2.5×10^5 cells/well. After 24 h, treat them with your test sample or controls for 24 h. Lyse the cells with PBS containing 1% Triton X-100 and 1% sodium deoxycholate for 30 min at -20 °C and centrifuge at 12,000×*g* for 15 min. Add 90 µL of cell lysate and 10 µL of 10 mM L-DOPA to each well, following a 20~60 min incubation at 37 °C in the dark, and detect the dopachrome at 490 nm. Calculate the tyrosinase activity of each sample and correct for the concentrations of proteins.

Step 5. Perform a melanin content assay by Western blot analysis.

Step 6. *Determination of intracellular cAMP levels*: Treat B16 melanoma cells with your test sample at 37 °C for 12 h. Measuring intracellular cAMP levels using a cAMP ELISA kit.

Diuretic/Anti-Diuretic Activity Test

Diuretics encourage animals to produce more urine. It is clear that sodium ion excretion controls both the volume and make-up of urine. In general, diuretics are used to treat a number of conditions that can be fatal, such as nephritic syndrome, congestive heart failure, kidney failure due to cirrhosis, pregnancy toxemia, diabetes, edema, and hypertension. Using the model below, you may determine whether your sample has diuretic or anti-diuretic effects.

Rodent Model

According to Kau et al. (1984) and Gabriel and Idu (2021):

Step 1. Collect male animals (e.g., mice or rats) and house them in standard conditions with free access to commercial chow and water *ad libitum*.

Step 2. Overnight fasted animals are randomly divided into the required groups with the required number of animals in each group.

Step 3. Before starting treatments, give all animals isotonic saline (0.9% NaCl) with an oral dose of 5% BW to impose a uniform water load. Thirty minutes later, orally administer your test sample or controls. As a positive control, you can use furosemide at a dose of 10 mg/kg.

Step 4. Place each animal individually in a metabolic cage, and determine the cumulative urine output at hourly intervals for 6 h. Collect the urine in graduated cylinder and measure it every 6 h, which is expressed as mL/100 g body weight per 6 h.

Additionally, we can perform the following tests.

Step 5. Perform electrolytes (Na^+, K^+ and Cl^-) concentrations and determine urine pH in the 6 h urine samples of the animals.

Step 6. By utilizing flame photometry, the concentrations of Na^+, K^+, and Cl^- in the urine can be determined. However, argentimetry can measure Cl- concentrations (titration). A pH meter or commercial kits can be used to measure the pH of fresh urine samples, and the results can be represented as mM/L. Remove debris and shedding from the samples before estimating the electrolyte content.

Step 7. *Assay of urea*: This test exploits the hydrolysis of urea to ammonia in the urease enzyme. Add 100 µL of reagent to 1 to 10 µL of serum samples in test tubes. Add 100 µL solution reagents to 1 to 10 µL of distilled water as a blank. Mix the solutions thoroughly for incubation for 10 min at 37 °C. Add 2.5 mL of reagents 2 and 3 into test tubes. Incubate the solutions properly for a further 10 min at 37 °C. Measure the absorbance of samples against a blank at 546 nm wavelength. Calculate the urea level as follows:

$$\text{Urea level (mg/dL)} = (\text{Absorbance}_{\text{sample}} \div \text{Absorbance}_{\text{standard}}) \times 80$$

Step 8. *Assay for creatinine level*: This test makes use of creatinine's interaction with an alkaline mixture containing picric acid to create a colorful complex. The complexity of the quantity produced and the concentration of creatinine are directly comparable. Test tubes should contain 0.2 mL of the sample macro and semi-micro. Add semi-micro to the standard solution tubes and an exact amount of 0.2 mL of standard macro to the 0.1 mL solution.

In a similar manner, combine 2 mL of standard macro solution, 1 mL of semi-micro solution, 2 mL of sample macro solution, and 1 mL of semi-micro solution in working reagent test tubes. The test tubes' solutions are blended. Determine the creatinine values as follows by measuring the absorbance of the samples and the standard at 492 nm:

$$\text{Creatinine level units (mg/dL)} = (\text{Absorbance}_{\text{sample}} \div \text{Absorbance}_{\text{standard}}) \times 2$$

Step 9. *Assay for electrolytes (Na^+, K^+, Cl^-, and HCO_3^-)*: The reaction of HCO_3^- with weak HCl to produce CO_2 is used in the assay for HCO_3^-. With the help of the phenol red indicator, excess acid is titrated into diluted NaOH. 200 μL of serum sample should be mixed with 0.01 N HCl and 1 drop of phenol red indicator. Brick red coloring, the endpoint, is achieved by titrating the solution with 0.01 N NaOH. Calculate HCO_3^- as follows:

Bicarbonate (μM/L) = 50 – Titre

Titre = Endpoint × 100

The test for Cl- takes advantage of the mercuric nitrate ($Hg_2(NO_3)_2$)-mediated production of Cl^- precipitate in a sample. Add Cl^- to the typical mercuric ion solution. In this situation, stable undissociated $HgCl_2$ is created. A violet colour results from the diphenylcarbazone and excess mercuric chloride nitrate reaction. 200 μL of serum sample should receive 2 mL of deionized water. Add 3 drops of the diphenylcarbazone indicator and 1 drop of HNO_3 after thoroughly combining the solutions. To reach a violet finish, the combination is then titrated using $Hg_2(NO_3)_2$. The same steps should be taken for the Cl^- standard solution. Calculate Cl^- using the formula:

$$\text{Chloride } (\mu M/L) = (\text{Titre}_{\text{sample}} \div \text{Title}_{\text{standard}}) \times 100$$

In order to dissociate neutral ground position, solutions containing components in flame are injected into the assay technique for Na^+ and K^+. The flame is stimulated by the atoms, which causes it to migrate to a spot with more energy. In the ground state, excited atoms will emit light with a different wavelength (590 and 770 nm for Na^+ and K^+, respectively). Measure the amount of light passing through an adequate filter in a photosensitive element while using a current meter to measure the amount of Na^+ and K^+ in the sample. Calculate the pH of urine using a pH meter that has been calibrated to measure the pH of fresh urine samples. Calculate the Na^+/K^+ ratio, Lipschitz value, diuretic index, and saliuretic index as follows:

Index of diuresis = (UVt/UVc)

Lipschitz's value = (UVt/UVr)
Index of saliuresis = (CUEt/CUEc)

Na^+/K^+ ratio = (UNa^+/UK^+)

where, UVt, UVc and UVr stand for mean urine volume of test, control, standard group, respectively. CUEt, CUEc, UNa^+ and UK^+ stand for concentration of electrolytes in urine of test, control, and concentration of Na^+ and K^+ in urine of a group, respectively.

References

Abeje, B. A., Bekele, T., Getahun, K. A., & Asrie, A. B. (2022). Evaluation of Wound Healing Activity of 80% Hydromethanolic Crude Extract and Solvent Fractions of the Leaves of *Urtica simensis* in Mice. *Journal of Experimental Pharmacology*, 221-241.

Abena, A. A., Diatewa, M., Gakosso, G., Gbeassor, M., Hondi-Assah, T. H., & Ouamba, J. M. (2003). Analgesic, antipyretic and anti-inflammatory effects of essential oil of *Lippia multiflora*. *Fitoterapia*, *74*(3), 231-236.

Abuduaini, A., Lu, X., Zang, D., Wu, T., & Aisa, H. A. (2021). Effects of a traditional caraway formulation on experimental models of vitiligo and mechanisms of melanogenesis. *Evidence-Based Complementary and Alternative Medicine*, *2021*, 1-17.

Aebi, H. (1984). [13] Catalase *in vitro*. In *Methods in Enzymology* (Vol. 105, pp. 121-126). Academic press.

Afroz, S., Alamgir, M., Khan, M. T. H., Jabbar, S., Nahar, N., & Choudhuri, M. S. K. (2006). Antidiarrhoeal activity of the ethanol extract of *Paederia foetida* Linn.(Rubiaceae). *Journal of Ethnopharmacology*, *105*(1-2), 125-130.

Aiyegoro, O. A., & Okoh, A. I. (2010). Preliminary phytochemical screening and *in vitro* antioxidant activities of the aqueous extract of Helichrysum longifolium DC. *BMC Complementary and Alternative Medicine*, *10*(1), 1-8.

Ajila, C. M., & Rao, U. P. (2008). Protection against hydrogen peroxide induced oxidative damage in rat erythrocytes by *Mangifera indica* L. peel extract. *Food and Chemical Toxicology*, *46*(1), 303-309.

Akah, P. A., & Offiah, V. N. (1992). Gastrointestinal effects of *Allamanda cathartica* leaf extracts. *International Journal of Pharmacognosy*, *30*(3), 213-217.

Akah, P. A., Orisakwe, O. E., Gamaniel, K. S., & Shittu, A. (1998). Evaluation of Nigerian traditional medicines: II. Effects of some Nigerian folk remedies on peptic ulcer. *Journal of Ethnopharmacology*, *62*(2), 123-127.

Akindele, A. J., & Adeyemi, O. O. (2007). Antiinflammatory activity of the aqueous leaf extract of *Byrsocarpus coccineus*. *Fitoterapia*, *78*(1), 25-28.
Akindele, A. J., & Adeyemi, O. O. (2007). Antiinflammatory activity of the aqueous leaf extract of *Byrsocarpus coccineus*. *Fitoterapia*, *78*(1), 25-28.
Albrahim, T., Alnasser, M. M., Al-Anazi, M. R., ALKahtani, M. D., Alkahtani, S., & Al-Qahtani, A. A. (2020). *In vitro* studies on the immunomodulatory effects of

Pulicaria crispa extract on human THP-1 monocytes. *Oxidative Medicine and Cellular Longevity, 2020.*

Alemu, A., Tamiru, W., Nedi, T., & Shibeshi, W. (2018). Analgesic and anti-inflammatory effects of 80% methanol extract of Leonotis ocymifolia (burm. F.) iwarsson leaves in rodent models. *Evidence-Based Complementary and Alternative Medicine, 2018.*

Alencar, M. V. O. B., Islam, M. T., de Lima, R. M. T., Paz, M. F. C. J., Dos Reis, A. C., da Mata, A. M. O. F., Filho, J. W. G. D. O., Cerqueira, G. S., Ferreira, P. M. P., e Sousa, J. M. D. C., & Melo-Cavalcante, A. A. D. C. (2019). Phytol as an anticarcinogenic and antitumoral agent: An *in vivo* study in *Swiss* mice with DMBA-Induced breast cancer. *IUBMB Life*, *71*(2), 200-212.

Allan, J. J., Pore, M. P., Deepak, M., Murali, B., Mayachari, A. S., & Agarwal, A. (2009). Reproductive and fertility effects of an extract of *Andrographis paniculata* in male Wistar rats. *International Journal of Toxicology*, *28*(4), 308-317.

Allchorne, A. J., Broom, D. C., & Woolf, C. J. (2005). Detection of cold pain, cold allodynia and cold hyperalgesia in freely behaving rats. *Molecular Pain*, *1*, 1744-8069.

Amorim, E. L., Nascimento, J. E., Monteiro, J. M., Peixoto Sobrinho, T. J. S., Araújo, T. A., & Albuquerque, U. P. (2008). A simple and accurate procedure for the determination of tannin and flavonoid levels and some applications in ethnobotany and ethnopharmacology. *Functional Ecosystems and Communities*, *2*(1), 88-94.

Amos, S., Adzu, B., Binda, L., Wambebe, C., & Gamaniel, K. (2001). Neuropharmacological effect of the aqueous extract of *Sphaeranthus senegalensis* in mice. *Journal of Ethnopharmacology*, *78*(1), 33-37.

Andrade-Cetto, A., Becerra-Jiménez, J., & Cárdenas-Vázquez, R. (2008). Alfa-glucosidase-inhibiting activity of some Mexican plants used in the treatment of type 2 diabetes. *Journal of Ethnopharmacology*, *116*(1), 27-32.

Akita, Y., Yang, Y., Kawai, T., Kinoshita, K., Koyama, K., Takahashi, K. and Watanabe, K., 1998. New assay method for surveying anti-emetic compounds from natural sources. *Natural Product Sciences*, *4*(2), 72-77.

Antolovich, M., Prenzler, P. D., Patsalides, E., McDonald, S., & Robards, K. (2002). Methods for testing antioxidant activity. *Analyst*, *127*(1), 183-198.

Apak, R. (2019). Current issues in antioxidant measurement. *Journal of Agricultural and Food Chemistry*, *67*(33), 9187-9202.

Apak, R., Güçlü, K., Özyürek, M., & Çelik, S. E. (2008). Mechanism of antioxidant capacity assays and the CUPRAC (cupric ion reducing antioxidant capacity) assay. *Microchimica Acta*, *160*, 413-419.

Ayoka, A. O., Akomolafe, R. O., Iwalewa, E. O., Akanmu, M. A., & Ukponmwan, O. E. (2006). Sedative, antiepileptic and antipsychotic effects of *Spondias mombin* L. (Anacardiaceae) in mice and rats. *Journal of Ethnopharmacology*, *103*(2), 166-175.

Banerjee, A., Ahmed, H., Yang, P., Czinn, S. J., & Blanchard, T. G. (2016). Endoplasmic reticulum stress and IRE-1 signaling cause apoptosis in colon cancer cells in response to andrographolide treatment. *Oncotarget*, *7*(27), 41432.

Baquer, N. Z., Kumar, P., Taha, A., Kale, R. K., Cowsik, S. M., & McLean, P. (2011). Metabolic and molecular action of *Trigonella foenum-graecum* (fenugreek) and trace metals in experimental diabetic tissues. *Journal of Biosciences*, *36*, 383-396.

Bashar, Q. M., & Albadrany, Y. M. (2022). Evaluation of the Antipyretic, Analgesic, and Anti-inflammatory Effects of Pregabalin in Chicks. *Egyptian Journal of Veterinary Sciences*, *53*(3), 323-328.

Bays, H., & Dujovne, C. (2002). Anti-obesity drug development. *Expert opinion on investigational drugs*, *11*(9), 1189-1204.

Begum, S., Gu, L. J., Lee, M. R., Li, Z., Li, J. J., Hossain, M. J., Wang, Y. B., & Sung, C. K. (2015). *In vivo* hair growth-stimulating effect of medicinal plant extract on BALB/c nude mice. *Pharmaceutical Biology*, *53*(8), 1098-1103.

Benzie, I. F., & Strain, J. J. (1996). The ferric reducing ability of plasma (FRAP) as a measure of "antioxidant power": the FRAP assay. *Analytical Biochemistry*, *239*(1), 70-76.

Benzie, I. F., & Strain, J. J. (1999). [2] Ferric reducing/antioxidant power assay: direct measure of total antioxidant activity of biological fluids and modified version for simultaneous measurement of total antioxidant power and ascorbic acid concentration. In *Methods in Enzymology* (Vol. 299, pp. 15-27). Academic press.

Bhinge, S. D., Jadhav, N. R., Randive, D. S., Bhutkar, M. A., Chavan, R., & Kumbhar, B. V. (2022). Isolation and identification of hair growth potential fraction from active plant extract of Blumea eriantha DC grown in Western Ghat of India: In silico study. *Journal of Ayurveda and Integrative Medicine*, *13*(2), 100542.

Bhushan, S., Rajput, S., Sharma, D., Kaur, T., Dhar, M. K., & Arora, S. (2021). *In vitro* Antioxidant, Antimutagenic and Anti-hemolytic Potency of Allyl Isothiocyanate: A Natural Molecule. *Journal of Biologically Active Products from Nature*, *11*(3), 228-241.

Bolla, S. R., Al-Subaie, A. M., Al-Jindan, R. Y., Balakrishna, J. P., Ravi, P. K., Veeraraghavan, V. P., Pillai, A. A., Gollapalli, S. S. R., Joseph, J. P., & Surapaneni, K. M. (2019). *In vitro* wound healing potency of methanolic leaf extract of *Aristolochia saccata* is possibly mediated by its stimulatory effect on collagen-1 expression. *Heliyon*, *5*(5).

Brenner, D. S., Golden, J. P., & Gereau IV, R. W. (2012). A novel behavioral assay for measuring cold sensation in mice. *PloS One*, *7*(6), e39765.

Carlton, S. M., Lekan, H. A., Kim, S. H., & Chung, J. M. (1994). Behavioral manifestations of an experimental model for peripheral neuropathy produced by spinal nerve ligation in the primate. *Pain*, *56*(2), 155-166.

Cascão, R., Vidal, B., Raquel, H., Neves-Costa, A., Figueiredo, N., Gupta, V., Fonseca, J. E., & Ferreira Moita, L. (2014). Potent anti-inflammatory and antiproliferative effects of gambogic acid in a rat model of antigen-induced arthritis. *Mediators of Inflammation*, *2014*.

Chan-Zapata, I., Canul-Canche, J., Fernández-Martín, K., Martín-Quintal, Z., Torres-Romero, J. C., Lara-Riegos, J. C., Ramírez-Camacho, M. A., & Arana-Argáez, V. E. (2018). Immunomodulatory effects of the methanolic extract from *Pouteria campechiana* leaves in macrophage functions. *Food and Agricultural Immunology*, *29*(1), 386-399.

Chew, Y. L., Goh, J. K., & Lim, Y. Y. (2009). Assessment of *in vitro* antioxidant capacity and polyphenolic composition of selected medicinal herbs from Leguminosae family in Peninsular Malaysia. *Food Chemistry*, *116*(1), 13-18.

Chitme, H. R., Chandra, R., & Kaushik, S. (2004). Studies on anti-diarrhoeal activity of *Calotropis gigantea* R. Br. in experimental animals. *Journal of Pharmacy and Pharmaceutical Science*, *7*(1), 70-5.

Choudhary, M., Kumar, V., Malhotra, H., & Singh, S. (2015). Medicinal plants with potential anti-arthritic activity. *Journal of Intercultural Ethnopharmacology*, *4*(2), 147.

Coelho, L. P., Reis, P. A., de Castro, F. L., Gayer, C. R. M., da Silva Lopes, C., e Silva, M. C. D. C., de Carvalho Sabino, K. C., Todeschini, A. R., & Coelho, M. G. P. (2005). Antinociceptive properties of ethanolic extract and fractions of *Pterodon pubescens* Benth. seeds. *Journal of Ethnopharmacology*, *98*(1-2), 109-116.

Coles, G. C., Bauer, C., Borgsteede, F. H. M., Geerts, S., Klei, T. R., Taylor, M. A., & Waller, P. J. (1992). World Association for the Advancement of Veterinary Parasitology (WAAVP) methods for the detection of anthelmintic resistance in nematodes of veterinary importance. *Veterinary Parasitology*, *44*(1-2), 35-44.

Coruzzi, G., Adami, M., Guaita, E., de Esch, I. J., & Leurs, R. (2007). Antiinflammatory and antinociceptive effects of the selective histamine H4-receptor antagonists JNJ7777120 and VUF6002 in a rat model of carrageenan-induced acute inflammation. *European Journal of Pharmacology*, *563*(1-3), 240-244.

Coulibaly, J. T., N'Goran, E. K., Utzinger, J., Doenhoff, M. J., & Dawson, E. M. (2013). A new rapid diagnostic test for detection of anti-Schistosoma mansoni and anti-*Schistosoma haematobium* antibodies. *Parasites & Vectors*, *6*, 1-8.

Demilew, W., Adinew, G. M., & Asrade, S. (2018). Evaluation of the wound healing activity of the crude extract of leaves of Acanthus polystachyus Delile (Acanthaceae). *Evidence-Based Complementary and Alternative Medicine*, *2018*.

Demsie, D. G., Yimer, E. M., Berhe, A. H., Altaye, B. M., & Berhe, D. F. (2019). Anti-nociceptive and anti-inflammatory activities of crude root extract and solvent fractions of *Cucumis ficifolius* in mice model. *Journal of Pain Research*, 1399-1409.

Deuis, J. R. & Vetter, I. (2016). The thermal probe test: a novel behavioral assay to quantify thermal paw withdrawal thresholds in mice. *Temperature*, *3*, 199-207.

Devi, R. C., Sim, S. M., & Ismail, R. (2011). Spasmolytic effect of citral and extracts of *Cymbopogon citratus* on isolated rabbit ileum. *Journal of Smooth Muscle Research*, *47*(5), 143-156.

Dilts, S. L., & Berry, C. A. (1967). Effect of cholinergic drugs on passive avoidance in the mouse. *Journal of Pharmacology and Experimental Therapeutics*, *158*(2), 279-285.

Doherty, N. S. (1981). Inhibition of arachidonic acid release as the mechanism by which glucocorticoids inhibit endotoxin-induced diarrhoea. *British Journal of Pharmacology*, *73*(2), 549.

Ebrahimzadeh, M. A., Nabavi, S. F., Nabavi, S. M., & Eslami, B. (2010). Antihemolytic and antioxidant activities of Allium paradoxum. *Central European Journal of Biology*, *5*, 338-345.

Eddy, N. B., & Leimbach, D. (1953). Synthetic analgesics. II. Dithienylbutenyl-and dithienylbutylamines. *Journal of Pharmacology and Experimental Therapeutics, 107*(3), 385-393.

Ellman, G. L. (1959). Tissue sulfhydryl groups. *Archives of biochemistry and biophysics, 82*(1), 70-77.

El-Saadani, M., Esterbauer, H., El-Sayed, M., Goher, M., Nassar, A. Y., & Jürgens, G. (1989). A spectrophotometric assay for lipid peroxides in serum lipoproteins using a commercially available reagent. *Journal of Lipid Research, 30*(4), 627-630.

Estrada-Soto, S., Rodríguez-Avilez, A., Castañeda-Ávila, C., Castillo-España, P., Navarrete-Vázquez, G., Hernández, L., & Aguirre-Crespo, F. (2007). Spasmolytic action of Lepechinia caulescens is through calcium channel blockade and NO release. *Journal of Ethnopharmacology, 114*(3), 364-370.

Falé, P. L., Borges, C., Madeira, P. J. A., Ascensão, L., Araújo, M. E. M., Florêncio, M. H., & Serralheiro, M. L. M. (2009). Rosmarinic acid, scutellarein 4′-methyl ether 7-O-glucuronide and (16S)-coleon E are the main compounds responsible for the antiacetylcholinesterase and antioxidant activity in herbal tea of *Plectranthus barbatus* ("falso boldo"). *Food Chemistry, 114*(3), 798-805.

Ferre, S., Guix, T., Prat, G., Jane, F., & Casas, M. (1990). Is experimental catalepsy properly measured?. *Pharmacology Biochemistry and Behavior, 35*(4), 753-757.

Ferrini, R., Miragoli, G., & Taccardi, B. (1974). Neuro-pharmacological studies on SB 5833, a new psychotherapeutic agent of the benzodiazepine class. *Arzneimittel-Forschung, 24*(12), 2029-2032.

Fogliano, V., Verde, V., Randazzo, G., & Ritieni, A. (1999). Method for measuring antioxidant activity and its application to monitoring the antioxidant capacity of wines. *Journal of Agricultural and Food Chemistry, 47*(3), 1035-1040.

Foyet, H. S., Tsala, D. E., Bodo, J. Z. E., Carine, A. N., Heroyne, L. T., & Oben, E. K. (2015). Anti-inflammatory and anti-arthritic activity of a methanol extract from *Vitellaria paradoxa* stem bark. *Pharmacognosy Research, 7*(4), 367.

Gabriel, B. O., & Idu, M. D. (2021). Anti-diuretic and anti-glycemic properties of *Jatropha gossypiifolia* L. leave extract on wistar rats. *Clinical Phytoscience, 7*(1), 1-12.

Ge, J., Liu, Z., Zhong, Z., Wang, L., Zhuo, X., Li, J., Ye, X. Y., Xie, T., & Bai, R. (2022). Natural terpenoids with anti-inflammatory activities: Potential leads for anti-inflammatory drug discovery. *Bioorganic Chemistry, 124*, 105817.

Ghayur, M. N., & Gilani, A. H. (2005). Pharmacological basis for the medicinal use of ginger in gastrointestinal disorders. *Digestive Diseases and Sciences, 50*, 1889-1897.

Ghiselli, A., Serafini, M., Maiani, G., Azzini, E., & Ferro-Luzzi, A. (1995). A fluorescence-based method for measuring total plasma antioxidant capability. *Free Radical Biology and Medicine, 18*(1), 29-36.

Girish, T. K., Vasudevaraju, P., & Rao, U. J. P. (2012). Protection of DNA and erythrocytes from free radical induced oxidative damage by black gram (Vigna mungo L.) husk extract. *Food and Chemical Toxicology, 50*(5), 1690-1696.

González, L. T., Minsky, N. W., Espinosa, L. E. M., Aranda, R. S., Meseguer, J. P., & Pérez, P. C. (2017). *In vitro* assessment of hepatoprotective agents against damage induced by acetaminophen and CCl4. *BMC Complementary and Alternative Medicine*, *17*(1), 1-10.

Goyal, R. K. (2003). Practical in Pharmacology. Vol 1. Ahemdabad, India: B. S. Shaha Prakashan, pp. 51-52.

Gundamaraju, R., Atigari, D. V., & Sheeba, D. S. (2012). Evaluation of anti-obesity activity of *Lantana camara* var Linn on butter induced Hyperlipidemia in Rats. *Research Journal of Pharmacology and Pharmacodynamics*, *4*(5), 315-318.

Gupta, B. D., Dandiya, P. C., & Gupta, M. L. (1971). A psycho-pharmacological analysis of behaviour in rats. *Japanese Journal of Pharmacology*, *21*(3), 293-298.

Habig, W. H., Pabst, M. J., & Jakoby, W. B. (1974). Glutathione S-transferases: the first enzymatic step in mercapturic acid formation. *Journal of Biological Chemistry*, *249*(22), 7130-7139.

Hanafy, A., Aldawsari, H. M., Badr, J. M., Ibrahim, A. K., & Abdel-Hady, S. E. S. (2016). Evaluation of hepatoprotective activity of Adansonia digitata extract on acetaminophen-induced hepatotoxicity in rats. *Evidence-Based Complementary and Alternative Medicine*, *2016*.

Handley, S. L. (1991). Evaluation of marble-burying behavior as a model of anxiety. *Pharmacology Biochemistry and Behavior*, *38*(1), 63-67.

Hargreaves, K., Dubner, R., Brown, F., Flores, C., & Joris, J. (1988). A new and sensitive method for measuring thermal nociception in cutaneous hyperalgesia. *Pain*, *32*(1), 77-88.

Hellon, R., & Townsend, Y. (1982). Mechanisms of fever. *Pharmacology & therapeutics*, *19*(2), 211-244.

Heo, H., Shin, Y., Cho, W., Choi, Y., Kim, H., & Kwon, Y. K. (2009). Memory improvement in ibotenic acid induced model rats by extracts of *Scutellaria baicalensis*. *Journal of Ethnopharmacology*, *122*(1), 20-27.

Hutner, S. H., Cury, A., & Baker, H. (1958). Microbiological assays. *Analytical Chemistry*, *30*(4), 849-867.

Idris, M. M., Mudi, S. Y., & Datti, Y. (2014). Phytochemical screening and mosquito repellent activity of the stem bark extracts of *Euphorbia balsamifera* (Ait). *ChemSearch Journal*, *5*(2), 46-51.

Islam, A. M. T., Uddin, M. E., Chowdhury, M. A. U., Rahman, M. M., Habib, M. R., & Rahman, M. A. (2013). *In vivo* antidiarrheal and cytotoxic potential of different fractions of *Pandanus foetidus* leaves. *American Journal of Biomedical Science*, *5*(3), 208-16.

Islam, M. T., Freitas, R. M., Oliveira, G. L. S., & Guha, B. (2014). Neuropharmacological screenings of hydroalcoholic fractions of *Urena lobata* L. *World J Pharm Pharmaceut Sci*, *3*(3), 62-71.

Jakoby, W. B. (1962). Enzymes of γ-Aminobutyrate Metabolism (Bacterial). Colowick SP, Kaplan, N. O., editor. New York: Academic Press; 1962. 765-778.

Jakoby, W. B. (1962). Enzymes of γ-Aminobutyrate Metabolism (Bacterial). Colowick SP, Kaplan, N. O., editor. New York: Academic Press, pp. 765-778.

Janssen, P. A., Niemegeers, C. J., & Dony, J. G. (1963). The inhibitory effect of fentanyl and other morphine-like analgesics on the warm water induced tail withdrawl reflex in rats. *Arzneimittel-forschung*, *13*, 502-507.

Jayawardene, K. D., Palombo, E. A., & Boag, P. R. (2021). Natural products are a promising source for anthelmintic drug discovery. *Biomolecules*, *11*(10), 1457.

Jocelyn, P. C. (1972). Biochemistry of the SH Group. Academic Press, London, pp. 10.

Jung, I. H., Kim, S. E., Lee, Y. G., Kim, D. H., Kim, H., Kim, G. S., Baek, N. I., & Lee, D. Y. (2018). Antihypertensive effect of ethanolic extract from Acanthopanax sessiliflorus fruits and quality control of active compounds. *Oxidative Medicine and Cellular Longevity, 2018.*

Kabouche, A., Kabouche, Z., Öztürk, M., Kolak, U., & Topçu, G. (2007). Antioxidant abietane diterpenoids from Salvia barrelieri. *Food Chemistry*, *102*(4), 1281-1287.

Kakkar, P., Das, B., & Viswanathan, P. N. (1984). A modified spectrophotometric assay of superoxide dismutase. *Indian Journal of Biochemistry and Biophysics*, 21, 131-132.

Kandsi, F., Conte, R., Marghich, M., Lafdil, F. Z., Alajmi, M. F., Bouhrim, M., Mechchate, H., Hano, C., Aziz, M., & Gseyra, N. (2021). Phytochemical analysis, antispasmodic, myorelaxant, and antioxidant effect of *Dysphania ambrosioides* (L.) mosyakin and clemants flower hydroethanolic extracts and its chloroform and ethyl acetate fractions. *Molecules*, *26*(23), 7300.

Karakaş, F. P., Yildirim, A., & Türker, A. (2012). Biological screening of various medicinal plant extracts for antibacterial and antitumor activities. *Turkish Journal of Biology*, *36*(6), 641-652.

Kasture, S. B. (2006). A Handbook of Experiments in preclinical pharmacology. Vol. 1. Nashik, India: Career Publications, pp. 43-110.

Kau, S. T., Keddie, J. R., & Andrews, D. (1984). A method for screening diuretic agents in the rat. *Journal of Pharmacological Pethods*, *11*(1), 67-75.

Khadayat, K., Marasini, B. P., Gautam, H., Ghaju, S., & Parajuli, N. (2020). Evaluation of the alpha-amylase inhibitory activity of Nepalese medicinal plants used in the treatment of diabetes mellitus. *Clinical Phytoscience*, *6*(1), 1-8.

Kikuzaki, H., Usuguchi, J., & NAKATANI, N. (1991). Constitutents of Zingiberaceae. I. Diarylheptanoids from the rhizomes of ginger (Zingiber officinale Roscoe). *Chemical and Pharmaceutical Bulletin*, *39*(1), 120-122.

Kiran, P. M., Raju, A. V., & Rao, B. G. (2012). Investigation of hepatoprotective activity of Cyathea gigantea (Wall. ex. Hook.) leaves against paracetamol–induced hepatotoxicity in rats. *Asian Pacific Journal of Tropical Biomedicine*, *2*(5), 352-356.

Kodama, T., FUKUI, K., & KOMETANI, K. (1986). The initial phosphate burst in ATP hydrolysis by myosin and subfragment-1 as studied by a modified malachite green method for determination of inorganic phosphate. *The Journal of Biochemistry*, *99*(5), 1465-1472.

Kohn, L. K., Foglio, M. A., Rodrigues, R. A., Sousa, I. D. O., Martini, M. C., Padilla, M. A., de Lima Neto, D. F., & Arns, C. W. (2015). In-vitro antiviral activities of extracts of plants of the Brazilian cerrado against the avian metapneumovirus (aMPV). *Brazilian Journal of Poultry Science*, *17*, 275-280.

Kooy, N. W., Royall, J. A., Ischiropoulos, H., & Beckman, J. S. (1994). Peroxynitrite-mediated oxidation of dihydrorhodamine 123. *Free Radical Biology and Medicine*, *16*(2), 149-156.

Kozak, W., Kluger, M. J., Tesfaigzi, J., Kozak, A., Mayfield, K. P., Wachulec, M., & Dokladny, K. (2000). Molecular mechanisms of fever and endogenous antipyresis. *Annals of the New York Academy of Sciences*, *917*(1), 121-134.

Kumar, A., D'Souza, P., & Bhargavan, D. (2013). Evaluation of renal protective activity of *Adhatoda zeylanica* (medic) leaves extract in wistar rats. *Journal of Health and Allied Sciences NU*, *3*(04), 045-056.

Kumar, M. R., Reddy, K. S., Reddy, A. G., Reddy, R. A., Anjaneyulu, Y., & Reddy, D. G. (2011). Lead-induced hepatotoxicity and evaluation of certain anti-stress adaptogens in poultry. *Toxicology International*, *18*(1), 62.

Kumar, S., Batra, C., Kataria, S. P., Arora, B., Singh, G., NayanRattan, K., & Ratan, S. (2007). Annals of Diagnostic. *Annals of Diagnostic Paediatric Pathology*, *11*(1-2), 21-23.

Kunchandy, E., & Rao, M. N. A. (1990). Oxygen radical scavenging activity of curcumin. *International Journal of Pharmaceutics*, *58*(3), 237-240.

Langford, D. J., Bailey, A. L., Chanda, M. L., Clarke, S. E., Drummond, T. E., Echols, S., Glick, S., Ingrao, J., Klassen-Ross, T., LaCroix-Fralish, M. L., & Mogil, J. S. (2010). Coding of facial expressions of pain in the laboratory mouse. *Nature Methods*, *7*(6), 447-449.

Lanza, G. A., Careri, G., & Crea, F. (2011). Mechanisms of coronary artery spasm. *Circulation*, *124*(16), 1774-1782.

Lasker, S. E., Iatropoulos, M. J., Hecht, S. S., Misra, B., Amin, S., Zang, E., & Williams, G. M. (1992). N-ethyl-N-nitrosourea induced brain tumors in rats monitored by nuclear magnetic resonance imaging, plasma proton nuclear magnetic resonance spectroscopy and microscopy. *Cancer Letters*, *67*(2-3), 125-131.

Li, Z., Liu, Y., Wang, L., Liu, X., Chang, Q., Guo, Z., Liao, Y., Pan, R., & Fan, T. P. (2014). Memory-enhancing effects of the crude extract of *Polygala tenuifolia* on aged mice. *Evidence-Based Complementary and Alternative Medicine*, *2014*.

Liu, X., & Huang, B. (2000). Heat stress injury in relation to membrane lipid peroxidation in creeping bentgrass. *Crop Science*, *40*(2), 503-510.

Lombardi, V. R., Carrera, I., & Cacabelos, R. (2017). *In vitro* screening for cytotoxic activity of herbal extracts. *Evidence-Based Complementary and Alternative Medicine*, *2017*.

Mahomoodally, M. F., Gurib-Fakim, A., & Subratty, A. H. (2007). Effect of exogenous ATP on *Momordica charantia* Linn. (Cucurbitaceae) induced inhibition of D-glucose, L-tyrosine and fluid transport across rat everted intestinal sacs *in vitro*. *Journal of Ethnopharmacology*, *110*(2), 257-263.

Makkar, H. P. S. (1999). Quantification of tannins in tree foliage. A laboratory manual for the FAO/IAEA coordinated research project on 'Use of nuclear and related techniques to develop simple tannin assay for predicting and improving the safety and efficiency of feeding ruminants on the tanniniferous tree foliage.' Joint FAO/IAEA Division of Nuclear Techniques in Food and Agric., Vienna, Austria, pp. 1-29.

Mans, D. R., Rocha, A. B., & Schwartsmann, G. (2000). Anti-cancer drug discovery and development in Brazil: targeted plant collection as a rational strategy to acquire candidate anti-cancer compounds. *The Oncologist*, *5*(3), 185-198.

Manzocco, L., Anese, M., & Nicoli, M. C. (1998). Antioxidant properties of tea extracts as affected by processing. *LWT-Food Science and Technology*, *31*(7-8), 694-698.

Mao, L. M., Qi, X. W., Hao, J. H., Liu, H. F., Xu, Q. H., & Bu, P. L. (2015). *In vitro*, ex vivo and *in vivo* anti-hypertensive activity of Chrysophyllum cainito L. extract. *International Journal of Clinical and Experimental Medicine*, *8*(10), 17912.

Marcocci, L., Maguire, J. J., Droylefaix, M. T., & Packer, L. (1994). The nitric oxide-scavenging properties of *Ginkgo biloba* extract EGb 761. *Biochemical and Biophysical Research Communications*, *201*(2), 748-755.

Matsuo, T., Shino, A., Iwatsuka, H., & Suzuoki, Z. (1970). Induction of overt diabetes in KK mice by dietary means. *Endocrinologia Japonica*, *17*(6), 477-488.

McCord, J. M., & Fridovich, I. (1969). Superoxide dismutase: an enzymic function for erythrocuprein (hemocuprein). *Journal of Biological Chemistry*, *244*(22), 6049-6055.

McLaughlin, J. L., Rogers, L. L., & Anderson, J. E. (1998). The use of biological assays to evaluate botanicals. *Drug Information Journal*, *32*(2), 513-524.

Meharie, B. G., Amare, G. G., & Belayneh, Y. M. (2020). Evaluation of hepatoprotective activity of the crude extract and solvent fractions of clutia abyssinica (euphorbiaceae) leaf against CCl4-induced hepatotoxicity in mice. *Journal of Experimental Pharmacology*, 137-150.

Mehta, A., Sethiya, N. K., Mehta, C., & Shah, G. B. (2012). Anti–arthritis activity of roots of *Hemidesmus indicus* R. Br.(Anantmul) in rats. *Asian Pacific Journal of Tropical Medicine*, *5*(2), 130-135.

Milano, J., Rossato, M. F., Oliveira, S. M., Drewes, C., Machado, P., Beck, P., Zanatta, N., Martins, M. A., Mello, C. F., Rubin, M. A., & Bonacorso, H. G. (2008). Antinociceptive action of 4-methyl-5-trifluoromethyl-5-hydroxy-4, 5-dihydro-1H-pyrazole methyl ester in models of inflammatory pain in mice. *Life Sciences*, *83*(21-22), 739-746.

Mizushima, Y., & Kobayashi, M. (1968). Interaction of anti-inflammatory drugs with serum proteins, especially with some biologically active proteins. *Journal of Pharmacy and Pharmacology*, *20*(3), 169-173.

Mohs, R. C., & Greig, N. H. (2017). Drug discovery and development: Role of basic biological research. *Alzheimer's & Dementia: Translational Research & Clinical Interventions*, *3*(4), 651-657.

Mondal, O. A., Haque, J., Haque, E., & Khan, A. R. (2012). Repellent activity of *Abroma augusta* extracts against *Tribolium castaneum* (herbst) adults. *Journal of Bio-Science*, *20*, 49-55.

Mopuri, R., Ganjayi, M., Banavathy, K. S., Parim, B. N., & Meriga, B. (2015). Evaluation of anti-obesity activities of ethanolic extract of *Terminalia paniculata* bark on high fat diet-induced obese rats. *BMC Complementary and Alternative medicine*, *15*, 1-11.

Mousa, Y. J. (2019). Analgesic, antipyretic and anti-inflammatory efficacy of ketorolac in the chicks. *Indian Journal of Animal Science*, *89*(10), 1086-1090.

Müller, T. D., Blüher, M., Tschöp, M. H., & DiMarchi, R. D. (2022). Anti-obesity drug discovery: advances and challenges. *Nature Reviews Drug Discovery*, *21*(3), 201-223.

Muruganandam, A. V., Kumar, V. I. K. A. S., & Bhattacharya, S. K. (2000). Status report on neuropharmacology. *Indian Journal of Pharmacology*, *32*(4), S119-S133.

Mythilypriya, R., Shanthi, P., & Sachdanandam, P. (2008). Salubrious effect of Kalpaamruthaa, a modified indigenous preparation in adjuvant-induced arthritis in rats—a biochemical approach. *Chemico-Biological Interactions*, *173*(2), 148-158.

Najam, R., & Anser, H. (2011). Behavioral and memory boosting effects of intellan and cyanocobalamin in mice. *Journal of Pharmacy and Nutrition Sciences*, *1*(1), 28-33.

Ndhlala, A. R., Muchuweti, M., Mupure, C., Chitindingu, K., Murenje, T., Kasiyamhuru, A., & Benhura, M. A. (2008). Phenolic content and profiles of selected wild fruits of Zimbabwe: Ximenia caffra, Artobotrys brachypetalus and Syzygium cordatum. *International Journal of Food Science & Technology*, *43*(8), 1333-1337.

Nemudzivhadi, V., & Masoko, P. (2014). *In vitro* assessment of cytotoxicity, antioxidant, and anti-inflammatory activities of *Ricinus communis* (Euphorbiaceae) leaf extracts. *Evidence-Based Complementary and Alternative Medicine*, *2014*.

Newbould, B. B. (1963). Chemotherapy of arthritis induced in rats by mycobacterial adjuvant. *British Journal of Pharmacology and Chemotherapy*, *21*(1), 127-136.

Nipanikar, S. U., Chitlange, S. S., & Nagore, D. (2017). Pharmacological evaluation of hepatoprotective activity of AHPL/AYTAB/0613 tablet in carbon tetrachloride-, ethanol-, and paracetamol-induced hepatotoxicity models in Wistar albino rats. *Pharmacognosy Research*, *9*(Suppl 1), S41.

Nishioka, T., Kawabata, J., & Aoyama, Y. (1998). Baicalein, an α-glucosidase inhibitor from *Scutellaria baicalensis*. *Journal of Natural Products*, *61*(11), 1413-1415.

Nolan, J. J., Ludvik, B., Baloga, J., Reichart, D., & Olefsky, J. M. (1997). Mechanisms of the kinetic defect in insulin action in obesity and NIDDM. *Diabetes*, *46*(6), 994-1000.

Noro, T., Oda, Y., Miyase, T., Ueno, A., & Fukushima, S. (1983). Inhibitors of xanthine oxidase from the flowers and buds of Daphne genkwa. *Chemical and Pharmaceutical Bulletin*, *31*(11), 3984-3987.

Obese, E., Biney, R. P., Henneh, I. T., Adakudugu, E. A., Anokwah, D., Agyemang, L. S., Woode, E., & Ameyaw, E. O. (2021). The Anticonvulsant Effect of Hydroethanolic Leaf Extract of *Calotropis procera* (Ait) R. Br.(Apocynaceae). *Neural Plasticity*, *2021*.

OECD. (2017). Test No. 402: acute dermal toxicity.

Ohkawa, H., Ohishi, N., & Yagi, K. (1979). Assay for lipid peroxides in animal tissues by thiobarbituric acid reaction. *Analytical Biochemistry*, *95*(2), 351-358.

Oliveira, G. L. D. S., Oliveira, F. R. D. A. M. D., Alencar, M. V. O. B. D., Gomes Junior, A. L., Souza, A. A. D., Cavalcante, A. A. D. C. M., & Freitas, R. M. D. (2014). Evaluation of antioxidant capacity of the aqueous extract of *Cynara scolymus* L. (Asteraceae) *in vitro* and in *Saccharomyces cerevisiae*. *African Journal of Pharmacy and Pharmacology*, *8*, 136-147.

Ottolenghi, A. (1959). Interaction of ascorbic acid and mitochondrial lipides. *Archives of Biochemistry and Biophysics*, *79*, 355-363.

Ou, B., Huang, D., Hampsch-Woodill, M., Flanagan, J. A., & Deemer, E. K. (2002). Analysis of antioxidant activities of common vegetables employing oxygen radical absorbance capacity (ORAC) and ferric reducing antioxidant power (FRAP) assays:

a comparative study. *Journal of Agricultural and Food Chemistry*, *50*(11), 3122-3128.

Oyedapo, O. O., & Famurewa, A. J. (1995). Antiprotease and membrane stabilizing activities of extracts of Fagara zanthoxyloides, Olax subscorpioides and *Tetrapleura tetraptera*. *International Journal of Pharmacognosy*, *33*(1), 65-69.

Oyeleke, M. B., Oni, H. T., Arokoyo, O. L., & Owoyele, B. V. (2022). Therapeutic effects of crude extracts of Bacopa floribunda on beta-amyloid 1-42-induced Alzheimer's disease via suppression of dyslipidemia, systemic inflammation and oxidative stress in male Wistar Rats. *Heliyon*, *8*(4).

Patel, S., Meldrum, B. S., & Fine, A. (1988). Susceptibility to pilocarpine-induced seizures in rats increases with age. *Behavioural Brain Research*, *31*(2), 165-167.

Patel, S., Sharma, V., Chauhan, N. S., Thakur, M., & Dixit, V. K. (2015). Evaluation of hair growth promoting activity of *Phyllanthus niruri*. *Avicenna journal of phytomedicine*, *5*(6), 512.

Patil, K. S., & Suryavanshi, J. (2007). Effect of Celastrus paniculatus Willd. seed on adjuvant induced arthritis in rats. *Pharmacognosy Magazine*, *3*(11), 177-181.

Pavlicevic, M., Marmiroli, N., & Maestri, E. (2022). Immunomodulatory peptides—A promising source for novel functional food production and drug discovery. *Peptides*, *148*, 170696.

Pellow, S., Chopin, P., File, S. E., & Briley, M. (1985). Validation of open: closed arm entries in an elevated plus-maze as a measure of anxiety in the rat. *Journal of Neuroscience Methods*, *14*(3), 149-167.

Pereira, W. S., da Silva, G. P., Vigliano, M. V., Leal, N. R., Pinto, F. A., Fernandes, D. C., Santos, S. V., Martino, T., Nascimento, J. R., de Azevedo, A. P. S., & Coelho, M. G. (2018). Anti-arthritic properties of crude extract from *Chenopodium ambrosioides* L. leaves. *Journal of Pharmacy and Pharmacology*, *70*(8), 1078-1091.

Peterson, G. L. (1983). Determination of total protein. *Methods in Enzymology*, *91*, 95-119.

Porsolt, R. D., Deniel, M., & Jalfre, M. (1979). Forced swimming in rats: hypothermia, immobility and the effects of imipramine. *European Journal of Pharmacology*, *57*(4), 431-436.

Porsolt, R. D., Le Pichon, M., & Jalfre, M. L. (1977). Depression: a new animal model sensitive to antidepressant treatments. *Nature*, *266*(5604), 730-732.

Prasad, S., Kashyap, R. S., Deopujari, J. Y., Purohit, H. J., Taori, G. M., & Daginawala, H. F. (2007). Effect of *Fagonia arabica* (Dhamasa) on *in vitro* thrombolysis. *BMC Complementary and Alternative Medicine*, *7*(1), 1-6.

Prieto, P., Pineda, M., & Aguilar, M. (1999). Spectrophotometric quantitation of antioxidant capacity through the formation of a phosphomolybdenum complex: specific application to the determination of vitamin E. *Analytical Biochemistry*, *269*(2), 337-341.

Prior, R. L., Hoang, H. A., Gu, L., Wu, X., Bacchiocca, M., Howard, L., Huang, D., Ou, B., & Jacob, R. (2003). Assays for hydrophilic and lipophilic antioxidant capacity (oxygen radical absorbance capacity (ORACFL)) of plasma and other biological and food samples. *Journal of Agricultural and Food Chemistry*, *51*(11), 3273-3279.

Rakotonirina, V. S., Bum, E. N., Rakotonirina, A., & Bopelet, M. (2001). Sedative properties of the decoction of the rhizome of *Cyperus articulatus*. *Fitoterapia*, *72*(1), 22-29.

Rao, B. K., Kesavulu, M. M., Giri, R., & Rao, C. A. (1999). Antidiabetic and hypolipidemic effects of *Momordica cymbalaria* Hook. fruit powder in alloxan-diabetic rats. *Journal of Ethnopharmacology*, *67*(1), 103-109.

Rees, D. A., & Alcolado, J. C. (2005). Animal models of diabetes mellitus. *Diabetic Medicine*, *22*(4), 359-370.

René, K., Vidal, P. K. E., Christine, F. M., Véronique, P. N. B., & Magloire, B. S. (2005). *Shigella dysenteriae* type 1-induced diarrhea in rats. *Japanese Journal of Infectious Diseases*, *58*(6), 335.

Robak, J., & Gryglewski, R. J. (1988). Flavonoids are scavengers of superoxide anions. *Biochemical Pharmacology*, *37*(5), 837-841.

Robert, A., Nezamis, J. E., Lancaster, C., Hanchar, A. J., & Klepper, M. S. (1976). Enteropooling assay: a test for diarrhea produced by prostaglandins. *Prostaglandins*, *11*(5), 809-828.

Rodrigues, M. R. A., Kanazawa, L. K. S., das Neves, T. L. M., da Silva, C. F., Horst, H., Pizzolatti, M. G., Santos, A. R. S., Baggio, C. H., & de Paula Werner, M. F. (2012). Antinociceptive and anti-inflammatory potential of extract and isolated compounds from the leaves of Salvia officinalis in mice. *Journal of Ethnopharmacology*, *139*(2), 519-526.

Roh, C., & Jung, U. (2012). Screening of crude plant extracts with anti-obesity activity. *International Journal of Molecular Sciences*, *13*(2), 1710-1719.

Ruch, R. J., Cheng, S. J., & Klaunig, J. E. (1989). Prevention of cytotoxicity and inhibition of intercellular communication by antioxidant catechins isolated from Chinese green tea. *Carcinogenesis*, *10*(6), 1003-1008.

Rumlová, M., & Ruml, T. (2018). *In vitro* methods for testing antiviral drugs. *Biotechnology Advances*, *36*(3), 557-576.

Sabino, K. C. C., Castro, F. A., Oliveira, J. C. R., Dalmau, S. R. A., & Coelho, M. G. P. (1999). Successful treatment of collagen-induced arthritis in mice with a hydroalcohol extract of seeds of Pterodon pubescens. *Phytotherapy Research: An International Journal Devoted to Pharmacological and Toxicological Evaluation of Natural Product Derivatives*, *13*(7), 613-615.

Sadasivudu, B., Rao, T. I., & Murthy, C. R. (1977). Acute metabolic effects of ammonia in mouse brain. *Neurochemical Research*, *2*, 639-655.

Sadraei, H., Ghanadian, M., Asghari, G., Madadi, E., & Azali, N. (2014). Antispasmodic and antidiarrhoeal activities of 6-(4-hydroxy-3-methoxyphenyl)-hexanonic acid from *Pycnocycla spinosa* Decne. exBoiss. *Research in Pharmaceutical Sciences*, *9*(4), 279.

Sancheti, S., Sancheti, S., Lee, S. H., Lee, J. E., & Seo, S. Y. (2011). Screening of Korean medicinal plant extracts for α-glucosidase inhibitory activities. *Iranian Journal of Pharmaceutical Research: IJPR*, *10*(2), 261.

Schiller, L. R. (2000). Diarrhea. *Medical Clinics of North America*, *84*(5), 1259-1274.

Scholz, G., Pohl, I., Genschow, E., Klemm, M., & Spielmann, H. (1999). Embryotoxicity screening using embryonic stem cells *in vitro*: correlation to *in vivo* teratogenicity. *Cells Tissues Organs*, *165*(3-4), 203-211.

Schotz, M. C., Garfinkel, A. S., Huebotter, R. J., & Stewart, J. E. (1970). A rapid assay for lipoprotein lipase. *Journal of Lipid Research*, *11*(1), 68-69.

Seeram, N. P., Henning, S. M., Niu, Y., Lee, R., Scheuller, H. S., & Heber, D. (2006). Catechin and caffeine content of green tea dietary supplements and correlation with antioxidant capacity. *Journal of Agricultural and Food Chemistry*, *54*(5), 1599-1603.

Sera, N. C. E., Aguilar, Y. M., Rosabal, A. E., & Dairon, M. Ã. (2017). Antidiarrheal Effects of *Anacardium occidentale* L. Leaf Powder on Newborn Chicks. *Revista de Producción Animal*, *29*(3), 47-54.

Shahed-Al-Mahmud, M., & Lina, S. M. M. (2017). Evaluation of sedative and anxiolytic activities of methanol extract of leaves of *Persicaria hydropiper* in mice. *Clinical Phytoscience*, *3*, 1-12.

Shamsa, F., Monsef, H., Ghamooshi, R., & Verdian-rizi, M. (2008). Spectrophotometric determination of total alkaloids in some Iranian medicinal plants. *The Thai Journal of Pharmaceutical Sciences*, *32*(1), 17-20.

Sharma, L. D., Bahga, H. S., & Srivastava, P. S. (1971). *In vitro* anthelmintic screening of indigenous medicinal plants against *Haemonchus contortus* (Rudolphi, 1803) Cobbold, 1898 of sheep and goats. *Indian Journal of Animal Research*, *5*(1), 33-38.

Shi, J., Weng, J. H., & Mitchison, T. J. (2021). Immunomodulatory drug discovery from herbal medicines: Insights from organ-specific activity and xenobiotic defenses. *Elife*, *10*, e73673.

Shinde, U. A., Phadke, A. S., Nair, A. M., Mungantiwar, A. A., Dikshit, V. J., & Saraf, M. N. (1999). Membrane stabilizing activity—a possible mechanism of action for the anti-inflammatory activity of *Cedrus deodara* wood oil. *Fitoterapia*, *70*(3), 251-257.

Singal, P. K., Kapur, N., Dhillon, K. S., Beamish, R. E., & Dhalla, N. S. (1982). Role of free radicals in catecholamine-induced cardiomyopathy. *Canadian Journal of Physiology and Pharmacology*, *60*(11), 1390-1397.

Singh, U., Tabibian, J., Venugopal, S. K., Devaraj, S., & Jialal, I. (2005). Development of an *in vitro* screening assay to test the antiinflammatory properties of dietary supplements and pharmacologic agents. *Clinical Chemistry*, *51*(12), 2252-2256.

Somani, R. R., Kadam, G., Vohra, R., Vijayaraghavan, S., & Shirodkar, P. Y. (2010). Studies of CNS activities of some mannich bases of 1, 3, 4-oxadiazole. *International journal of Pharmacology*, *6*(5), 696-704.

Stein, R. L. (1985). Catalysis by human leukocyte elastase: III. Steady-state kinetics for the hydrolysis of p-nitrophenyl esters. *Archives of Biochemistry and Biophysics*, *236*(2), 677-680.

Stepek, G., Buttle, D. J., Duce, I. R., Lowe, A., & Behnke, J. M. (2005). Assessment of the anthelmintic effect of natural plant cysteine proteinases against the gastrointestinal nematode, *Heligmosomoides polygyrus*, *in vitro*. *Parasitology*, *130*(2), 203-211.

Stern, S., & Bayes de Luna, A. (2009). Coronary artery spasm: a 2009 update. *Circulation*, *119*(18), 2531-2534.

Sunilson, J. A. J., Anandarajagopal, K., Kumari, A. V. A. G., & Mohan, S. (2009). Antidiarrhoeal activity of leaves of *Melastoma malabathricum* Linn. *Indian Journal of Pharmaceutical Sciences*, *71*(6), 691.

Tadesse, W. T., Hailu, A. E., Gurmu, A. E., & Mechesso, A. F. (2014). Experimental assessment of antidiarrheal and antisecretory activity of 80% methanolic leaf extract of Zehneria scabra in mice. *BMC Complementary and Alternative Medicine*, *14*, 1-8.

Takagi, K., Watanabe, M., & Saito, H. (1971). Studies of the spontaneous movement of animals by the hole cross test; effect of 2-dimethyl-aminoethanol and its acyl esters on the central nervous system. *The Japanese Journal of Pharmacology*, *21*(6), 797-810.

Tang, X. C., Lin, Z. G., Cai, W., Chen, N., & Shen, L. (1984). Anti-inflammatory effect of 3-acetylaconitine. *Zhongguo yao li xue bao= Acta Pharmacologica Sinica*, *5*(2), 85-89.

Taniguchi, N., Kanai, S., Kawamoto, M., Endo, H., & Higashino, H. (2004). Study on application of static magnetic field for adjuvant arthritis rats. *Evidence-Based Complementary and Alternative Medicine*, *1*, 187-191.

Tesfaye, B. A., Berhe, A. H., Wondafrash, D. Z., & Berhe, D. F. (2021). Cardioprotective effect of crude extract and solvent fractions of Urtica simensis leaves on cyclophosphamide-induced myocardial injury in rats. *Journal of Experimental Pharmacology*, 147-160.

Tessema, Z., & Molla, Y. (2021). Evaluation of the wound healing activity of the crude extract of root bark of Brucea antidysentrica, the leaves of *Dodonaea angustifolia* and Rhamnus prinoides in mice. *Heliyon*, *7*(1).

Than, A., Kulkarni, H. J., Hmone, W., & Tha, S. J. (1989). Anti-diarrhoeal efficacy of some Burmese indigenous drug formulations in experimental diarrhoeal test models. *International Journal of Crude Drug Research*, *27*(4), 195-200.

Toda, M., Kawabata, J., & Kasai, T. (2000). α-Glucosidase inhibitors from clove (Syzgium aromaticum). *Bioscience, Biotechnology, and Biochemistry*, *64*(2), 294-298.

Tokofai, B. M., Idoh, K., Oke, O. E., & Agbonon, A. (2021). Hepatoprotective effects of Vernonia amygdalina (Astereaceae) extract on CCl4-induced liver injury in broiler chickens. *Animals*, *11*(12), 3371.

Torres-González, L., Cienfuegos-Pecina, E., Perales-Quintana, M. M., Alarcon-Galvan, G., Muñoz-Espinosa, L. E., Pérez-Rodríguez, E., & Cordero-Pérez, P. (2018). Nephroprotective effect of *Sonchus oleraceus* extract against kidney injury induced by ischemia-reperfusion in wistar rats. *Oxidative Medicine and Cellular Longevity*, *2018*.

Tran, N., Pham, B., & Le, L. (2020). Bioactive compounds in anti-diabetic plants: From herbal medicine to modern drug discovery. *Biology*, *9*(9), 252.

Turner, R. A. (1965). Screening Methods in pharmacology. Academy Press, New York. Vol. 11, pp. 113.

Tyler, T. D., & Tessel, R. E. (1979). A new device for the simultaneous measurement of locomotor and stereotypic frequency in mice. *Psychopharmacology*, *64*, 285-290.

Várady, M., Bjørn, H., Craven, J., & Nansen, P. (1997). *In vitro* characterization of lines of *Oesophagostomum dentatum* selected or not selected for resistance to pyrantel, levamisole and ivermectin. *International Journal for Parasitology*, *27*(1), 77-81.

Vianna, R. M. J., Ongali, B., Regoli, D., Calixto, J. B., & Couture, R. (2003). Up-regulation of kinin B1 receptor in the lung of streptozotocin-diabetic rat: autoradiographic and functional evidence. *British Journal of Pharmacology*, *138*(1), 13-22.

Viswanatha, G. L., Venkataranganna, M. V., Prasad, N. B. L., & Ashok, G. (2016). Evaluation of anti-epileptic activity of leaf extracts of *Punica granatum* on experimental models of epilepsy in mice. *Journal of Intercultural Ethnopharmacology*, *5*(4), 415.

Vogel, H. (2007). Drug Discovery and Evaluation: Pharmacological Assays. Berlin: Springer Science and Business Media 2007.

Warnick, J. E., Huang, C. J., Acevedo, E. O., & Sufka, K. J. (2009). Modelling the anxiety-depression continuum in chicks. *Journal of Psychopharmacology*, *23*(2), 143-156.

Warriar, P., Barve, K., & Prabhakar, B. (2019). Anti-arthritic effect of garcinol enriched fraction against adjuvant induced arthritis. *Recent Patents on Inflammation & Allergy Drug Discovery*, *13*(1), 49-56.

Wibbenmeyer, L., Sevier, A., Liao, J., Williams, I., Latenser, B., Lewis, R., Kealey, P., & Rosenquist, R. (2011). Evaluation of the usefulness of two established pain assessment tools in a burn population. *Journal of Burn Care & Research*, *32*(1), 52-60.

Williams, A. R., Fryganas, C., Ramsay, A., Mueller-Harvey, I., & Thamsborg, S. M. (2014). Direct anthelmintic effects of condensed tannins from diverse plant sources against *Ascaris suum*. *PloS one*, *9*(5), e97053.

Willoughby, L. F., Schlosser, T., Manning, S. A., Parisot, J. P., Street, I. P., Richardson, H. E., Humbert, P. O., & Brumby, A. M. (2013). An *in vivo* large-scale chemical screening platform using Drosophila for anti-cancer drug discovery. *Disease Models & Mechanisms*, *6*(2), 521-529.

Wood, J. L. (1970). In: Fishman, W. H. (Ed.), In: *Metabolic Conjugation and Metabolic Hydrolysis,* vol. II. Academic Press, New York, pp. 61-299.

World Health Organization. (1981). Instructions for determining the susceptibility or resistance of adult mosquitoes to organochlorine, organophosphate and carbamate insecticides: diagnostic test. Geneva: WHO/VBC/, pp.81-807.

World Health Organization. (2009). *Guidelines for efficacy testing of mosquito repellents for human skins*. WHO/HTM/NTD/ WHOPES/2009.WHO: Gevena, pp. 4-18.

WS, R. (2006). Rasband, WS, ImageJ, US National Institutes of Health, Bethesda, Maryland, USA.

Xu, J., Song, X., Yin, Z. Q., Cheng, A. C., Jia, R. Y., Deng, Y. X., Ye, K. C., Shi, C. F., Lv, C., & Zhang, W. (2012). Antiviral activity and mode of action of extracts from neem seed kernel against duck plague virus *in vitro*. *Poultry Science*, *91*(11), 2802-2807.

Yahaya, T. A., Okhale, S. E., & Adeola, S. O. (2014). Neuropharmacological effects of standardized aqueous stem bark extract of *Parkia biglobossa* in Wistar rats. *Avicenna Journal of Phytomedicine*, *4*(1), 59.

Yang, Z. G., Sun, H. X., & Fang, W. H. (2005). Haemolytic activities and adjuvant effect of Astragalus membranaceus saponins (AMS) on the immune responses to ovalbumin in mice. *Vaccine*, *23*(44), 5196-5203.

Yemitan, O. K. (2008). *Pharmacological and Toxicity Studies of the Aqueous Root Extract of Dalbergia Saxatilis Hook, F. (Papilionaceae)* (Doctoral dissertation, University of Lagos (Nigeria)).

Yoshiyama, Y., Sugiyama, T., & Kanke, M. (2005). Experimental diabetes model in chick embryos treated with streptozotocin. *Biological and Pharmaceutical Bulletin*, *28*(10), 1986-1988.

Yuan, L., Wang, Y., Lu, C., & Li, X. (2013). Angiotensin-converting enzyme 2 deficiency aggravates glucose intolerance via impairment of islet microvascular density in mice with high-fat diet. *Journal of Diabetes Research*, *2013*.

Yuan, X., Wang, J., Yao, H., & Chen, F. (2005). Free radical-scavenging capacity and inhibitory activity on rat erythrocyte hemolysis of feruloyl oligosaccharides from wheat bran insoluble dietary fiber. *LWT-Food Science and Technology*, *38*(8), 877-883.

Zafar, F., Jahan, N., Khan, A., & Akram, W. (2015). Cardioprotective potential of polyphenolic rich green combination in catecholamine induced myocardial necrosis in rabbits. *Evidence-Based Complementary and Alternative Medicine*, *2015*.

Zhang, J., & Kirkham, M. B. (1994). Drought-stress-induced changes in activities of superoxide dismutase, catalase, and peroxidase in wheat species. *Plant and Cell Physiology*, *35*(5), 785-791.

Zhong, W., Shahbaz, O., Teskey, G., Beever, A., Kachour, N., Venketaraman, V., & Darmani, N. A. (2021). Mechanisms of nausea and vomiting: current knowledge and recent advances in intracellular emetic signaling systems. *International journal of molecular sciences*, *22*(11), 5797.

Zimmerman, M. (1983). Ethical guidelines for investigations of experimental pain in conscious animals. *Pain*, *16*(2), 109-110.

Chapter 10

Biopharmaceutical Studies

10.1. Absorption Assays

10.1.1. *In Vitro* Permeation Test (Franz Diffusion Model)

The Franz diffusion cells (Figure 10.1) consist of glass (contact area: 4.7 cm^2) prepped with a silanizing chemical. A membrane separates the donor (A) and the receptor compartment (B). A clamp holds these compartments together. Diffusion media are housed in the 37-mL-sized receptor compartment. Running water through an outer water jacket is required to keep the temperature at 37 °C. A specified amount of test drug or sample is kept in compartment A. It is done after 30 minutes of acclimatization of the separating membrane to the receptor solution. To stop the solvent from evaporating, parafilm is then placed over compartment A. A bar magnet that spins constantly (at 400 rpm) agitates the receptor solution. At various times, 2.0 mL aliquots of receptor solution samples are collected using the receptor compartment's sampling port. To maintain a constant volume of receptor solution within compartment B, the cells are replenished with the solution (Bhise et al. 2010).

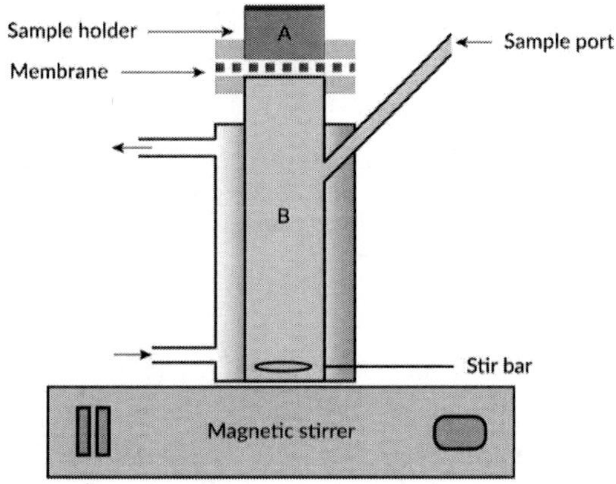

Figure 10.1. Franz diffusion chamber instrumentation

Step 1. Prepare a suitable receptor solution, for example, Sorensen's phosphate buffer-Solution A: 3.5% disodium hydrogen phosphate. Solution B: 2.76% sodium dihydrogen phosphate. Mix 40.5 mL of solution A with 9.5 mL of solution B and adjust the volume to 100 mL.

Step 2. Create a calibration standard curve.

Step 3. Place a cellophane membrane between compartments A and B.

Step 4. 37 mL of receptor solution should be placed in the receptor compartment (pH 7.4). By pumping the contents of a thermostatic water bath through the cell's outer layer, one can maintain a constant temperature (37 ^{o}C) within the cell. Throughout the experiment, place a Teflon-coated magnetic bar inside the cell to stir compartment B's contents at 600 rpm. The membrane should touch the receptor medium properly.

Step 5. Keep the required amount of your test sample in compartment A and cover it with aluminum foil. This will prevent the evaporation of the solvent. At regular intervals, take 2 mL of the receptor sample out of compartment B and replace it right away with 2 mL of the receptor solution kept at a constant temperature.

Step 6. Dilute the withdrawn samples if required and analyze them spectrophotometrically at a specified wavelength (at which the test sample shows maximum absorbance).

Step 7. Determine the amount of your test sample diffused by using the standard calibration curve.

Step 9. Make permeability coefficient calculations using the formula below.

$$K_p = J_{ss} \div C_v$$

where, K_p = permeability coefficient (cm/h), J_{ss} = flux (mg/cm /hr), C_v = initial concentration of the drug in the donor compartment (mg).

10.1.2. Percutaneous Absorption Test (Multiple Membrane Model)

Molecules with low MW and lipophilicity can easily pass through the ellophane membrane. Therefore, you should avoid using it. You can use a number of natural membranes for this purpose. Medications that are hydrophilic will easily pass through onion membranes, whereas drugs that are lipophilic will easily pass through egg membranes. Natural membranes can be employed for diffusion research because they include hydrophilic pores and channels that allow tiny to medium-sized hydrophilic medicines to infiltrate and disperse in a manner akin to that of human skin (Panchagnula and Thomas 2000; Bhise et al. 2010).

Step 1. For this purpose, use 0.05 M PBS (pH 7.4).
Step 2. Prepare a standard calibration curve.
Step 3. Prepare the membrane(s) as follows:

1. Shave the rat's belly hair, then cut the skin samples to their full thickness. Wash the rat's skin off with water. Fat and connective tissues should be carefully removed, and the skin should be exposed to receptor liquid (0.05 M PBS; pH 7.4) for 60 minutes.
2. *Allium cepa* L. (onion)'s central membrane should be carefully peeled off to create a consistent membrane measuring at least 10 cm without any cracks or openings.
3. *Gallus domesticus* eggs have a calcified outer shell membrane (inside the shell). You can make this membrane by soaking the egg in a 0.01 N HCl solution for 6 hrs. This will dissolve the calcified layer. Carefully cut the membrane to release the egg's contents, then rinse it with a regular saline solution.
4. Examine the membrane's consistency and integrity under a microscope.

Step 4. Release and permeation test:

1. By using various membranes constructed as described above, calculate the amount of your test sample molecules diffused by using the dialysis cell technique.
2. Put a rat's skin over the tube. 50 mL of the receptor phase should be added to a 100 mL beaker in which the tube should be submerged (0.05 M PBS; pH 7.4).
3. Throughout the trials, stir the receptor phase continually with a tiny magnetic bar at a speed of 100 rpm in order to maintain homogeneity and a temperature of 37 °C.
4. Apply a predetermined amount of the formulation to the membrane. Remove the sample and measure the absorbance spectrophotometrically at 320 nm at predefined intervals.
5. Use egg membrane, onion, and cellophane for the same study.
6. Utilize the standard calibration curve to calculate the amount of MTD dispersed.

7. Determine the slope of the linear component of the graph by plotting it against time and the amount of drug dispersed per unit area.
8. Make permeability coefficient calculations using the formula below.

$$K_p = J_{ss} \div C_v$$

where, K_p = permeability coefficient (cm/h), J_{ss} = flux (mg/cm /hr), C_v = initial concentration of the drug in the donor compartment (mg).

10.2. Protein Binding Assays

Protein-binding may change at the point of action, the effective concentration, and/or the rate of elimination of the drug molecule, thus affecting the length of time for which effective concentrations are maintained. Protein binding capacity also refers to a drug molecule's ability to bind to its specific receptor, which is responsible for the desired therapeutic effect (Panchagnula and Thomas 2000; Bhise et al. 2010). An example of a popular protein-binding assay is given below.

10.2.1. Filter Paper Assay

According to Makkar (1999):

Step 1. Prepare the following reagents:

1. *Tannic acid solution*: It's 0.1 mg ascorbic acid containing 0.1% tannic acid solution in 50% methanol.
2. *Acetate buffer* (0.05 M, pH 5.0): It is a 0.36% (v/v) glacial acetic acid solution at pH 5.0 maintained by using a 4 N NaOH solution.
3. *Bovine serum albumin (BSA) solution*: It is 0.2% BSA in 100 mL of acetate buffer (pH 5.0, 0.05 M).
4. *Dye solution*: It is a 3% (w/v) trichloroacetic acid (TCA) solution containing 0.2 g of Ponceau S dye.

5. *Acetic acid solution* (0.2%): It is a 2% (v/v) glacial acetic acid solution.
6. *NaOH (sodium hydroxide) solution* (0.1 N): It is a 0.4% (w/v) NaOH solution.
7. *Acetic acid solution* (10%): It is a 10% (v/v) aqueous solution.

Step 2. Prepare the plant extract

Use acetone for this purpose, as it does not interfere with this method. Take 200 mg of finely crushed, dried (e.g., plant) material in a glass beaker (capacity: approximately 25 mL). 20 minutes are spent with the beaker suspended in an ultrasonic water bath after adding 10 mL of 70% aqueous acetone. If a chilled centrifuge is not available, cool the contents by storing the centrifuge tube on ice before centrifuging the mixture for 10 minutes at about 3000×*g* using a standard clinical centrifuge. Gather the supernatant and store it in the freezer. Transfer the pellet that is still in the centrifuge tube to the beaker using two portions of five milliliters of 70% aqueous acetone, and then repeat the ultrasonic treatment procedure for the remaining 20 minutes. As said before, centrifuge the mixture and collect the supernatant.

Step 3. Assay procedure

Cut a sheet of 1 MM Whatman paper for chromatography to the proper size and required number. On this sheet, make squares of roughly 1.5 - 2 cm with a light lead pencil. Apply several aliquots (5 - 25 µL, each containing 5 - 25 µg Hg tannic acid) to the sheet, at least three times, on various squares. Apply 10 - 50 µL of sample (e.g., plant extract) in the center of the squares on the chromatography sheet. After letting the spots dry, quickly mist the paper with the BSA solution until it is saturated. To get rid of the unbound BSA, wash the paper three times for 10 minutes each with the acetate buffer (pH 5, 0.05 M) after 30 minutes. After leaving the strips in the stain solution for 10 minutes, add 0.2% Ponceau S dye solution to stain the paper. Repeated tests shouldn't use the staining solution. Wash the soiled strips in a solution of 0.2% acetic acid until no more color comes off the strips. Typically, three washes are necessary to make the background visible. Cut the discoloured portions after letting the strips air dry. A chromatography sheet should be simultaneously stained and washed in the same way as other samples to prepare a comparable blank. Slice the stained region into small pieces, add 3 mL of 0.1 N sodium hydroxide solution, and vortex. Next, add

0.3 mL of 10% acetic acid, and centrifuge at around 2500 g to elute the color. Measure the color's 525 nm absorbance against the equivalent blank. Use a calibration standard curve to convert the absorbance to determine protein content. Apply various BSA concentrations (5 - 50 μg; 5 - 50 μL of 1 mg/mL BSA solution in the acetate buffer) as distinct spots (triplicated for each concentration) on a chromatography sheet and cut into strips. This will create a standard curve. Apply the dye solution to these strips, wash them, and then read the color as you would for the samples.

Note: Ascorbic acid can be added to the solvent used to extract phenols and tannins because it does not interfere with the test.

10.3. Drug Metabolism Assays

Drugs that are non-polar, lipophilic, and water-insoluble undergo the metabolic process in order to become polar, water-soluble compounds that are simple for the kidneys to eliminate. In this way, detoxification is a process of metabolism. Drug biotransformation enzymes can be broadly categorized into two types: microsomal and non-microsomal enzymes. You can isolate the microsomes from the liver homogenate's endoplasmic reticulum. Numerous oxidative, reductive, hydrolytic, and glucuronidation processes are catalyzed by the diverse array of microsomal enzymes. The cytoplasmic enzymes known as non-microsomal enzymes include those that catalyze conjugation reactions other than glucuronidation, a variety of reductive and hydrolytic processes, and a limited number of oxidation processes (Bhise et al. 2010).

10.3.1. *In Vitro* Metabolism Test

Step 1. Rats can be killed by being struck (blow) in the head, and the livers must be removed as soon as possible (25 g of liver is needed) and placed in a beaker with ice and KCl/0.01 M buffer.

Step 2. Weigh the liver and continue adding KCl/0.01 M buffer until the liver is 25% suspended in water (approx. 100 mL).

Step 3. On a cold tile or in the tared beaker beneath the buffer, cut or chop the liver into small pieces.

Take a small amount at a time and homogenize in a tissue homogenizer while exposing each fraction to 6 or 8 vertical excursions. Additionally, use an ice bucket to keep everything chilled. The suspension should be centrifuged at 10,000×*g* for 20 minutes at 4 °C. Typically, 2 × 50 mL will be adequate, and the tubes ought to be as full and evenly distributed as possible.

Step 4. To be utilized on the day of preparation, extract the supernatant (10,000×g) and store it on ice. 250 mg of liver are contained in 1 mL.

Step 5. Centrifuge the 10,000×*g* supernatant in 4 × 14 mL batches for 1 h at 100,000×*g*. Expel the supernatants by decanting them. The pellets should be resuspended in 10 mL of KCl/PBS (0.01M, pH 7.6) in the centrifuge tubes before being filled.

Step 6. Decant the supernatant after a 0.5-hour centrifugation. Pour 1 mL (or more, if necessary) of 0.05 M PBS (pH 7.6) over the pellets before storing them. Keep it at -18 °C for further research.

Step 7. Prepare a series of tests for the concentration of your test sample. Because preliminary incubation can render microsomal enzymes inactive, make these solutions using ice-cold reagents and keep the mixtures ice-cold until the experiment is started.

Step 8. Only two flasks should be kept on ice for the 0.5-hour incubation period at 37 °C with gentle shaking. After 0.5 h, bring the reaction flasks' temperature to 4 °C. If required, keep the eight flasks at -18 °C.

Step 9. Add 0.5 mL aliquots of these solutions to screw-capped tubes containing 10 mL of n-heptane containing 1.5% amyl alcohol and 1 mL of 0.5 M citrate buffer (pH 5.5) saturated with NaCl. Centrifuge after 10 minutes of shaking. Use pipettes to entirely remove the watery layer. In the same tubes, add 1.5 mL of the citrate buffer. Centrifuge after another 10 minutes of shaking. 8 mL of the heptane layer should be transferred to a new tube with 4 mL of 0.8 M PBS (pH 11.0). Centrifuge after proper shaking and measure the aqueous layer's spectrum at a specified wavelength (recommended for your test sample or standard).

10.3.2. Food Interference Test

The mixed-function oxidase (MFO) system, which is located in the liver's endoplasmic reticulum, is principally responsible for the biotransformation of medicines. It is commonly known that an animal's ability to digest medications is correlated with its nutritional state. A diet high in protein stimulates the production of the enzyme cytochrome p450 (CYP), which increases the metabolism of medicines. It has been demonstrated that dietary deficiencies in Ca, Zn, Fe, vitamin C, or thiamin can change how quickly drugs are metabolized. Additionally, some diets and dietary components may prevent your medicine from acting as intended in the body's physiological system. Food typically remains in your stomach for 40 minutes to more than 2 hours. The time spent in the small bowel should then be multiplied by 40 to 120 minutes. A medicine is absorbed into the bloodstream in the stomach and intestines after oral delivery, which typically takes 1 - 6 hours. The effects of food on drug action can be monitored by using the following method:

Example for a neurologically active test sample:

Step 1. Collect experimental animals (e.g., mice, rats, and rabbits) and maintain them in a standard environment with standard food and water ad libitum. Acclaim the animals 3 - 7 days prior to this study.

Step 2. Fasten the animals overnight (12 h) with only free access to water before starting this research. Randomly distribute the required number of animals in the control (vehicle), positive control (test sample), and 3 test groups (sample + carbohydrate diet, sample + protein diet, and sample + lipid diet). In this case, you can use food products like gluten-free, casein-free, etc.

Step 3. Give the respective treatment to the control and positive control groups orally. Do not supply food or water to these animals during the observation period.

Step 4. Give foods to the respective test groups 10 minutes prior to administering the test drug.

Step 5. Observe various neuropharmacological parameters (see the Neuropharmacological Study section) after administration of controls or a diet + sample. Compare the data among various groups and diet groups to see the effect of food interference on your sample's neurological effects.

10.4. Drug Excretion Assays

Drugs and their metabolites are expelled from the body without undergoing any chemical change through a process called urinary excretion. Therefore, molecules are excreted in their free form or their conjugates in urine, and these can be estimated spectrophotometrically. This can be assayed by using the following method (Bhise et al. 2010).

10.4.1. Urinary Excretion Test (Rat Model)

Step 1. Collect Wistar rats (average b.w.: 200 - 230 g) and maintain as mentioned above. Acclaim the animals 3 - 7 days prior to this study.

Step 2. After an overnight fast, water loading should be done by giving 10 mL of water to each rat over 1 hour. Place the individual rat in a separate metabolic cage and collect a drug-free urine sample as a blank.

Step 3. Prepare a standard calibration curve with your test sample at different concentrations. Then administer the test drug (a specified dose) with 5 mL of water to the rats. Give 5 mL of water every time to get a sufficient urine sample.

Step 4. Administer your sample orally to the animals. Collect urine samples from the laboratory animals at 30, 60, 90, 120, 180, 240, 360, and 600th minutes. Note the total amount of each urine sample that was thrown up during the period. Additionally, note the urine pH and store it at -20 ^{o}C until analysis. The amount of conjugated drug can be determined from the difference between the total drug administered and excreted total free drug in each sample collection point (period) measured in comparison to the calibration curve.

10.5. Assay of Pharmacokinetic Parameters

When a pharmacological dose is administered via an extravascular route, the drug molecules must first pass across a biological membrane for absorption. Since a drug's delivered dose is not completely absorbed at once, the plasma profile acquired after extravascular delivery of a drug differs from the plasma profile acquired when the same drug is administered as a quick intravenous bolus injection. Very recently, it has been introduced that the pharmacokinetic parameters of a drug candidate can be measured by using *in silico* models. However, you can perform this study by using animal models. An example of this study (Beconi et al. 2011) is given below.

Step 1. Prior to the administration of the dose, the animals (such as rats) should become acclimated to the research setting for 16 - 21 days. They should be kept in individual cages made of hanging wire and are generally kept on a 12-hour cycle of light and darkness. Maintain an average room temperature of 18 to 29 °C, a relative humidity of 30 to 70%, and an airflow of more than 10 fresh air changes per hour on a daily basis. Give access to regular food and water at all times, with the exception of when the animal is fasting before receiving a dose.

Step 2. Administer your test drug to the required groups (consisting of the required number of animals in each group) and routinely check body weights, perform clinical observations, and collect plasma and brain samples. Take blood samples (to make plasma) and brain samples at Collect blood (for preparation of plasma) and brain samples at 0.08, 0.25, 0.5, 1, 2, 4, 8, and 24th hours post-dose.

Step 3. Utilize the WinNonlin application (version 5.2) to determine the mean drug concentrations at each time point using non-compartmental analysis. Use either the intravascular (i.v. bolus) or extravascular (p.o. or S.C.) administration routes in this case. Then back-extrapolate the plasma concentration at time zero for the intravenous route using the first two post-dose plasma concentrations that are observed. Assume that the concentration is zero for both the p.o. and S.C. routes at time zero. For the purposes of determining the C_{mean} values or PK parameters, treat tissue and plasma concentrations that are below the limit of quantification as absent samples.

Step 4. Use the linear trapezoidal method to determine the area under the plasma concentration curve (AUC) (linear interpolation). A minimum of the final three recorded concentrations should be used to estimate the terminal elimination phase of the PK profile based on the best fit (r^2). Determine the dosing schedule, the AUC, the terminal elimination phase rate constant (k_{el}), the observed (rather than expected) plasma/brain levels, and the PK variables for each group that describe the systemic exposure to your test sample in plasma and brain. Using the equation C_t/k_{el}, where C_t stands for the last detectable concentration, calculate the percentage of the AUC from C_t to infinity. $AUC_{0-\infty}$ was calculated using the extrapolated component of the AUC. Divide the dose-normalized extravascular plasma $AUC_{0-\infty}$ by the dose-normalized intravenous plasma $AUC_{0-\infty}$ by 100 to get the percent bioavailability (%F). Make the assumption that the levels are linear. First-pass metabolism refers to the quantity of a drug that is processed or transported through absorption in the intestine and liver and does not enter systemic circulation.

Step 5. Animal plasma and brain drug concentrations are measured using an LC-MS/MS technique. Drugs are added to control brain homogenate or control plasma taken from the animals to create calibration standards. The concentrations of 1.00 - 5000 ng eq/mL for plasma, 0.500 - 2500 ng eq/mL for the brain (1 and 1.22 mg eq/kg doses), and 1.00 - 5000 ng eq/mL for the brain (10 mg eq/kg doses) are used to create three calibration curves. The lower limit of quantification (LLOQ), which is 5.58 and 9.76 nM for rat plasma and brain, respectively, is the lowest acceptable calibration standard for each experiment. In the LC-MS/MS test, use an appropriate internal standard, such as econazole nitrate.

Step 6. How to calculate the half-life ($t_{1/2}$): Pooled male rat liver microsomes (purchased commercially) are mixed with the test drug (1 M), and then the mixture is incubated at 37 °C in 0.1 M PBS. The addition of NADPH starts reactions after warming the mixture for 5 minutes (1 mM). At 0, 5, 10, 20, and 40 min, aliquots (80 L) are obtained, and the reaction is stopped right away by adding 80 µL of an analytical internal standard (for example, acetonitrile) containing (IS). Centrifuge the samples and use LC-MS/MS with multiple reaction monitoring to examine the supernatant fractions (MRM). Every incubation should be done twice. Use testosterone as a positive control. The relative decline in MRM area ratio intensity over time compared with that of the control (percent parent drop) is used to calculate the half-life ($t_{1/2}$) of your drug in the incubation. The MRM area response ratio of the analyte over IS for Time = 0 (control) is set to 100%. Half-life values are derived from the following relationships:

$$t_{1/2}\ (\text{min}) = -0.693/\lambda$$

where, λ is the slope of the Ln concentration *vs* time curve.

The intrinsic clearance (Cl_{int}) is calculated as:

$$Cl_{int} = (0.693 \text{ x incubation volume } (\mu L))/(t_{1/2} \text{ (min) x mg of microsomal protein})$$

Step 7. Drug metabolites are identified after being incubated in a mixture of rat liver microsomes. Use the identical incubation conditions as above, with the exception that the drug concentration is 10 µM, liver microsomal protein is utilized at a concentration of 1 mg/mL, and the metabolites are identified 60 minutes after incubation. Incubations of testosterone are employed as a positive control, and control incubations (T = 0 min) are used as a reference. ToF-MS collects full-scan mass spectra as precise mass. Software called Waters MassLynx™ version 4.1 (SCN 714) is used to manage the devices and collect data from them. Waters MetaboLynx™ XS software is used to query the TOF-MS spectra and produce metabolite reports.

Step 8. This can be achieved by using CacoReady TM 24-transwell plates with plated Caco cells. In Hanks' Balanced Salt Solution with 25 mM HEPES, test drugs and reference compounds (such as propranolol, digoxin, and vinblatine) are introduced at a concentration of 10 μM to either the apical or basolateral chambers of the transwell plate assembly (pH 7.4). In order to determine the viability of the cell layer, Lucifer Yellow (LY) is added to the donor buffer in each well. When a high level of LY transport (>100 nm/s) is seen, results are disregarded because LY cannot freely pass through lipophilic barriers. Aliquots from both chambers are taken after a 1-hour incubation at 37 °C and added to acetonitrile in a 96-well plate that also contains an analytical internal standard. (HPLC-MS/MS) is used to determine the chemical concentrations in the samples. P_{app} values are derived from the following relationship:

$$P_{app} = ([\text{compound}]_{\text{acceptor final}} \times V_a) \div (A \times \text{time} ([\text{compound}]_{\text{donor initial}})$$

where,

V_a = Volume in acceptor compartment
A = Surface area on the cell membrane

The efflux ratio (Er) is calculated as

$$Er = P_{app} (B \text{ to } A) / P_{app} (A \text{ to } B)$$

The following assay acceptance criteria are used:

Propranolol: P_{app} (A>B) value $\geq 20(\times 10^{-6}$cm/s)
Vinblastine: P_{app} (A>B) value < 5 $(\times 10^{-6}$cm/s) with Efflux ratio ≥ 5.
Lucifer yellow permeability: $\leq$100nm/s

Step 9. The human OATP2B1 (OATP-B), OCT1, OCT2, OAT3, PEPT1, and PEPT2 uptake transporters, in order to ascertain whether your medicine is a substrate of those transporters. By contrasting the drug's absorption into cells expressing the chosen uptake transporter with its uptake into control cells, it is possible to determine the drug's potential to be a substrate of an uptake transporter. Cells expressing transporters and control cells are introduced to cells expressing transporters and control cells at two concentrations (PEPT1 and PEPT2 at 100 and 300 μM, OCT1 and OCT2 at 50 and 100 μM, and OATP2B1 at 100 and 300 μM), and cells are then incubated for 2 and 20 min at 37 ± 1 °C (75 L final incubating volume). The IC50 of reporter substrate transport inhibition determined in the indirect transporter assay and a factor of one lower are used as the final drug doses (for example, memantine). The probe substrate, drug, and solvent are added to 200 μL of Krebs-Henseleit buffer, which is then incubated at 37 °C. The LC-MS/MS technique is used to determine medication concentration.

10.6. Bioavailability Assay

The phrase "bioavailability" describes how well a medicine or nutrient reaches the action site or the biological fluid that has access to the site of action, such as blood. A reference product is used to evaluate "relative bioavailability," and an IV is used to calculate "absolute bioavailability" as 100%. The bioavailability of your test sample can be determined by using the following animal model:

10.6.1. Plasma Sampling Model (Mouse Model)

Step 1. Create a standard calibration curve using various test drugs' concentrations.

Step 2. Collect and fasten (only with free access to water *ad libitum*) twenty albino mice (either sexes, avg. b.w.: 24 - 30 gm) and distribute them into four groups: Then administer your test drug (two different doses) via oral and intraperitoneal routes. Groups I and II receive oral administration, while Groups III and IV receive intraperitoneal administration of the drug.

Step 3. Collect blood samples from Groups I and III at 30th minutes, and from Groups II and IV at 60th minutes after sacrificing the animals without using an anesthetic agent.

Step 4. Centrifuge the blood sample and submit the collected serum for UV-Vis analysis at the specified wavelength.

Step 5. Determine the plasma concentration of the drug from the previously prepared calibration curve to estimate the percentage of bioavailable drugs at 30 and 60th minutes.

References

Beconi, M. G., Howland, D., Park, L., Lyons, K., Giuliano, J., Dominguez, C., Munoz-Sanjuan, I., & Pacifici, R. (2011). Pharmacokinetics of memantine in rats and mice. *PLoS Currents, 3*.

Bhise, S. B., Dias, R. J., Dhawale, S. C., & Mali, K. K. (2010). *Laboratory manual of biopharmaceutics and pharmacokinetics.* Trinity Publishing House, India, *1*, 1-66.

Makkar, H. P. S. (1999). Quantification of tannins in tree foliage. A laboratory manual for the FAO/IAEA coordinated research project on 'Use of nuclear and related techniques to develop simple tannin assay for predicting and improving the safety and efficiency of feeding ruminants on the tanniniferous tree foliage.' Joint FAO/IAEA Division of Nuclear Techniques in Food and Agric., Vienna, Austria, pp. 1-29.

Panchagnula, R., & Thomas, N. S. (2000). Biopharmaceutics and pharmacokinetics in drug research. *International Journal of Pharmaceutics, 201*(2), 131-150.

Chapter 11

Toxicity Analysis

11.1. Toxicity Analysis

Toxicity testing determines whether the test substance has the potential for toxic responses towards biological systems and, if so, to what extent. Toxicity studies are crucial in order to determine the potential negative consequences brought on by biological or chemical compounds. For instance, with prolonged chemical exposure, people typically experience genotoxicity, immunotoxicity, carcinogenicity, reproductive and developmental impacts, and harmful effects on organs. To evaluate the risk posed by a chemical or drug candidate, toxicity assessment requires *in vitro*, *in vivo*, and *in silico* techniques. The ultimate aim is to ensure the safety of nutrients, drugs, or drug-like products for humans. Some widely used toxicity testing modalities include:

11.1.1. Acute and Sub-Acute Toxicity Study (Animal Model)

Oral *acute* toxicity studies are done using the 'Up-and-Down' approach in animals (e.g., mice and rats) in accordance with the Organization for Economic Co-operation and Development's (OECD's) guideline no. 425 at single dosages of 175, 500, and 2000 mg/kg.

Step 1. Take five female animals (e.g., rats or mice) and treat them with the respective dose orally.

Step 2. Check each animal for symptoms of regurgitation and keep them in a metal cage for the first 5 minutes after dosing. According to OECD guidelines, monitor each animal every 15 min for the first 4 h following dosing, every 30 min for 6 h, and every day for 48 h to look for behavioral signs of toxicity (such as changes in the skin, hair, eyes, mucous membranes, respiratory, circulatory, ANS, and CNS activities, motor activity, convulsions, tremors, salivation, diarrhea, lethargy, or sleep) (2001).

Step 3. Measure the animals' body weights on days 1, 7, and 14 while keeping records of any long-term potential deadly effects.

For *sub-acute* studies, follow the following steps (Gornall et al. 1949; Baravalle et al. 2006):

Step 1. Randomly assign male and female animals (e.g., mice or rats) into 4 groups (n = 12/group: 6/6 male:female).

Step 2. Treat Groups I–III with 150, 300, and 600 mg/kg of your test sample (e.g., crude extract), respectively, and give vehicle (5–10 mL/kg) to the control group orally for 28 days.

Step 3. Record daily food and water intake, stool weight, urine volume, etc. Measure the body weights and analyze the urine parameters of all animals weekly.

Step 4. Take weight and sacrifice the animals on day 29. To obtain blood samples for biochemical and hematological analysis, pierce the heart. For histological investigation, weigh, trim, and fix in Bouin's solution after removing different organs such as the heart, liver, kidneys, spleens, ovaries, and testes.

Step 5. Calculate the percentage weight gain following the below-mentioned equation:

$$\text{Weight gain (\%)} = [W_f - (W_i \div W_i)] \times 100$$

where W_f and W_i are the final and initial weights, respectively.

Step 6. Use the following equation to get the proportionate organ weight of each harvested organ:

$$\text{Relative organ weight (\%)} = (\text{Organ weight} \div \text{Body weight}) \times 100$$

Step 7. Place the blood samples for hematological analysis in vials with ethylene diamine tetraacetic acid, an anticoagulant (e.g., EDTA). Using an automated haematology analyzer, check the following parameters: red distribution width (RDW), mean platelet volume (MPV), platelet distribution width (PDW), mean corpuscular volume (MCV), total and differential leukocytes (WBC), erythrocytes (RBC), hemoglobin (Hgb), haematocrit (HCT), platelet count (PLT), mean corpuscular hemoglobin (MCH), and mean corpuscular volume (MCV).

Step 8. To prevent hemolysis of the blood cells, carefully place the blood sample for biochemical examination in plain bottles. After 5 minutes of centrifugation at 4000×*g*, collect the blood serum. Utilize an automated ion selective electrode machine to perform an analysis of serum electrolytes (such as sodium, potassium, chloride, and bicarbonate ions) as well as the enzymes aspartate aminotransferase (AST), alanine aminotransferase (ALT), total and conjugated bilirubin, total protein, albumin, urea, and creatinine.

Step 9. To estimate the protein concentration, use a piece of each organ. Prepare each organ's homogenate in normal saline (0.9% NaCl) at 10%. (i.e., 10 g of organ in 100 mL of solution).

Step 10. Assessment of albumin, globulins, and serum total protein:

This can be accomplished using one of several methods, including the sulfite approach developed by Campbell and Hanna, the alcohol method developed by Pillemer and Hutchinson, or the modified sulfate method developed by Majoor. For the Biuret method, follow the steps mentioned below:

1. Dissolve 1.50 g of $CuSO_4.5H_2O$ and 6.0 g $C_4H_4O_6KNa{\cdot}4H_2O$ in 500 mL of distilled water. Add 300 mL of 10% NaOH solution and mix properly. Store in an amber or paraffin-lined bottle.
2. Mark the required cuvettes as Cuvettes B for blank, T for total protein, or A for albumin. Take 2 mL of a 22.6% Na_2SO_4 solution in Cuvette B as a blank.
3. Take 0.5 mL of serum into a centrifuge tube and add 9.5 mL of 22.6% $NaSO_4$ to it. Mix them using the inversion technique. Transfer only 2.0 mL of the mixture to Cuvette T. And add 3 mL of ether to the remaining serum-sulfate mixture, mix for 30 seconds, and centrifuge. Transfer 2.0 mL of the aqueous phase to Cuvette A by slanting the tube. Add 8.0 mL of the biuret reagent to each cuvette and swirl to completely combine.
4. Keep the mixture at room temperature for 30 minutes. With the "blank" Cuvette B in place, set the photoelectric calorimeter or spectrophotometer to transmit at 100% of its maximum at 540 nm. Cuvettes 1 and A should be used in place of Cuvette B, and you should note each one's percentage transmission (or optical density).
5. By using the calibration curve, determine the concentrations of total protein, albumin, and globulin (= total protein + albumin). 5.0 mL of clear, normal serum should be pipetted into a graduated cylinder with a stopper before being diluted with isosaline solution to make 50 mL.
6. Prepare nine cuvettes (or test tubes) in duplicate, and pipette successive amounts of 0.9% saline into each one: 2.0, 1.85, 1.70, 1.55, 1.40, 1.20, 1.00, 0.80, and 0.60 mL. Add the dilute serum in

the following amounts, in identical order: 0, 0.15, 0.30, 0.45, 0.60, 0.80, 1.00, 1.20, and 1.40 mL. Pipette 8.0 mL of biuret reagent into each cuvette, stir, and read the results as before after 30 minutes. The residual diluted serum can be used for Kjeldahl nitrogen analyses. When non-protein nitrogen from a separate analysis of the original serum is subtracted from the total nitrogen content of 100 mL of serum, protein nitrogen remains, which is multiplied by 6.25 to get the standard protein concentration. Plot the observed transmission or density values against the standard serum's protein concentration at 0, 15, 30, 45, 60, 80, 1.0, 1.2, and 1.4 times.

Step 11. Dehydrate the frozen tissues in a succession of progressively stronger alcohols, clarify them in xylene, and embed them in paraffin wax that is melted at 60 °C for histological investigation. By using a microtome to slice through the imbedded tissue, section the organs (5 m thick), mount them on slides coated in 3-aminopropyltriethsilane, and let them dry for 24 hours at 37 °C. Use xylene to deparaffinize the portions on the slides, then hydrate them with progressively stronger alcohols. Use Mayer's haematoxylin and eosin dyes to stain the slides, let them dry, and then mount them for histopathological analysis under a light microscope (X40, 100, or 200).

11.1.1.1. Contact Insecticidal Activity

Step 1. Place the filter paper, sprayed with the test sample, inside a cylindrical or conical flask (approx. area of 23.8 cm^2).

Step 2. Set the flask aside so the solvent can evaporate.

Step 3. Place 20 adult *Callosobruchus maculatus* (commonly known as the cowpea weevil or cowpea seed beetle) in the treated flask and monitor for 24 h to observe the mortality.

Step 4. As a control and positive control, use a vehicle and a suitable reference insecticidal agent.

11.1.1.2. Piscicidal Activity

According to Sukari et al. (1992):

Step 1. Use the fish *Labistes reticulates* (Cyrinodontiadae) or *Tilapia mossambica* (Cichlidae) for this study.

Step 2. They are bred and grown in concrete tanks and acclimated there for a few days before testing.

Step 3. Small plastic aquariums (19.0 × 11.5 cm) with 1.6 or 4 L of water should each accommodate 10 *L. reticulates* (average length: 2.5 cm) or 5 *T. mossambica* (average length: 7.0 cm).

Step 4. Before using it as dilution water, aerate the tap water. Fish must be restrained for 24 hours prior to testing and during the entire 72-hour test period.

Step 5. Blend 100 mg (or the required amount to attain the desired concentration) of the test sample in 1 L of water and squeeze through a muslin cloth after filtering. You will receive a stock solution with a concentration of 100,000×*g* from which to produce five test solutions with concentrations of 5,000, 1,000, 500, 100, and 10 ppm.

Step 6. Observe fish deaths frequently during the course of 72 hours. It duplicates the study with a suitable standard and vehicle as a control group.

11.1.1.3. Allium cepa Test

According to Konuk et al. (2007):

Step 1. Collect fresh medium-sized (approx. diameter: 1.5 to 2.0 cm) onions for this study and soak them in tap water for 20 minutes.

Step 2. In order to promote root growth, carefully remove the outermost layers and sprouting parenchyma from the center crown of onions.

Step 3. After 20 minutes of tap water rinsing, soak the bulbs' roots for the first 60 hours at 25 ± 1 °C in the dark in plastic vials with a capacity of 15-20 mL.

Step 4. Transfer five onions (five for each concentration) with satisfactory root growth to the control (vehicle) and test the sample (recommended concentrations) for up to another 72 h.

Step 5. Measure root growth in every 24 h exposure period in mm and keep the record.

Step 6. By inhibiting root growth, evaluate the test sample's toxicity in onions compared to the control (vehicle) group. Take $CuSO_4$ at 0.6–1.2 mg/L as a standard.

Step 7. Determine the half-maximal inhibitory concentration (IC_{50}) for the test sample or standard at each exposure time.

11.1.1.4. Allium sativum Test

According to Islam (2021):

Step 1. Collect large-sized and fresh garlic and carefully remove the outer cloves (only the big cloves) of *A. sativum* for this study.

Step 2. Each clove's central crown should have its outer peel and budding parenchyma carefully removed in order to promote root growth.

Step 3. Then, immerse the root section of the cloves for up to 72 hours at 28 ± 1°C in the dark after thoroughly rinsing them with tap water for 5 min.

Step 4. Measure root growth in every 24 h exposure period in mm and keep the record.

Step 5. Follow steps 4 - 7 of the *A. cepa* test to complete this study.

11.1.1.5. Cicer arietinum Test

According to Bhattacharya et al. (2012):

Step 1. Collect fresh (not more than 90 days old) large chickpea seeds, rinse the seeds three times, and soak them for 10 minutes in distilled water.

Step 2. Prepare two-layered seedling beds with sanitary napkins (tissue paper) in clean plastic cups (capacity: 15-20 mL). Wet the first (lower portion) bed with the test sample or controls and keep five seeds carefully on the bed (n = 5), maintaining an optimal distance between them.

Step 3. Carefully place tared tissue paper to cover the seeds in the second bed (upper bed) and wet it with the same sample as before.

Step 4. Cover the cups with paper or plastic covers and keep them in a 12-hour dark-light cycle for 72 hours at room temperature. Wet each treatment bed with the respective sample or controls every 24 hours.

Step 5. Use a vehicle (e.g., distilled water) and $CuSO_4$ (50 μM) as control and standard, respectively.

Step 6. Measure the shoot and root lengths and calculate the IC_{50} as mentioned above.

11.1.1.6. Artemia salina Test

According to Meyer et al. (1982):

Step 1. Collect fresh shrimp eggs from an authentic source and hatch them in artificial salt water (39.35 mM of NaCl, 18.66 mM of $MgCl_2.6H_2O$,

28.16 mM of Na_2SO_4, 8.84 mM of $CaCl_2.2H_2O$, or 5.93 mM of $CaCl_2.6H_2O$ and 9.38 mM of KCl in 1000 mL of distilled water) at 25 - 30 °C.

Step 2. Utilize $NaHCO_3$ as a buffer to raise the brine solution's pH to 9.0.

Step 3. Hatch the eggs for 36 - 48 hours.

Step 4. Transfer 10 live nauplii to the tube containing test samples or controls and adjust the final volume of 5 mL in each tube with mineral water and brine solution (1:1).

Step 5. Keep the tubes at room temperature and count live nauplii after 24 h.

Step 6. Use $K_2Cr_2O_7$ and the vehicle as the standard and negative controls, respectively.

Step 7. Calculate percentage mortality and IC_{50} to see or compare toxicity among the test sample and control groups.

11.2. Cytotoxicity Analysis

11.2.1. *Allium cepa* Test

This test is followed by a toxicity study of the previously discussed A. cepa test. After step 7:

Step 8. Cut the roots of all bulbs under each sample or concentration and fix in a carnoy solution (ethanol and glacial acetic acid (3:1, v/v)) for 24 h at 4°C and preserve in 70% ethanol until the test commences.

Step 9. The roots are then hydrolyzed with 1 N HCl at room temperature for 11 minutes after being washed with distilled water three times for 5 minutes each.

Step 10. In a jar colored amber, soak the roots in Schiff's dye. After 2 hours, rinse the roots under running distilled water to remove the dye.

Step 11. Section the meristematic regions manually with the help of surgical blades, add 2% acetic carmine solution to it, and observe it under a microscope at 100X magnification.

Step 12. Count 1000 cells for each concentration and determine the state of cell division, i.e., the mitotic index (MI), to determine the cytotoxic effects of the test substances.

Figure 11.1 shows the experimental steps of the *Allium cepa* study.

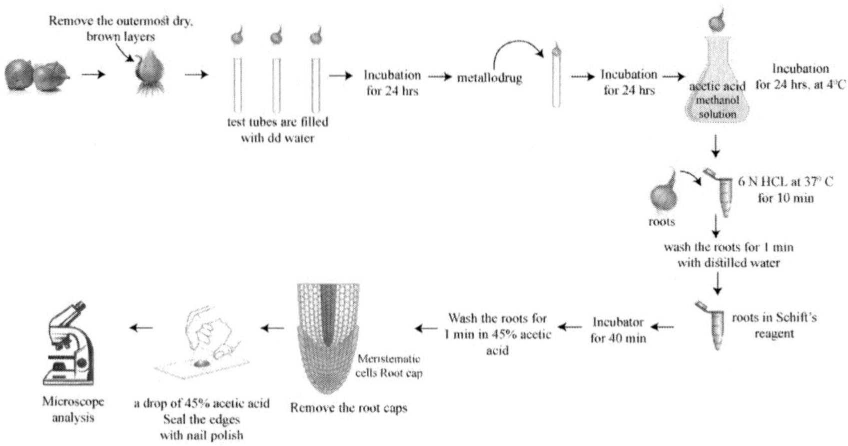

Figure 11.1. Experimental steps of *Allium cepa* assay (Islam et al. 2016)

11.2.2. Hemolysis test (rat erythrocyte model)

According to Girish et al. (2012):

Step 1. Prepare a 10% RBC suspension in PBS (pH 7.4) from the collected blood of a Wistar rat anesthetized by sodium pentobarbital (35 mg/kg, intraperitoneal).

Step 2. Add 0.15 mL of hydrogen peroxide (200 mM in PBS at pH 7.4) and 0.2 mL of the test sample to 0.5 mL of the RBC (10%) suspension.

Step 3. Centrifuge the reaction mixture's constituents for 180 sec at 2,500×*g* after 30 min of incubation at 37 °C.

Step 4. Mix 0.2 mL of supernatant with 2.8 mL of PBS (pH 7.4) and measure the absorbance at 475 nm.

Step 5. Use 0.2 mL of vehicle and Triton X-100 as a control and positive control for this study.

Step 6. Calculate the percentage hemolysis by using the following formula:

$$\text{Hemolysis (\%)} = [(A_{\text{Samle/Standard}} - A_{\text{Vehicle}}) \times 100] \div A_{\text{Samle/Standard}}$$

11.2.3. MTT [3-(4,5 dimethylthiazol-2-yl)-2,5-diphenyltetrazolium bromide] Assay

This technique is frequently used to evaluate the chemosensitivity of tumor cell lines *in vitro*. The assay is founded on the idea that only cells with active metabolisms can convert the water-soluble MTT salt into its formazan byproduct. The levels of MTT absorbance are unaffected by the dead cells. Succinate dehydrogenase, a mitochondrial enzyme, transforms the water-soluble, yellow substrate MTT into the spectrophotometrically quantifiable, insoluble, purple formazan result in living cells. The mitochondrial activity per cell and the number of cells present are factors in the MTT experiment. Only metabolically active cells can reduce MTT, and the level of activity indicates how viable the cells are. Follow the instructions below to complete this study (Kasthuri and Ramesh 2018):

Step 1. Collect the required cell line and grow it in its specified medium. Keep the cells at 37 °C, 5% CO_2, 95% air, and 100% relative humidity (RH). The culture medium is switched out twice a week, and the maintained cultures are passed every 7 days.

Step 2. By separating the monolayer cells with trypsin-EDTA, you create single-cell suspensions. Achieve a final density of 1×10^5 cells/mL by counting the number of surviving cells using a hemocytometer and dilution with media containing 5% FBS.

Step 3. To promote cell attachment, distribute the cell suspension onto 96-well plates at a density of 10,000 cells per well and maintain it for 24 h at 37 °C, 5% CO_2, 95% air, and 100% RH.

Step 4. Remove the cell medium and treat it with your test sample at different concentrations.

Step 5. Re-incubate the cells for 5 days at 37°C with 5% CO_2. A volume of 30 L of MTT (a stock solution of 5 mg/mL in PBS) should be added to each well before the plates are incubated for 4 h at 37 °C.

Step 6. Discard the medium with caution using an aspirator, and then add 50 μL of DMSO to each well to dissolve the MTT crystals into formazan.

Step 7. Utilize a microplate reader to determine the absorbance, which is proportional to the amount of MTT decreased at 570 nm. Utilizing a linear regression equation and the concentration of your test sample that causes a 50% decrease in absorbance compared to that of untreated cells, determine

LD_{50} values. Express LD_{50} values as the average of four independent triplicate assays and four separate triplicate assays, respectively.

11.3. Genotoxicity Analysis

Certain substances exert toxic effects on genetic materials (e.g., DNA and RNA). Genotoxicity tests aim to identify if a substance can damage DNA and RNA, causing mutations and genotoxicity. Permanent genotoxic effects are responsible for causing cancer. In contrast, genotoxicity studies also aim to use agents for cancer cell destruction. Some widely used genotoxic study protocols have been given below.

11.3.1. Plant Model

11.3.1.1. Allium cepa Test

This test is followed by a toxicological and cytotoxic study of the previously discussed *A. cepa* test. For this, the chromosomal aberrations (CA), i.e., chromosomal bridges, chromosomal fragments/loose, chromosomal tackiness/stickiness, and micronuclei formation, are evaluated to determine the genotoxic effects of the test substances (Islam et al. 2016).

11.3.2. Animal Models

11.3.2.1. Alkaline comet assay (Mouse model)

Step 1. After giving the respective treatment for a specified period, euthanize the animals (mice) by using an i.p. dose (150 mg/kg, i.p.) of pentobarbital sodium and sacrificing them. Then perform the alkaline comet assay as follows:

Step 2. Collect the bones and mix the 10 mL bone marrow sample with 90 mL of 0.75% w/v low-melting agarose (MP: 37 °C).

Step 3. Cover the prepared observation sample with coverslips (24 × 60 mm) after spreading 0.75% (w/v) of normal melting point agarose on a slide that has already been coated. To solidify, keep the slides at room temperature.

Step 4. Remove the coverslips and treat the slides with lysis solution (2.5 M NaCl, 100 mM EDTA, 10 mM Tris, 1% Triton X-100, 10% DMSO, pH 10) at 4 °C and keep them in a dark place for 3 days.

Step 5. Perform electrophoresis at 4 °C for 20 min at 25 V and 300 mA using the electrophoresis medium of 300 mM EDTA, 1 mM NaOH, and pH >13.

Step 6. For 5 minutes, the slides must be treated with a neutralizing solution (0.4 M Tris, pH 7.5), after which they must be exposed for 10 minutes to a fixing solution comprising trichloroacetic acid (15%), zinc sulphate heptahydrate (5%), and glycerol.

Step 7. Dry the slides, apply a 0.02% solution of $AgNO_3$, and then wash them three times with distilled water. Slides should be dipped into the stop solution (acetic acid) for 5 minutes. Then wash the slides three times with distilled water and dry them at room temperature.

Step 8. Conduct photomicrography at 40X by counting 100 cells on each slide (2 per animal) using an optical microscope and classifying the damage into the following 5 categories: class 0 (no damage to genetic materials); class 1-3 (low to medium damage); and class 4 (highest damage).

Step 9. Determine the damage index and damage frequency.

11.3.2.2. Micronucleus Test

11.3.2.2.1. Allium cepa Model

After treatment with Schiff's reagent.

Step 1. Wash the tips of all roots for 60 seconds in 45% acetic acid after incubating them for 40 minutes at 37 °C.

Step 2. With a razor blade, cut the root caps off the well-stained root tips. Roots that have been treated should be between 0.5 and 2.0 cm long.

Step 3. On a clean microscope slide, submerge 1 mm of the meristematic region in a drop of 45% acetic acid. In order to prevent air bubbles, place a coverslip on the mounting solution, with one edge touching the solution first. Let the mounting solution completely cover the coverglass. Apply pressure with a pencil's eraser end to squash into single cells. Use nail polish to seal the slip's edges. The slide is now prepared for examination with a fluorescence microscope.

Step 4. Calculate and determine the percentage (%) of micronuclei in 1,000 cells.

11.3.2.2.2. Mouse Model

Follow the alkaline comet assay (as mentioned before) for this purpose (Morais et al. 2016). Briefly,

Step 1. On the previously coded slides, collect bone marrow cell suspension (25 mL) and combine it with 0.3 mL of fetal bovine serum (20%).

Step 2. Stain the slides using 10% Giemsa in 0.2 M PBS (pH 5.8).

Step 3. After photomicrography, count the number of normochromatic erythrocytes (NCE), polychromatic erythrocytes (PCE), and micronuclei in polychromatic erythrocytes (MNPCE) at 1000 for every 400 cells treated.

Step 4. Determine the PCE/NCE ratio.

11.3.2.2.3. Fish (Oreochromis niloticus) Model

According to Hartmann and Speit (1997):

Step 1. Transfer the fish into the previously cleaned aquariums while maintaining the same conditions at 29 ± 2 °C (pH: 7.8 ± 0.3). Three samples, each with an exposure time (ET) of three days, are placed in each tank. Cytotoxic and mutagenic standard cyclophosphamide (CPA) is administered at a dose of 4 mg/L (i.p.). After the ET, the fish are kept in a vessel for profound anesthesia, drowsiness, and death before blood (0.5 mL) is obtained by gill incision with the help of heparinized syringes to conduct the comet assay.

Step 2. Then, combine 100 mL of low-melting agarose (0.5%) with 5 mL of fish blood at 37 °C. Cover the slide with a coverslip after spreading the mixture on a slide that had already been coated with 1.5% normal melting point agarose.

Step 3. Remove the coverslips after allowing them to set for 10 minutes in the refrigerator. The slides should be shielded from light before being submerged vertically for at least 12 h in a cold lysis solution (89% stock lysis solution, 1% Triton X-100, 10% DMSO, pH 10; stock lysis solution, 2.5 M NaCl, 100 mM EDTA, 10 mM Tris, pH 10).

Step 4. Slides should be subjected to electrophoresis in an alkaline solution (1 mM EDTA, 300 mM NaOH, pH >13) as follows: After 20 V (0.74 V cm^{-1}), 300 mA, and 20 min in a dimly lit environment, neutralization with Tris-HCl (0.4 M, pH 7.5), washing with ice-cold distilled water, and air drying are performed.

Step 5. After air drying for 180 seconds, fix the slides with cold absolute methanol, and then use $AgNO_3$ solution to stain them.

Step 6. Count 200 cells per fish (i.e., 600 cells/group) under an optical microscope while performing photomicrography at 40×, identifying 5 classes of damage as mentioned above.

Step 7. Calculate the damage index (ID) as follows: ID: 0 × (C0) + 1 × (C1) + 2 × (C2) + 3 × (C3) + 4 × (C4). Score every image as per the extent of DNA migration using a visual analysis of 100 cells per slide. Calculate damage frequency (FD) (range: 0 to 100%) as follows: FD: 100 - C0, where, C0 stands for class 0 (C0) cell numbers among the 100 cells evaluated.

Step 8. Analyze the damage index and damage frequency (600 cells/group).

11.4. Mutagenicity Analysis

11.4.1. Ames Test

Step 1. Isolate a Salmonella typhimurium strain that is auxotrophic for histidine.

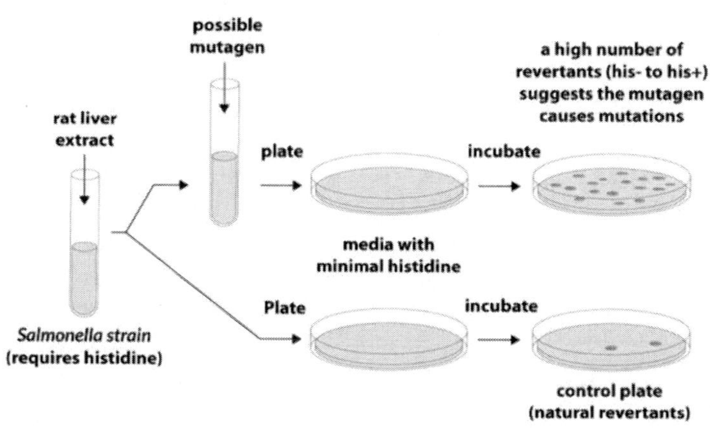

Figure 11.2. *Steps of Ames test*

Step 2. Prepare the S. typhimurium test suspension in a simple buffer containing a test chemical (e.g., 2-aminofluorene). Histidine can be used sparingly to begin the bacterial growth process. Only bacteria that have been altered to have the ability to synthesize histidine can establish colonies after histidine levels have been low.

Step 3. Make a suspension with the organism for control purposes (without your test sample).

Step 4. Incubate the suspensions for 20 minutes at 37 °C.

Step 5. Get the two agar plates ready and spread the suspension over them.

Step 6. Incubate the plates for 2 days at 37 °C and count the colony numbers on each plate.

Figure 11.2 presents the general steps of the Ames test.

11.4.2. Salmonella Assay

According to Ntuli et al. (2018):

Step 1. Choose and gather mutant Salmonella species. Perform this test both with and without the rat liver metabolic activation (S9). An Aroclor 1254-induced S9 homogenate (0.7 nM cytochrome P450/mg protein) was produced from male Fischer rats and added to the S9 mixture at a level of 2 mg protein/mL, causing metabolic activation.

Step 2. At 45 °C, combine 0.1 mL of the test sample with 0.1 mL of bacterial culture, 0.5 mL of S9, and 2 mL of top agar. Let it sit overnight.

Step 3. Mix the reaction mixture through vortexing, transfer to a minimum glucose agar plate, and incubate for 2 days at 37 °C without light. Make a negative control using DMSO as the solvent, both with and without the S9 combination and without the diagnostic mutagens.

Step 4. Use concentrations that are ten times lower than the cytotoxic dosages for the study. For every concentration, use at least five replicates and run every experiment in duplicate.

References

Baravalle, C., Salvetti, N. R., Mira, G. A., Pezzone, N., & Ortega, H. H. (2006). Microscopic characterization of follicular structures in letrozole-induced polycystic ovarian syndrome in the rat. *Archives of Medical Research*, *37*(7), 830-839.

Bhattacharya, S., De Sarkar, N., Banerjee, P., Banerjee, S., Mukherjee, S., Chattopadhyay, D., & Mukhopadhyay, A. (2012). Effects of arsenic toxicity on germination, seedling growth and peroxidase activity in Cicer arietinum. *Int J Agric Food Sci*, 2(4), 131-137.

Girish, T. K., Vasudevaraju, P., & Rao, U. J. P. (2012). Protection of DNA and erythrocytes from free radical induced oxidative damage by black gram (Vigna mungo L.) husk extract. *Food and Chemical Toxicology*, *50*(5), 1690-1696.

Gornall, A. G., Bardawill, C. J., & David, M. M. (1949). Determination of serum proteins by means of the biuret reaction. *The Journal of Biological Chemistry*, *177*(2), 751–766.

Hartmann, A., & Speit, G. (1997). A simple technique for quantification of low levels of DNA damage in individual cells. *Toxicology Letters*, *90*, 183-188.

Islam, M. T. (2022). Toxicity study of *Urena lobata* using *Allium sativum*: a new eukaryotic biomonitoring test system. *Khulna University Studies*, 35-40.

Islam, M. T., Streck, L., Silva, S. W. C., Paz, M. F. C. J., Júnior, A. L. G., Alencar, M. V. O. B., Mata, A. M. O. F., Silva-Junior, A. A., Dantas, S. M. M. M., & Melo-Cavalcante, A. A. C. (2016). Evaluation of toxic, cytotoxic, genotoxic and mutagenic effects of phytol and its nanoemulsion: Data-in-brief. *World J. Pharm. Pharm. Sci*, *5*, 410-418.

Kasthuri, O. R., & Ramesh, B. (2018). Toxicity studies on leaf extracts of Alternanthera brasiliana (L.) Kuntze and Alternanthera bettzickiana (Regel) Voss. *Journal of Applied Pharmaceutical Science*, *8*(10), 082-089.

Konuk, M. U. H. S. İ. N., Liman, R. E. C. E. P., & Cigerci, I. H. (2007). Determination of genotoxic effect of boron on Allium cepa root meristematic cells. *Pakistan Journal of Botany*, *39*(1), 73.

Meyer, B. N., Ferrigni, N. R., Putnam, J. E., Jacobsen, L. B., Nichols, D. E. J., & McLaughlin, J. L. (1982). Brine shrimp: a convenient general bioassay for active plant constituents. *Planta medica*, *45*(05), 31-34.

Moraes, G. P. D., Alencar, M. V. O. B. D., Islam, T., Araújo, L. D. S., Gomes, D. C. V., Carvalho, R. M. D., Correia, D., Ferreira, P. M. P., Picada, J. N., Ferraz, A., & Picada, J. N. (2016). Toxicogenetic profile of rats treated with aqueous extract from *Morinda citrifolia* fruits. *Journal of Medicinal Plant Research*, *10*(2), 18-28.

Ntuli, S. S., Gelderblom, W. C., & Katerere, D. R. (2018). The mutagenic and antimutagenic activity of Sutherlandia frutescens extracts and marker compounds. *BMC Complementary and Alternative Medicine*, *18*(1), 1-10.

Organization for Economic Development. 2001. Guideline for Testing of Chemicals. Guideance, no. 425.

Sukari, A., Rahmani, M. A. W. A. R. D. I., Manas, R., & Takahashi, S. (1992). Toxicity studies of plant extracts on insects and fish. *Pertanika*, *15*, 41-41.

Chapter 12

Computer-Aided Drug Design (*In Silico* Study)

12.1. Computational Drug Analysis

Computational analysis (CADD: computer-aided drug design) or *in silico* analysis is part of drug discovery in the field of medicinal chemistry. Generally, new drugs are discovered from natural plant and animal sources, depending on accidental observation and analysis or traditional uses. In CADD, the entire process has been performed through bioinformatics and computer science. Through this computerized experimental method, researchers predict the binding interactions between drug candidates and proteins, enzymes, receptors, etc. Sometimes CADD is used for the screening of small natural compounds, and sometimes it's used to claim the pharmacological effect of an *in vitro* or *in vivo* study result. Sometimes researchers utilize this CADD for the identification of protein structure via bioinformatics and genome sequences. All of these strategic approaches are well-suited and appropriate for drug discovery. As a result, CADD has recently played an important role in drug discovery and development. In the CADD section, two approaches are available: structure-based drug design and ligand-based drug design. This chapter covers basic *in silico* design and methods for claiming the pharmacological effect of *in vitro* and *in vivo* study results.

12.2. Structure-Based Drug Design

Structure-based drug design (SBDD) is a multi-sectoral, iterative, and mathematical process that is well recognized as a method in research and pharmaceuticals. SBDD played a tremendous role in the discovery and development of a number of established drugs and clinical ligands, e.g., zanamivir, nelfinavir, and aleglitazar. In this part of the drug discovery section, a plethora of databases, computational programs, and software are used. Among all the ligand and protein databases and software, the acceptable databases and resources are enumerated in the table below (Table 12.1). Figure 12.1 presents an outline of structure-based drug design.

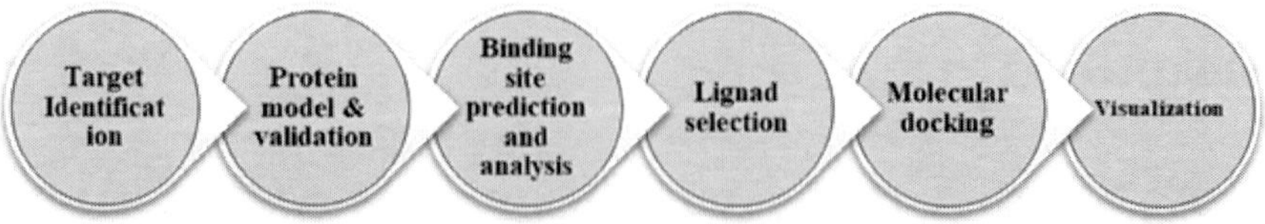

Figure 12.1. Outline of structure-based drug design.

12.3. Ligand-Based Drug Design

If the protein structure is not known, the properties of the compound can be predicted in advance using only the drug structure of the compound. QSAR: Since the structure of a compound is related to its activities, it is assumed that compounds with similar structures will exhibit similar activities. Finding common patterns through data accumulated through experiments and predicting active values through them. Figure 12.2 presents an outline of ligand-based drug design.

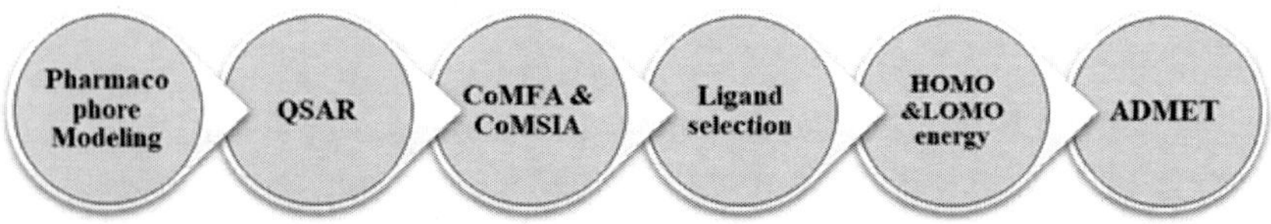
Pharmaco phore Modeling
QSAR
CoMFA & CoMSIA
Ligand selection
HOMO &LOMO energy
ADMET

Figure 12.2. Outline of ligand-based drug design.

12.4. Total Process of Structure-Based Drug Design

12.4.1. Target Identification

The identification and confirmation of drug targets is the first phase of the drug discovery process. It is a macromolecule with a known function in the pathophysiology of a disease. Proteins, including receptors and enzymes, nucleic acids (DNA and RNA), carbohydrates, and fat are the four principal pharmacological targets found in organisms. The bulk of medications on the market target proteins as therapeutic targets. However, because of the decoding of various diseases, nucleic acids may become very important as medicinal targets in the near future. Choosing prospective therapeutic targets from thousands of candidate macromolecules is a difficult undertaking.

Genomic and proteomic methods are the most essential tools for target identification in the post-genomic age. In addition, advances in high-throughput omics technology have resulted in a massive amount of data on host-pathogen interactions.

12.4.2. Protein *(Target)* Structure Modeling, Energy Minimization and Validation

Homology modeling (also known as comparative modeling) is, to date, the most reliable and well-established computational approach for predicting protein structures. Structural bioinformatics models of three-dimensional crystal protein (target) structures in PDB format were acquired from the Protein Data Bank (PDB) (https://www.rcsb.org/), and homology modeling of human protein (target) was conducted using the *Swiss* model (Schwede et al. 2003). Before modeling, the sequence was obtained from UniProt (Bairoch et al. 2005), and the template was chosen by BLAST analysis with the NCBI BLAST (Johnson et al. 2008) tool. After finishing the target structure, we used the Swiss-PDB Viewer software tool to minimize and optimize structural energy, and then all heteroatoms and water molecules in proteins were eliminated using PyMOL before docking (Yuan et al. 2017). PROCHECK (Laskowski et al. 2006) was used to validate the homology model and PDB file. As a result, compound molecular docking was used to provide information on how targets bind. Figure 12.3 shows the step-by-step process of protein (target) structure modeling, energy minimization, and validation.

12.4.3. Binding Site Prediction and Analysis

It is not a simple undertaking to choose binding sites; academics have proposed several crucial criteria for picking a binding site. The functional activity of any protein is thought to be determined by a highly conserved cluster of amino acid residues found in binding site pockets. CASTp (Tian et al. 2018) was used to approximate viral receptor active sites for effective docking, and PyMol (V.2.4) was utilized to define the Cartesian coordinates x, y, and z (active sites). These areas were also employed by Auto Dock Vina to generate grid boxes for molecular docking. The highest-scoring active sites were found to be a necessary precursor for the formation of a grid in identified viral and vector receptors. CASTp was utilized to characterize and quantify active sites, binding sites, inaccessible interior cavities, surface-accessible structural pockets and structures, and protein cavities.

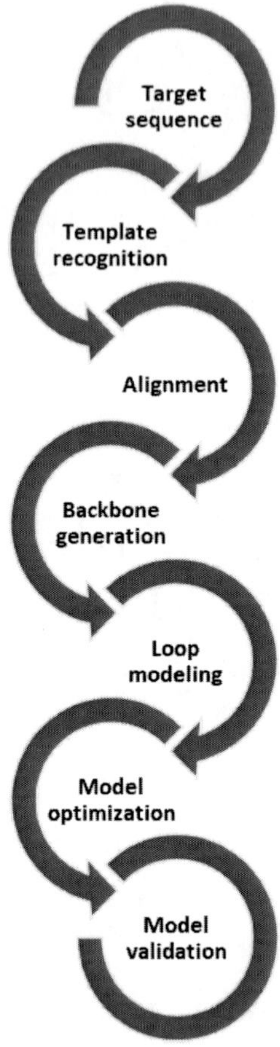

Figure 12.3. Step-by-step of protein (target) structure modeling, energy minimization and validation

12.4.4. Ligand Selection

Ligand selection is also an important CADD step, just like target identification and protein structure building. A plethora of databases are available for finding appropriate ligands.

Table 12.1. The accessibility of significant compound databased platforms for ligand discovery

Sl No	Database	Description	Availability	References
1	ZINC	Freely accessible database of commercially available compounds for molecular docking and virtual screening.	https://zinc.docking.org/	Irwin and Shoichet, 2005
2	PubChem	A database of small chemical molecules their biological activities	https://pubchem.ncbi.nlm.nih.gov/	Kim et al. 2016
3	ChemSpider	A chemical structure database used for drug discovery	http://www.chemspider.com/	Pence and Williams, 2010.
4	ChEMBL	A small molecule database that contains information about ADMET and binding for a huge number of bioactive compounds	https://www.ebi.ac.uk/chembl/	Gaulton et al. 2017
5	DrugBank	A comprehensive database resource containing information about drugs, their targets and other useful information	https://go.drugbank.com/	Wishart et al. 2018

12.4.5. Molecular Docking, Virtual Screening and Visualization

Molecular docking is a numerical technique for drug discovery in medicinal chemistry. This method is used by several tools to forecast the pharmacodynamic profile of drug candidates by ranking and orienting them to receptor binding sites. The docking result describes the degree of ligand interaction with the active site of the requested protein. The active binding sites of the target protein are the positions of the ligand in the original target protein grids (40 × 40 × 40), which are examined using the visualization software Biovia Discovery Studio and LigPlot Plus. Table 12.2 presents a summary of the highly cited molecular docking programs used in drug discovery.

12.4.6. Molecular Dynamics (MD) Simulation

MD modeling is currently regarded as a critical stage in computer-aided drug discovery research at the atomic level. Many unknown biological roles of proteins and their deep dynamic processes can be uncovered by analyzing their internal mobility (Al-Khafaji et al. 2020). In terms of the dynamically changing time scale, we may utilize it to determine if the protein-ligand combination is stable (Bekker and Kamiya 2021). On a time, scale of 100 ns, we ran MD simulations on four proteins with docked ligands as well as cocrystal ligands created via molecular binding. To execute the MD simulation, we utilized the GROMACS package (Van Der Spoel et al. 2005). The CHARMM 27 force field (MacKerell et al. 2000) was utilized to parameterize the whole ligand-protein combination. The solvent was selected to be the intermolecular three-point transfer potential (TIP3P), with Na^+ or Cl^- ions added to modify the charge to replicate the physiological milieu. Then, to reduce the energy of these systems, we employed the steepest descent method with an acceptable value of 1000 kJ/mol. The NVT and NPT pools then balanced out the positionally constrained complexes on the protein molecule in 0.1 ns. The stability was determined within 100 ns using MD simulations with no limitations on protein molecules or ligands. Finally, GROMACS modules such as gmx rms, gmxrmsf, and gmxh bond were utilized to examine MD trajectories.

Table 12.2. A summary of the highly cited molecular docking programs used in drug discovery

Sl No	programs	Description	Availability	References
01	AutoDock4	Used for molecular docking. It predicts the binding affinity and poses of a small molecule to a 3D structure target protein	https://autodock.scripps.edu	Bitencourt-Ferreira et al. 2019
02	Autodock vina	Used for virtual screening and molecular docking	http://vina.scripps.edu/index.html	Seeliger and de Groot, 2010
03	Glide Schrodinger	A complete package for molecular modeling and CADD	http://www.schrodinger.com/	Bhachoo and Beuming, 2017
04	Hex	Used for docking studies	http://hex.loria.fr/	Bagali and Gowrishankar, 2016
05	Molecular operating environment (MOE)	A complete package for molecular modeling and CADD	http://www.chemcomp.com/	Vilar et al. 2008
06	PyRx	Used for docking studies	https://pyrx.sourceforge.io/	Dallakyan and Olson, 2015.

12.4.7. Molecular Mechanics/Poisson-Boltzmann Surface Area (MM-PBSA) Calculations

Utilization of the g_mmpbsa tool to estimate the binding free energies of the protein-ligand systems (Kumari et al. 2014). One of the popular methods to estimate the interaction energies is the Molecular Mechanics Poisson–Boltzmann Surface Area (MM-PBSA) analysis (Homeyer and Gohlke 2012). This method uses molecular dynamics simulation trajectories to predict binding free energies (ΔEMMPBSA) of protein-protein, protein-ligand, or protein–DNA systems. We performed the MMPBSA analysis on the last 20 ns of the MD trajectory of each protein-ligand system at an interval of 50 ps.

12.4.8. ADMET Analysis

ADME (Adsorption, Distribution, Metabolism, and Excretion) is important to analyze the pharmacodynamics of the proposed molecule that could be used as a drug. The SWISS-ADME tool (Daina et al. 2017) is a website (https://www.swissadme.ch) that allows the user to draw their respective ligand or drug molecule or include SMILES data from PubChem and provides the parameters, such as lipophilicity (iLOGP, XLOGP3, WLOGP, MLOGP, SILICOS-IT, Log P0/w), water solubility-Log S (ESOL, Ali, SILICOS-IT), drug-likeness rules (Lipinski, Ghose, Veber, Egan, and Muegge), and Medicinal Chemistry (PAINS, Brenk, Leadlikeness, Synthetic accessibility) (Daina et al. 2017). Data from PubChem, which consists of SMILES of diterpene ligands (https://pubchem.ncbi.nlm.nih.gov/compound) was entered into the search bar and analyzed.

For identification of the drug likeliness of diterpene ligands, a study has been utilized similar to the way that Lipinski's rule of five (Lipinski et al. 2004), Ghose filters (Ghose et al. 2006), the CMC 50 like rule (Sneader et al. 1990), Veber filters (Veber et al. 2002), the MDDR like rule (Averbukh et al. 2014), BBB likeness (Clark, 2003), and QED (Bickerton et al. 2012) were used to gauge the compounds. Lipinski's filter was used to measure hydrophobicity. Many of the ligands in the active compounds had the pharmacokinetic profile and physicochemical descriptors expected. In drug development, these guidelines have been used to preselect bioactive molecules (Leeson et al. 2004).

Toxicology prediction of small compounds is critical for predicting the acceptability of small molecules before they are consumed by human and animal models. pkCSM is an online database where tiny molecules may be virtually drawn or evaluated by inputting their SMILES. The website may give information on toxicological consequences such as human MTD, LD50, hepatotoxicity, and Minnow toxicity. The website was accessed, and SMILES of diterpene ligand data from PubChem was searched and entered into the website, as well as the toxicity mode (Pires et al. 2015).

12.4.9. Network Pharmacology

Three main stages are included in network pharmacology assessment: (a) target estimation for selected bioactive ligands; (b) amplification studies for predicted targets; and (c) network construction and analysis for selected ligands, targets, and pathways. Briefly, targets of chosen drugs were predicted using DIGEP-Pred (Lagunin et al. 2013) at a pharmacological activity (Pa) of 0.5. Next, the predicted proteins of the chosen drugs were enriched using STRING (Szklarczyk et al. 2019) to generate the protein-protein interaction. All proteins that are obtained from the STRING database were submitted to the Enricher database (https://maayanlab.cloud/Enrichr/) to enrich their biological processes, molecular function, cellular components, and KEGG pathways. Finally, the network between the chosen drugs, their targets, and pathways was constructed using Cytoscape (Smoot et al. 2011).

In summary, the discovery of active chemical targets is primarily reliant on computerized methodologies for complicated biological screening systems. Furthermore, such software and its uses are potential growth areas for molecular modeling and drug development. Furthermore, more computational research is needed to eliminate human bias in the design and evaluation of molecular property spaces for lead optimization and ADME analysis. For the future of computational drug discovery, more focus should be placed on the creation of new tools with greater accuracy, as well as the refinement of existing molecular modeling methodologies. Furthermore, these methodologies have a high potential for widespread usage in drug development processes, which is a precondition for success.

References

Al-Khafaji, K., & Tok, T. T. (2020). Molecular dynamics simulation, free energy landscape and binding free energy computations in exploration the anti-invasive activity of amygdalin against metastasis. *Computer Methods and Programs in Biomedicine*, *195*, 105660.

Averbukh, I., Ben-Zvi, D., Mishra, S., & Barkai, N. (2014). Scaling morphogen gradients during tissue growth by a cell division rule. *Development*, *141*(10), 2150-2156.

Bagali, S. S., & Gowrishankar, B. S. (2016). Molecular Docking of Antipain Inhibitor Using Hex Software. *International Journal of Computational Biology and Bioinformatics*, *2*(1), 3-8.

Bekker, G. J., & Kamiya, N. (2021). Dynamic docking using multicanonical molecular dynamics: Simulating complex formation at the atomistic level. *Protein-ligand Interactions and Drug Design*, 187-202.

Bhachoo, J., & Beuming, T. (2017). Investigating protein–peptide interactions using the Schrödinger computational suite. *Modeling Peptide-protein Interactions: Methods and Protocols*, 235-254.

Bitencourt-Ferreira, G., Pintro, V. O., & de Azevedo, W. F. (2019). Docking with autodock4. *Docking Screens for Drug Discovery*, 125-148.

Clark, D. E. (2003). In silico prediction of blood–brain barrier permeation. *Drug discovery today*, *8*(20), 927-933.

Daina, A., Michielin, O., & Zoete, V. (2017). SwissADME: a free web tool to evaluate pharmacokinetics, drug-likeness and medicinal chemistry friendliness of small molecules. *Scientific Reports*, *7*(1), 42717.

Dallakyan, S., & Olson, A. J. (2015). Small-molecule library screening by docking with PyRx. *Chemical Biology: Methods and Protocols*, 243-250.

Gaulton, A., Hersey, A., Nowotka, M., Bento, A. P., Chambers, J., Mendez, D., Mutowo, P., Atkinson, F., Bellis, L. J., Cibrián-Uhalte, E., & Leach, A. R. (2017). The ChEMBL database in 2017. *Nucleic Acids Research*, *45*(D1), D945-D954.

Ghose, A. K., Herbertz, T., Salvino, J. M., & Mallamo, J. P. (2006). Knowledge-based chemoinformatic approaches to drug discovery. *Drug Discovery Today*, *11*(23-24), 1107-1114.

Homeyer, N., & Gohlke, H. (2012). Free energy calculations by the molecular mechanics Poisson− Boltzmann surface area method. *Molecular Informatics*, *31*(2), 114-122.

Irwin, J. J., & Shoichet, B. K. (2005). ZINC− a free database of commercially available compounds for virtual screening. *Journal of Chemical Information and Modeling*, *45*(1), 177-182.

Johnson, M., Zaretskaya, I., Raytselis, Y., Merezhuk, Y., McGinnis, S., & Madden, T. L. (2008). NCBI BLAST: a better web interface. *Nucleic Acids Research*, *36*(suppl_2), W5-W9.

Kim, S., Thiessen, P. A., Bolton, E. E., Chen, J., Fu, G., Gindulyte, A., Han, L., He, J., He, S., Shoemaker, B. A., & Bryant, S. H. (2016). PubChem substance and compound databases. *Nucleic Acids Research*, *44*(D1), D1202-D1213.

Kumari, R., Kumar, R., Open Source Drug Discovery Consortium, & Lynn, A. (2014). g_mmpbsa- A GROMACS tool for high-throughput MM-PBSA calculations. *Journal of Chemical Information and Modeling*, *54*(7), 1951-1962.

Lagunin, A., Ivanov, S., Rudik, A., Filimonov, D., & Poroikov, V. (2013). DIGEP-Pred: web service for in silico prediction of drug-induced gene expression profiles based on structural formula. *Bioinformatics*, *29*(16), 2062-2063.

Laskowski, R. A., MacArthur, M. W., & Thornton, J. M. (2012). PROCHECK: validation of protein-structure coordinates. International tables for crystallography. *Volume F chapter*, *21*(4), 684-687.

Leeson, P. D., Davis, A. M., & Steele, J. (2004). Drug-like properties: guiding principles for design–or chemical prejudice? *Drug Discovery Today: Technologies*, *1*(3), 189-195.

Lipinski, C. A. (2004). Lead-and drug-like compounds: the rule-of-five revolution. *Drug discovery today: Technologies*, *1*(4), 337-341.

MacKerell Jr, A. D., Banavali, N., & Foloppe, N. (2000). Development and current status of the CHARMM force field for nucleic acids. *Biopolymers: Original Research on Biomolecules*, *56*(4), 257-265.

Pence, H. E., & Williams, A. (2010). ChemSpider: an online chemical information resource.

Pires, D. E., Blundell, T. L., & Ascher, D. B. (2015). pkCSM: predicting small-molecule pharmacokinetic and toxicity properties using graph-based signatures. *Journal of Medicinal Chemistry*, *58*(9), 4066-4072.

Schwede, T., Kopp, J., Guex, N., & Peitsch, M. C. (2003). SWISS-MODEL: an automated protein homology-modeling server. *Nucleic Acids Research*, *31*(13), 3381-3385.

Seeliger, D., & de Groot, B. L. (2010). Ligand docking and binding site analysis with PyMOL and Autodock/Vina. *Journal of Computer-Aided Molecular Design*, *24*(5), 417-422.

Smoot, M. E., Ono, K., Ruscheinski, J., Wang, P. L., & Ideker, T. (2011). Cytoscape 2.8: new features for data integration and network visualization. *Bioinformatics*, *27*(3), 431-432.

Sneader, W. A. L. T. E. R. (1990). Chronology of drug introductions. *Comprehensive Medicinal Chemistry*, *1*, 7-80.

Szklarczyk, D., Gable, A. L., Lyon, D., Junge, A., Wyder, S., Huerta-Cepas, J., Simonovic, M., Doncheva, N. T., Morris, J. H., Bork, P., & Mering, C. V. (2019). STRING v11: protein–protein association networks with increased coverage, supporting functional discovery in genome-wide experimental datasets. *Nucleic Acids Research*, *47*(D1), D607-D613.

Tian, W., Chen, C., & Liang, J. (2018). CASTp 3.0: computed atlas of surface topography of proteins and beyond. *Biophysical Journal*, *114*(3), 50a.

Van Der Spoel, D., Lindahl, E., Hess, B., Groenhof, G., Mark, A. E., & Berendsen, H. J. (2005). GROMACS: fast, flexible, and free. *Journal of Computational Chemistry*, *26*(16), 1701-1718.

Veber, D. F., Johnson, S. R., Cheng, H. Y., Smith, B. R., Ward, K. W., & Kopple, K. D. (2002). Molecular properties that influence the oral bioavailability of drug candidates. *Journal of Medicinal Chemistry*, *45*(12), 2615-2623.

Vilar, S., Cozza, G., & Moro, S. (2008). Medicinal chemistry and the molecular operating environment (MOE): application of QSAR and molecular docking to drug discovery. *Current topics in Medicinal Chemistry*, *8*(18), 1555-1572.

Wishart, D. S., Feunang, Y. D., Guo, A. C., Lo, E. J., Marcu, A., Grant, J. R., Sajed, T., Johnson, D., Li, C., Sayeeda, Z., & Wilson, M. (2018). DrugBank 5.0: a major update to the DrugBank database for 2018. *Nucleic Acids Research*, *46*(D1), D1074-D1082.

Wu, C. H., Apweiler, R., Bairoch, A., Natale, D. A., Barker, W. C., Boeckmann, B., Ferro, S., Gasteiger, E., Huang, H., Lopez, R., & Suzek, B. (2006). The Universal Protein Resource (UniProt): an expanding universe of protein information. *Nucleic Acids Research*, *34*(suppl_1), D187-D191.

Yuan, S., Chan, H. S., & Hu, Z. (2017). Using PyMOL as a platform for computational drug design. *Wiley Interdisciplinary Reviews: Computational Molecular Science*, *7*(2), e1298.

Chapter 13

Reagent Preparation

13.1. Reagents

These are chemical substances that are added to a system to cause a specific reaction or to identify the presence or absence of certain compounds. These are substances used in various scientific and analytical processes to facilitate reactions, detect specific compounds, or perform tests. They play a crucial role in analysis across different fields, including chemistry, biology, environmental science, medicine, and many others (Cheng et al. 1992; Boström et al. 2011). They can be categorized into several types:

1. *Analytical reagents*: These are high-purity substances used in precise measurements to detect or quantify specific analytes in a sample. They have strict quality standards to ensure accurate and reliable results.
2. *Indicator reagents*: These substances change color or produce a visible signal when a specific chemical reaction occurs. They help to determine the endpoint of a reaction, identify the presence of particular substances, or monitor changes during an analysis.
3. *Solvents*: Solvents are used to dissolve other substances and create solutions for various tests and experiments. They act as a medium for reactions and are often crucial for extracting specific compounds from a mixture.
4. *Buffer solutions*: Buffers help maintain a stable pH in a solution, preventing drastic changes in acidity or alkalinity during a reaction. This is crucial for ensuring the accuracy and reproducibility of many analytical techniques.
5. *Reducing and oxidizing agents*: These reagents are used in redox (reduction-oxidation) reactions to transfer electrons between reactants. They are essential in many chemical analyses and titrations.

13.2. Importance of Reagents in Analysis

Reagents and chemicals are of paramount importance in analysis for the following reasons:

1. *Specificity*: Reagents are carefully selected to react only with the target analyte of interest, ensuring that the analysis yields accurate and specific results.
2. *Sensitivity*: Analytical reagents are often designed to detect very low concentrations of a substance, making it possible to analyze trace amounts or impurities.
3. *Reproducibility*: The use of high-quality reagents with consistent compositions ensures that the analysis can be replicated by different researchers or in various laboratories.
4. *Precision*: Analytical reagents are precisely formulated to have a known and defined chemical composition, allowing for accurate measurements and calculations.
5. *Safety*: Reagents often come with handling instructions and safety precautions to protect researchers from potential hazards during their use.
6. *Standardization*: In many fields, there are established standards for reagents that researchers use to ensure consistency and comparability of results across different studies.
7. *Quantification*: Some reagents are essential for quantitative analysis, enabling the determination of concentrations or amounts of specific substances in a sample.

Thus, reagents are indispensable tools in scientific analysis, enabling researchers to gain insights into the composition and properties of various materials, environmental samples, biological specimens, and much more. Their careful selection and proper use are critical to obtaining accurate and reliable data, which forms the foundation of scientific advancements and discoveries.

13.3. Chemicals

Chemicals are substances that have a distinct molecular composition and are often used in various scientific, industrial, and everyday applications. They can be either elements or compounds composed of multiple elements bonded together. Chemicals can exist in various physical states, such as solid, liquid, or gas, depending on factors like temperature and pressure (Ames et al. 1990).

13.4. Importance of Chemicals in Analysis

In the context of analysis, chemicals play a crucial role in a wide range of scientific fields, including chemistry, biology, medicine, environmental science, and more. Their importance in analysis can be summarized as follows:

1. *Identification*: Chemicals are used as reference standards to identify unknown substances. Through various analytical techniques, researchers can compare the properties of an unknown sample with those of known chemicals to determine its identity.
2. *Quantification*: In quantitative analysis, chemicals are used to calibrate instruments and establish standard curves. These standards help determine the concentration or amount of a specific substance in a sample.
3. *Separation*: Chemicals, especially solvents, are used to dissolve and separate mixtures of substances. Techniques like chromatography and electrophoresis rely on specific chemicals to separate and analyze components in complex mixtures.
4. *Reaction and detection*: Chemicals are used as reagents in various chemical reactions to detect and analyze specific compounds. For instance, reagents can react with certain substances to produce a color change, indicating the presence of a target compound.
5. *Quality control*: In industries such as pharmaceuticals and food production, chemicals are used to assess the quality and purity of products. Analytical techniques ensure that products meet specific standards and regulatory requirements.
6. *Environmental monitoring*: Chemical analysis is essential for monitoring pollutants and contaminants in air, water, and soil. Identifying and quantifying these substances helps assess environmental risks and develop appropriate remediation strategies.
7. *Research and development*: In scientific research and development, chemicals are indispensable for studying new materials, developing

innovative products, and advancing our understanding of various phenomena.

8. *Forensic analysis*: Chemical analysis is vital in forensic investigations to determine the presence of substances in evidence and identify their role in a crime.
9. *Health and safety*: Chemical analysis plays a crucial role in assessing the safety of products and materials, ensuring compliance with health regulations, and identifying potential hazards.

Thus, chemicals are fundamental tools in analytical processes, providing valuable insights into the composition, properties, and behavior of substances, which, in turn, contributes to advancements in science, technology, and various industries.

13.5. Difference between Chemicals and Reagents

The terms "reagents" and "chemicals" are closely related and sometimes used interchangeably, but they have distinct meanings in the context of chemistry and laboratory work.

1. *Chemicals*: The term "chemicals" refers to any substance that has a defined chemical composition and properties. Chemicals can be either pure substances or mixtures, and they can be natural or synthetic. They can exist in various physical states, such as solids, liquids, or gases. In a laboratory setting, chemicals are the broad category of substances used in experiments or processes to bring about chemical reactions, analyze samples, or perform various tasks. This includes substances like acids, bases, solvents, salts, and many other compounds that chemists and researchers use in their work.
2. *Reagents*: Reagents are a specific subset of chemicals used in chemical reactions to detect, analyze, or produce other substances. They are typically selected based on their specific chemical properties and their role in the reaction being carried out. Reagents are crucial in laboratory experiments as they enable scientists to identify the presence of certain compounds, quantify substances, or trigger specific reactions. Reagents can be classified into different categories, such as analytical reagents (used for analysis and identification), synthetic reagents (used to facilitate specific

chemical reactions), and diagnostic reagents (used in medical and biological testing).

Briefly, chemicals encompass a wide range of substances with defined chemical properties, while reagents specifically refer to chemicals used in laboratory reactions and processes to achieve particular outcomes. All reagents are chemicals, but not all chemicals are reagents unless they are being used in a specific chemical reaction or analytical procedure.

13.6. Reagent Preparation

Prepare all of the reagents according to the formula below and store them in an amber-colored glass container at a suitable temperature or storage conditions (e.g., dark and cool). Also, tag a label containing the manufacturer's name, date of preparation, etc. on the container.

$(NH_4)_6Mo_7O_{24}$ (4 mM) solution: Its molecular weight (MW) is 1235.86 g/mole. Thus, you should dissolve 1235.86 × 4 or 4943.44 mg of $(NH_4)_6Mo_7O_{24}$ (4 mM) in 1000 mL of distilled water.

1-chloro-2, 4-dinitrobenzene (1 M): Its MW is 202.55 g/mole. Thus, you should dissolve 202.55 g in 1000 mL of it in chloroform, ether, hot alcohol, or benzene.

2,4,6 tripyridyl-s-triazine (10 mM) solution: Its MW is 312.33 g/mole. Thus, you should dissolve 312.34 × 10 or 3123.4 mg of it, in 1000 mL of methanol.

2-deoxy-Dribose (28 mM): Its molecular MW is 134.13 g/mole. Thus, you should dissolve 134.13 × 28 or 3755.64 mg of it in 1000 mL of distilled water.

3-isobutyl-1-methylxanthine (0.5 mM): Its MW is 222.3 g/mole. Thus, you should dissolve 222.3 ÷ 2 or 111.15 mg of it in 1000 mL of aqueous NaOH solution.

4-nitrophenyl-α-D-glucopyranoside (0.5 mM): Its MW is 301.25 g/mole. Add 301.25 ÷ 2 or 150.625 mg of it in 1000 mL of water, warm ethanol, or methanol.

5,5′-dithiobis(2-nitrobenzoic acid) (3 mM): Its MW is 396.35 g/mole. Add 396.35 × 3 or 1189.05 mg of it in 1000 mL of methanol.

5-HT (2 µM): Its MW is 176.215 g/mole. Thus, you should dissolve 176.215 × 2 or 352.43 µg of it in 1000 mL of methanol or acetic acid (2%).

7-Ethoxyresorufin (2.5 µM): Its MW is 241.24. Dissolve MW × 2.5 µg of it in a 1000 mL vehicle containing DMSO or ethanol.

ABTS (5 mM) solution: Its MW is 514.62 g/mole. Therefore, add 514.62 × 5 or 2573.1 mg of ABTS. Prepare the ABTS solution by mixing an equal volume of a 5 mM ABTS stock solution with a 2.45 mM potassium persulfate solution. Store the mixture in the dark at room temperature for 12–16 h. You should dilute with methanol during your antioxidant test.

Acetate buffer (0.05 M): It is a 0.36% (v/v) glacial acetic acid solution at pH 5.0 maintained by using a 4 N NaOH solution.

Acetate buffer (300 mM or 0.3 M): Add sodium acetate 231.643 mg and acetic acid 10.58 mg in 800 mL distilled water. Adjust the desired pH using HCl or NaOH and final volume by adding distilled water up to 1000 mL.

Acetic acid (0.2 M) solution: Its MW is 60.052 g/mole. Thus, add 60.052 × 0.2 or 12.0104 g (eq. volume) of it and adjust the final volume up to 1000 mL with distilled water.

Acetic acid (0.2%) solution: Add 0.2 mL of acetic acid to 99.8 mL of distilled water.

Acetic acid (0.7-1%) solution: Add 0.7-1 mL of acetic acid to 99.3-99 mL of distilled water.

Acetic acid (10%) solution: Add 10 mL of acetic acid to 90 mL of distilled water.

Acetic acid (20%) solution: Add 20 mL of acetic acid to 80 mL of distilled water.

Acetic acid (30%) solution: Add 30 mL of acetic acid to 70 mL of distilled water.

Acetic acid (50 mM) solution: Add 60.052 × 50 or 3,002.6 mg (eq. volume) of it and adjust the final volume up to 1000 mL with distilled water.

Aceto-orcein (1%) solution: It is used to stain biological samples such as formol- and Carnoy-fixed tissues, coloring mast cells, nuclei, basophilic cytoplasm, cerebral corpora amylacea, and cartilage strongly; keratin and erythrocytes moderately; muscle and collagen weakly. Add 1 g of orcein powder to 55 mL of boiling glacial acetic acid. Then cool the solution, add 45 mL of distilled water, and filter it.

ACh (0.5 μM): Its MW is 146.2074 g/mole. Add 146.2074 × 0.5 or 73.1037 μg of it to distilled water or alcohol and adjust the final volume up to 1000 mL.

$AgNO_3$ (0.5 mM): Its MW is 169.87 g/mole. Dissolve 169.87 × 0.5 or 84.935 mg of it in 1000 mL distilled water.

$AgNO_3$ (5 mM): Dissolve 169.87 × 5 or 849.35 mg of it in 1000 mL of distilled water.

Aniline (10%) solution: Dissolve 10 mL of it in 90 mL of carbon tetrachloride or ligroin.

APAP (2, 4, or 8 mM): Its MW is 151.163 g/mole. Therefore, add the required amount of mg to distilled water and adjust to a final volume of 1000 mL.

Ascorbic acid (1 mM): It is vitamin C. Its MW is 176.12 g/mole. Dissolve 176.12 mg in 1000 mL of distilled water.

Bacto-peptone (2%): Mix 2 g of it with 98 gm of the culture medium.

Barfoed's reagent: Add a 0.33 molar solution of neutral cupric (II) acetate to a 1% acetic acid solution.

Barium sulphate (15%) solution: Add 15 g $BaSO_4$ in 100 mL of distilled water.

Benedict's reagent: Mix 17.3 g of $CuSO_4.5H_2O$, 100 g Na_2CO_3, and 173 g of sodium citrate in distilled water (required quantity).

Bovine serum albumin (BSA) solution: It is 0.2% BSA in 100 mL of acetate buffer (pH 5.0, 0.05 M).

Brewer's yeast (20%) (aq. susp.): Add 20 g of it to distilled water and adjust the volume up to 100 mL.

BSA (0.5%): It is a 0.5 g mixture in 100 mL of distilled water. Invert or vortex the tube to completely dissolve the BSA.

BSA (1%): In this case, mix only 1 g of BSA and prepare similarly.

Butylated hydroxytoluene (10 μM): Its MW is 220.35 g/mole. Add 220.35 × 10 or 2203.5 μg to distilled water and adjust a final volume of 1000 mL.

$C_{11}H_{12}N_2O$ (2%) solution: Add 2 g of it to distilled water and make a final volume of 100 mL.

C_2H_5OH (20%): Know the potency of your supplied ethanol at first. If it is 100%, add 20 mL of ethanol to 80 mL of distilled water.

C_2H_5OH (4%): Know the potency of your supplied ethanol at first. If it is 100%, add 4 mL of ethanol to 94 mL of distilled water.

C_2H_5OH (75%): Know the potency of your supplied ethanol at first. If it is 100%, add 75 mL of ethanol to 25 mL of distilled water.

C_2H_5OH (95%): Know the potency of your supplied ethanol at first. If it is 100%, add 95 mL of ethanol to 5 mL distilled water.

$C_4H_6NiO_4$ (1 mM): Its MW is 176.78. Add 176.78 mg to 1000 mL of distilled water.

$C_4H_6O_3$ (20%) solution: Add acetic anhydride 20 mL to 80 mL of distilled water.

$CaCl_2$ (0.03 to 30.0 mM): Its MW is 110.98 g/mole. Add the required amount of mg to 1000 mL of distilled water.

$CaCl_2.2H_2O$ (5.93 or 8.84 mM) solution: Its MW is 147.015 g/mole. Add the required amount of mg to 1000 mL of distilled water.

Carbachol (10^{-6} M): Its MW is 147.196 g/mole. Dissolve 147.196 × 6/1000000 or 0.000883176 g of it in 1000 mL of distilled water.

CCl_4 (20, 30, or 40 mM): Its MW is 153.82 g/mole. Dissolve the required amount of mg in 1000 mL of ethanol.

CDNB (2 mM): 2,4-Dinitrochlorobenzene's MW is 202.55. Add 202.55 × 2 or 405.10 mg of it to 1000 mL of ether or benzene.

CH_3OH (50%) solution: First, you need to know the potency of your supplied methanol. For this, add 50 mL of methanol to 50 mL of distilled water.

CH_3OH (70%) solution: Add 70 mL methanol to 30 mL distilled water.

Charcoal (3%) solution: Add 3 g of charcoal to 100 mL of distilled water.

Chlorose (1%) solution: Add 1 g of it to charcoal to 100 mL of suitable solvent.

Citrate buffer (0.5 M): Add 25.703 g of sodium citrate dihydrate to 800 mL of distilled water. Then add 2.421 g of citric acid to the mixture. Adjust the solution to the final desired pH using HCl or NaOH. Then, add distilled water until the volume is 1000 mL.

Co (II) (230 μM): Its MW is 168.991 g/mole. Add 38,867.93 μg of it to 100 μg of picolinic acid in 100 mL of distilled water.

Co (II) (4.6 mM) solution: Mix 15.7 mg of $CoF_2.4H_2O$ with 20 mg of picolinic acid in 20 mL of distilled water.

CO_2 (5%): 5% CO_2 means 50000 ppm.

Crystal violet (0.05%) solution: Add 0.05 g of crystal violet to 25 mL of 100% methanol and 75 mL of distilled water.

Crystal violet (0.5%) solution: Add 0.5 g of crystal violet to 25 mL of 100% methanol and 75 mL of distilled water.

$CuCl_2$ (0.01 M): Its MW is 134.45 g/mole. Dissolve 134.45 × 0.01 or 1.3445 g of it in 1000 mL of distilled water.

CuOOH (50 μM) solution: Its MW is 96.553. Dissolve 96.553 × 50 or 4,827.65 μg of it, in 1000 mL of distilled water.

$CuSO_4$ (0.1 mM): Its MW is 159.609 g/mole. Dissolve 159.609 × 0.1 or 15.9609 mg of it in 1000 mL of distilled water.

$CuSO_4$ (2%) solution: Dissolve 2 g of it in 100 mL of distilled water.

$CuSO_4$ (5 μM) solution: Dissolve MW × 5 μg of it in 1000 mL distilled water.

$CuSO_4$ (50 μM) solution: Dissolve MW × 50 μg of it in 1000 mL distilled water.

Dexamethasone (2.5 μM): Its MW is 392.464 g/mole. Dissolve MW × 2.5 μg of it in 1000 mL of distilled water.

Dextrose (5.5 mM): Its MW is 180.156 g/mole. Dissolve MW × 5.5 μg of it in 1000 mL of distilled water.

D-glucose solution (10%): Dissolve 10 g of it in 100 mL of distilled water.

Diethylcarbamazine (25 mM): Its MW is 199.293 g/mole. Dissolve MW × 25 mg of it in 1000 mL of distilled water.

Dihydroxyrhodamine 123 (5 μM) solution: Dissolve MW × 5 μg of it in 1000 mL of distilled water.

Dihydroxyrhodamine 123 (5 mM) solution: Dissolve MW × 5 mg of it in 1000 mL of distilled water.

DMPD (200 mM) solution: Its MW is 209.11. Dissolve MW × 200 mg of it, in 1000 mL of distilled water.

DMSO (0.05%): Add 0.05 mL of it to 99.95 mL distilled water.

DMSO (0.1%): Add 0.1 mL of it to 99.9 mL of distilled water.

DMSO (10%): Add 10 mL of it to 90 mL of distilled water.

DMSO (5%): Add 5 mL of it to 95 mL distilled water.

DPPH (0.5 mM) solution: Its MW is 394.32 g/mole. Dissolve MW × 0.5 mg of it in 1000 mL of ethanol. Keep in dark.

Dragendorff's reagent: Pour 0.5 g of $Bi(NO_3)_3$ into an empty beaker. Add 10 mL of concentrated HCl. Pour 4 g of KI into another beaker, add a little distilled water, and stir until KI is completely dissolved. Mix the two solutions. Observe the formation of a dark orange solution.

Dye solution: It is a 3% (w/v) trichloroacetic acid (TCA) solution containing 0.2 g Ponceau S dye.

EDTA (0.1 mM): Its MW is 292.2438 g/mole. With the help of a magnetic stirrer, dissolve MW × 0.1 mg of it in 1000 mL of distilled water.

EDTA (0.5 mM) solution: Dissolve MW × 0.5 mg of it in 1000 mL of distilled water with the help of a magnetic stirrer.

EDTA (1 mM) solution: Dissolve MW × 1 mg of it in 1000 mL of distilled water with the help of a magnetic stirrer.

EDTA (1.04 mM) solution: Dissolve MW × 1.04 mg of it in 1000 mL of distilled water with the help of a magnetic stirrer.

EDTA (10%) solution: Dissolve 10 g of it in 100 mL of distilled water with the help of a magnetic stirrer.

EDTA (100 μM) solution: Dissolve MW × 100 μg of it in 1000 mL of distilled water with the help of a magnetic stirrer.

EDTA (100 mM) solution: Dissolve MW × 100 mg of it in 1000 mL of distilled water with the help of a magnetic stirrer.

EDTA (15%) solution: Dissolve 15 g of it in 100 mL of distilled water with the help of a magnetic stirrer.

EDTA (30 mM) solution: Dissolve MW × 30 mg of it in 1000 mL of distilled water with the help of a magnetic stirrer.

EDTA (300 mM) solution: Dissolve MW × 300 mg of it in 1000 mL of distilled water with the help of a magnetic stirrer.

EDTA (5 mM) solution: Dissolve MW × 5 mg of it in 1000 mL of distilled water with the help of a magnetic stirrer.

EDTA (6.29 mM) solution: Dissolve MW × 6.29 mg of it in 1000 mL of distilled water with the help of a magnetic stirrer.

Ellman's reagent: 5,50 -dithiobis-2- nitrobenzoic acid (0.1 mM) prepared in 0.3 M phosphate buffer with 1% of sodium citrate solution.

ENU (0.1 mM/kg): Its MW is 117.11. It is a dose of 11.711 mg/kg of N-ethyl-N-nitrosourea in a suitable vehicle.

Eosin Y stain (1%) solution: *Eosin Y stock solution*: Add 1 g of it to 20 mL of distilled water and mix until dissolved. Then add 80 mL of 95% ethanol, and mix. Store it at room temperature. *Eosin Y working solution*: Add 100 mL of eosin Y stock solution to 300 mL of 80% ethanol and mix well. While working in a fume hood, add 4 mL of glacial acetic acid and mix well. Store it covered at room temperature.

FBS (10%): 10 g should be supplemented with the recommended culture medium.

$FeCl_2$ (0.02 M) solution: Dissolve MW × 0.02 mg of it in 1000 mL distilled water.

$FeCl_2.6H_2O$ (20 mM) solution: Its MW is 166.038. Dissolve MW × 20 mg of it in 1000 mL of distilled water.

$FeCl_3$ (0.05 M) solution: Its MW is 162.2 g/mole. Dissolve MW × 0.05 mg of it, in 1000 mL of distilled water.

$FeCl_2$ (0.01 M): Its MW is 126.751 g/mole. Dissolve MW × 0.01 mg of it in 1000 mL of distilled water.

$FeCl_3$ (0.1%) solution: Dissolve MW × 0.1 mg of it in 1000 mL distilled water.

$FeCl_3$ (20 mM) solution: Dissolve MW × 20 mg of it in 1000 mL distilled water.

$FeCl_3$ (5%) solution: Dissolve 5 g of it in 100 mL of distilled water.

Fehling solution A: It is a mixture of 7 g $CuSO_4.5H_2O$ and 2 drops of dil. H_2SO_4 with up to 100 mL distilled water.

Fehling solution B: Mix 35 g of potassium tartrate and 12 g of NaOH, and adjust the final volume to 100 mL with distilled water.

Ferrozine (0.25 mM) solution: Its MW is 514.4. Dissolve MW × 0.25 mg of it in 1000 mL of distilled water.

$FeSO_4$ (0.02 M) solution: Its MW is 151.908 g/mole. Dissolve MW × 0.02 mg of it in 1000 mL of distilled water.

$FeSO_4$ (0.1 mM) solution: Dissolve MW × 0.1 mg of it in 1000 mL distilled water.

Finasteride (2%) solution: Add 2 g of it to a suitable vehicle and properly mix it before use.

Fluorescein (60 nM): Its MW is 332.31 g/mole. Dissolve MW × 60 ng of it in 1000 mL of distilled water.

Folin-Coilett-Phenol Reagent: Dissolve 10 g of sodium tungstate and 2.5 g of sodium molybdate in 70 mL of distilled water. Add 5 mL of 85% phosphoric acid and 10 mL of conc. HCl. Reflux for ten hours.

Formaldehyde (3.7%) solution: Add 3.7 mL of it to 96.3 mL of distilled water.

Formalin (1.35%) solution: A 100% formalin solution is equivalent to 37 to 40% formaldehyde. It is a 0.5% formaldehyde solution.

Formalin (10%): It is 1 part of the stock formalin with 9 parts distilled water.

Furfural (1%): Dissolve 1 g of furfural in 100 mL of ethanol or ether.

GABA (873 mM): Its MW is 103.12 g/mole. Dissolve MW × 873 mg of it in 1000 mL suitable vehicle.

Giemsa (10%): Dissolve 7.6 g of Giemsa powder into 250 mL of methanol. Heat the solution from to ~60 °C. Slowly add 250 mL of glycerin to it. Filter the solution and let it stand for a while prior to use.

Glucose (2%): Dissolve 2 g glucose in 100 mL of distilled water.

Glucose (20%) solution: Dissolve 20 g glucose in 100 mL of distilled water.

Glutamate (1 μM): Its MW is 147.13 g/mole. Dissolve MW × 1 μg of it in 1000 mL of distilled water. For proper mixing, apply gentle heat.

Griess reagent: 1.0 mL of sulfanilic acid reagent (0.33% in 20% glacial acetic acid at room temperature for 5 min with 1 mL of naphthylethylenediamine dichloride (0.1% w/v).

GSH (5 mM): Its MW is 48772.195. Dissolve MW × 5 mg of it in 1000 mL of distilled water.

GSH (60 mM): Dissolve MW × 60 mg of it in 1000 mL distilled water.

GSSG (1.0 mM): Its MW is 612.6. Dissolve MW × 1 mg of it in 1000 mL of distilled water.

GST (1 nM) solution: Its MW is 25.8 kDa. Dissolve MW × 1 ng of it in 1000 mL distilled water.

Gum acacia (2%): Add 2 g of it to 100 mL of distilled water and mix by using a magnetic stirrer.

H_2DCF-DA (10^{-5}M): Its MW is 487.29. Dissolve MW × 10^{-5} mg of it in 1000 mL of a suitable vehicle containing DMSO or ethanol.

H_2O_2 (0.55 M): Its MW is 34.0147 g/mole. Dissolve MW × 0.55 g of it, in 1000 mL of distilled water. It is light sensitive, therefore prepare and preserve it in a dark condition. Also use a freshly prepared solution for each study.

H_2O_2 (0.82 M): Dissolve MW × 0.82 g of it in 1000 mL distilled water. Follow the above-mentioned instruction.

H_2O_2 (1 mM): Dissolve MW × 1 mg of it in 1000 mL distilled water. Follow the above-mentioned instructions.

H_2O_2 (2 mM): Dissolve MW × 2 mg of it in 1000 mL distilled water. Follow the above-mentioned instructions.

H_2O_2 (200 mM): Dissolve MW × 200 mg of it in 1000 mL distilled water. Follow the above-mentioned instructions.

H_2O_2 (27.5 mM): Dissolve MW × 27.5 mg of it in 1000 mL distilled water. Follow the above-mentioned instructions.

H_2O_2 (40 mM): Dissolve MW × 40 mg of it in 1000 mL distilled water. Follow the above-mentioned instructions.

H_2O_2 (5%): Add 5 mL of it to 95 mL of distilled water. Follow the above-mentioned instructions.

H_2O_2 (7.5 mM): Dissolve MW × 7.5 mg of it in 1000 mL of distilled water. Follow the above-mentioned instructions.

H_2PtCl_6 (0.5 mM): Its MW is 517.91. Dissolve MW × 0.5 mg of it in 1000 mL of distilled water.

H_2SO_4 (0.6 M) solution: Its MW is 98.079 g/mole. Add MW × 0.6 g (eq. volume) of it to distilled water and adjust the final volume up to 1000 mL. Slowly add water side-by-side. Do not pipette by direct mouth.

H_2SO_4 (80%) solution: It contains 80 mL of pure (conc.) acid and 20 mL of distilled water.

H_3PO_4 (5%) solution: It contains 5 mL of pure (conc.) acid and 95 mL of distilled water. Slowly add water side-by-side. Pipette by mouth is not recommended.

Hager's reagent: Dissolve 1 g of picric acid in 100 mL of distilled water.

$HAuCl_4$ (1 mM) solution: Its MW is 339.785 g/mole. Dissolve MW × 1 mg of it, in 1000 mL of distilled water.

HCl (0.01 N) solution: Its MW is 36.458 g/mole. Dissolve MW × 0.01 g of it in 1000 mL of distilled water. Slowly add water side-by-side. Pipette by mouth is not recommended.

HCl (0.04 N) solution: Dissolve MW × 0.04 g of it, in 1000 mL of distilled water. Follow the above-mentioned precautions.

HCl (0.6%) solution: It contains 0.6 mL of pure (conc.) acid and 99.4 mL of distilled water. Follow the above-mentioned precautions.

HCl (1 M) solution: Dissolve MW × 1 g of it in 1000 mL of distilled water. Follow the above-mentioned precautions.

HCl (1 N) solution: Dissolve MW × 1 g of it in 1000 mL of distilled water. Follow the above-mentioned precautions.

HCl (2 N) solution: Dissolve MW × 2 g of it in 1000 mL of distilled water. Follow the above-mentioned precautions.

HCl (3.5%) solution: It contains 3.5 mL of pure (conc.) acid and 96.5 mL of distilled water. Follow the above-mentioned precautions.

HCl (40 mM) solution: Dissolve MW × 40 mg of it in 1000 mL of distilled water. Follow the above-mentioned precautions.

Hemoglobin (0.0016%): It contains 0.0016 g of Hb in the 100 mL solution.

$Hg_2(NO_3)_2$ (3%) solution: It contains 3 g $Hg_2(NO_3)_2$ in the 100 mL aqueous solution (distilled water).

Hippuryl-histidyl-leucine (6.5 mM): Its MW is 429.5. Dissolve MW × 6.5 mg of it in 1000 mL of a suitable vehicle.

I_2 (5%) solution: Dissolve 10 g of potassium iodide in 100 mL of distilled water. While shaking, slowly add 5 g of iodine crystals.

K_2CO_3 (0.1 M) solution: Its MW is 138.205 g/mole. Dissolve MW × 0.1 g of it, in 1000 mL of distilled water.

$K_3Fe(CN)_6$ (1%): It contains 1 g of $K_3Fe(CN)_6$ in the 100 mL of distilled water.

K_3PO_4 (0.1 N) solution: Its MW is 212.27 g/mole. Dissolve MW × 0.1 g of it, in 1000 mL distilled water.

KCl (120 mM) solution: Its MW is 74.5513 g/mole. Dissolve MW × 120 mg of it in 1000 mL of distilled water.

KCl (154 mM) solution: Dissolve MW × 154 mg of it in 1000 mL of distilled water.

KCl (5 mM) solution: Dissolve MW × 5 mg of it in 1000 mL of distilled water.

KCl (9.38 mM) solution: Dissolve MW × 9.38 mg of it in 1000 mL of distilled water.

KH_2PO_4-KOH buffer (20 mM): Prepare 800 mL of distilled water in a suitable container. Add 2.721.72 g of K_2HPO_4 to the solution. Add 1.122112 g of KOH to the solution. Add distilled water until the volume is 1 L.

KI (10%) solution: It contains 10 g of KI in 100 mL of distilled water.

$KMnO_4$ (10%) solution: It contains 10 g of $KMnO_4$ in 100 mL of distilled water.

Krebs–Henseleit buffer: It contains NaCl 118 mM + KCl 4.7 mM + $CaCl_2$ 2.5 mM + $MgSO_4$ 1.2 mM + $NaHCO_3$ 25 mM + KH_2PO_4 1.2 mM + Glucose 10 mM.

L-DOPA (10 mM): Its MW is 197.1879 g/mole. Dissolve MW × 10 mg of it, in 1000 mL of PBS.

L-glutamine (2 mM): Its MW is 146.14 g/mole. Dissolve MW × 2 mg of it in 1000 mL of distilled water.

Linoleic acid (1 mM) emulsion: Its MW is 280.4472 g/mole. Emulsify MW × 1 mg of it in 1000 mL of suitable emulsifying agent containing vehicle.

Linoleic acid (2.51%) solution: Emulsify 2.51 mL of it in 97.49 mL of suitable emulsifying agent containing vehicle.

L-NAME (1 μM): Its MW is 269.69. Dissolve MW × 1 μg of it, in 1000 mL of distilled water.

Maltose (3.5 mM): Its MW is 342.3 g/mole. Dissolve MW × 3.5 mg of it in 1000 mL of distilled water.

Mayer's reagent: Dissolve 1.36 g of $HgCl_2$ and 5 g of KI in 100 mL of distilled water.

MeO-Suc-Ala-Ala-Pro-Val-pNA (700 μM): Its MW is 590.6. Dissolve MW × 700 μg of it in 1000 mL of a suitable vehicle.

$MgCl_2$ (5 mM) solution: Its MW is 95.211 g/mole. Dissolve MW × 5 mg of it, in 1000 mL of distilled water.

$MgCl_2.6H_2O$ (18.66 mM) solution: Its MW is 203.30. Dissolve MW × 18.66 mg of it in 1000 mL of distilled water.

Millon's reagent: Dissolve 160 g of $Hg(NO_3)_2$ and 160 g of $HgNO_3$ in 400 mL conc. HNO_3 solution. Adjust to a 1000 mL final volume by the addition of distilled water.

Minoxidil (1%) suspension: Dissolve 1 g of it in 100 mL of distilled water.

N-(1-naphthyl) ethylenediamine dihydrochloride (0.1%): Dissolve 0.1 g of it in 100 mL of distilled water.

Na/K buffer (75 mM): Use 0.1 M KH_2PO_4 and 0.1 M Na_2HPO_4. Mix one volume of the KH_2PO_4 stock solution with four volumes of the Na_2HPO_4 stock solution. Dilute two volumes of the 0.1 M K-Na phosphate buffer from Step 1 with one volume of water (i.e., to a final concentration of 75 mM).

Na_2CO_3 (200 mM) solution: Its MW is 105.9888 g/mole. Dissolve MW × 200 mg of it, in 1000 mL of distilled water.

Na_2CO_3 (35%) solution: It contains 35 g of Na_2CO_3 in 100 mL aqueous (distilled water) solution.

Na_2EDTA (0.15 mM) solution: Its MW is 336.21. Dissolve MW × 0.15 mg of it in 1000 mL of distilled water.

Na_2EDTA (1 mM) solution: Dissolve MW × 1 mg of it in 1000 mL of distilled water.

Na_2SO_4 (22.6%) solution: It contains 22.6 g of Na_2SO_4 in 100 mL of distilled water.

Na_2SO_4 (28.16 mM) solution: Its MW is 142.04 g/mole. Dissolve MW × 28.16 mg of it, in 1000 mL of distilled water.

Na_3N (0.12 M) solution: Its MW is 82.98 g/mole. Dissolve MW × 0.12 g of it in 1000 mL of distilled water.

Na_3PO_4 (28 mM) solution: Its MW is 163.94 g/mole. Dissolve MW × 28 mg of it, in 1000 mL of distilled water.

Na_3PO_4 (50 mM) solution: Dissolve MW × 50 mg of it in 1000 mL of distilled water.

$NaCH_3COO$ buffer (0.1 M): Prepare 800 mL of distilled water in a suitable container. Add 5.772 g of $NaCH_3COO$ to the solution. Add 1.778 g of CH_3COOH to the solution. Adjust the solution to the desired pH using 10 N HCl. Add distilled water until the volume is 1000 mL.

NaCl (0.2 M) solution: Its MW is 58.44 g/mole. Dissolve MW × 0.2 g of it in 1000 mL of distilled water.

NaCl (0.9%) solution: It contains 0.9 g NaCl in 100 mL of distilled water.

NaCl (1 M) solution: Dissolve MW × 1 g of it in 1000 mL of distilled water.

NaCl (10%) solution: It contains 10 g NaCl in 100 mL of distilled water.

NaCl (150 mM) solution: Dissolve MW × 150 mg of it in 1000 mL of distilled water.

NaCl (154 mM) solution: Dissolve MW × 154 mg of it in 1000 mL of distilled water.

NaCl (2.5 M) solution: Dissolve MW × 2.5 g of it in 1000 mL of distilled water.

NaCl (39.35 mM) solution: Dissolve MW × 39.35 mg of it in 1000 mL of distilled water.

NaCl (50 mM) solution: Dissolve MW × 50 mg of it in 1000 mL of distilled water.

NaCl (90 mM) solution: Dissolve MW × 90 mg of it in 1000 mL of distilled water.

Na-CMC (1%): It contains 1 g of Na-CMC in 100 mL of distilled water.

$NaCO_3$ (10%) solution: It contains 10 g $NaCO_3$ in 100 mL of distilled water.

NADH (0.936 mM): Its MW is 663.43 g/mole. Dissolve MW × 0.936 mg of it in 1000 mL of distilled water.

$NADP^+$ (26.1 mM): Its MW is 744.413 g/mole. Dissolve MW × 26.1 mg of it in 1000 mL of distilled water.

NADPH (0.1 mM): Its MW is 744.413 g/mole. Dissolve MW × 0.1 mg of it, in 1000 mL of distilled water.

NADPH (0.25 mM): Dissolve MW × 0.25 mg of it in 1000 mL of distilled water.

NADPH (1 μM): Dissolve MW × 1 μg of it in 1000 mL of distilled water.

NADPH (3 mM) solution: Dissolve MW × 3 mg of it in 1000 mL of distilled water.

$NaHCO_3$ (0.1 M) solution: Its MW is 84.007 g/mole. Dissolve MW × 0.1 g of it, in 1000 mL of distilled water.

NaOH (0.01 M or 0.01N) solution: Its MW is 39.997 g/mole. Dissolve MW × 0.01 g of it in 1000 mL of distilled water.

NaOH (0.1 N) solution: Dissolve MW × 0.1 g of it in 1000 mL of distilled water.

NaOH (1 mM) solution: Dissolve MW × 1 mg of it in 1000 mL of distilled water.

NaOH (1 M) solution: Dissolve MW × 1 g of it in 1000 mL of distilled water.

NaOH (10%) solution: It contains 10 g of NaOH in 100 mL of distilled water.

NaOH (20%) solution: It contains 20 g NaOH in 100 mL distilled water.

NaOH (300 mM): Dissolve MW × 300 mg of it in 1000 mL of distilled water.

Neocuproine (0.0075 M): Its MW is 208.26 g/mole. Dissolve MW × 0.0075 g of it in 1000 mL of methanol or hydro-methanol.

Neutral-buffered formalin (4%): For 1000 mL of 4% rormaldehyde, add 800 mL of 1× PBS to a glass beaker on a stir plate in a ventilated hood. Heat while stirring to approximately 60 °C. Take care that the solution does not boil.

NH_3 (10%) solution: Add 10 mL of liquid NH_3 to 90 mL distilled water.

NH_3 (20%) solution: Add 20 mL of liquid NH_3 to 80 mL distilled water.

NH_4CH_3COO (1 M) solution: Its MW is 77.082. Dissolve MW × 1 g of it, in 1000 mL of distilled water.

NH_4SCN (30%) solution: It contains 30 g of NH_4SCN in 100 mL of alcohol or other suitable solvents.

Nitroblue tetrazolium (0.3 mM): Its MW is 817.64 g/mole. Dissolve MW × 0.3 mg of it in 1000 mL of distilled water or other suitable solvents.

O_2 (95%): It means the gaseous environment contains 95% O_2.

Oil Red O (0.5%): It contains 0.5 g of dye in 100 mL of distilled water.

$Pb(C_2H_3O_2)_2$ (10%) solution: It contains 10 g of $Pb(C_2H_3O_2)_2$ in 100 mL of deionized water.

$Pd(NO_3)_2$ (0.5 mM): Its MW is 230.43 g/mole. Dissolve MW × 0.5 mg of it in 1000 mL of distilled water.

$PdCl_2$ (0.226 M): Its MW is 177.33 g/mole. Dissolve MW × 0.226 g of it in 1000 mL of distilled water.

Perchloric acid (0.1 M): Its MW is 100.46 g/mole. Mix MW × 0.1 g (eq. vol.) of it with 1000 mL of distilled water.

Perchloric acid (70%): Mix 70 mL of it with 30 mL of distilled water.

Phenazine methosulfate (0.12 mM) solution: Its MW is 306.34. Dissolve MW × 0.12 mg of it in 1000 mL of distilled water.

Phosphate-Buffered Saline (PBS) (0.1 M, pH 7.4): Mix 40 mL of 0.2 M Na_2HPO_4 with 10 mL of NaH_2PO_4. Add 0.9 g of NaCl and stir until dissolved. Bring the volume to 100 mL with distilled water and adjust the pH to 7.4.

Potassium Phosphate Buffer (1 M, pH 6.5): Prepare 800 mL of distilled water in a suitable container. Add 95 g of KH_2PO_4 to the solution. Add

52.5 g of K_2HPO_4 to the solution. Adjust the pH to 6.5. Add distilled water until the volume is 1 L.

Pyrogallol (2 mM): Its MW is 126.11 g/mole. Dissolve MW × 2 mg of it in 1000 mL of ethanol or other suitable solvent.

RBC (1, 4, 5 and 10%) suspension: Collect blood from the animal following the appropriate procedure and centrifuge it. Separate the RBC (erythrocytes). Add 10 mL of this RBC to 90 mL of ***Alsever's solution*** (2.05% dextrose, 0.8% sodium citrate, 0.055% citric acid, and 0.42% NaCl in 100 mL of distilled water).

RPMI medium (10%): This medium contains glucose (2 g), pH indicator (phenol red, 5 mg), salts (6 g NaCl, 2 g $NaHCO_3$, 1.512 g Na_2HPO_4, 400 mg KCl, 100 mg $MgSO_4$, and 100 mg $Ca(NO_3)_2$). Add 10 gm of this medium to the other required components of your culture plate (to adjust to 100 g or 100 mL).

RPMI medium (5%): Add 5 gm of this medium to other required components of your culture plate (to adjust 100 g or 100 mL).

Saline (0.5%) solution (*isotonic solution*): It contains 0.5 g of NaCl in 100 mL of distilled water.

Saline (0.9%) solution (*hypotonic solution*): It contains 0.9 g of NaCl in 100 mL of distilled water.

Schiff's dye: Add 1 g fuchsin, 1.9 g $Na_2S_2O_5$ to 100 mL of 0.15 N HCl. Shake the mixture at intervals or mechanically for 2 h, decolorize with charcoal and filter.

SDS-polyacrylamide (12%): It contains 12 g of it in 100 mL of distilled water.

Sodium deoxycholate (1%): It contains 1 g of $C_{24}H_{41}NaO_5$ in 100 mL of distilled water.

Sodium dodecyl sulfate (8.1%) solution: It contains 8.1 g of $NaC_{12}H_{25}SO_4$ in 100 mL of distilled water.

Sodium nitroprusside (10 mM): Its MW is 297.95. Dissolve MW ×10 mg of it in 1000 mL of distilled water and filter it.

Sodium phosphate buffer (0.1 M): Prepare 800 mL of distilled water in a suitable container. Add 20.214 g of $H_{15}Na_2O_{11}P$ to the solution. Add 3.394 g of H_4NaO_5P to the solution. Adjust the solution to the final desired pH using HCl or NaOH. Add distilled water until the volume is 1000 mL.

Sorensen's phosphate buffer: Solution A: 3.5% disodium hydrogen phosphate. Solution B: 2.76% sodium dihydrogen phosphate. Mix 40.5

mL of solution A with 9.5 mL of solution B and adjust the volume up to 100 mL.

Sucrose (0.25 M): Its MW is 342.3 g/mole. Dissolve MW × 0.25 g of it, in 1000 mL of distilled water.

Sucrose (1%) solution: It contains 1 g of sucrose in 100 mL of distilled water.

Sucrose (56 mM): Dissolve MW × 56 mg of it in 1000 mL of distilled water.

Sulphanilamide (1%): It contains 1 g of sulphanilamide in 100 mL of distilled water or other suitable solvents.

Tannic acid (10%) solution: Add 10 mL of tannic acid to 90 mL of distilled water.

Tannic acid solution: Its 0.1 mg of ascorbic acid and contains 0.1% tannic acid solution in 50% methanol.

TBA (0.5%): It contains 0.5 g of TBA dissolved in ethanol or other suitable solvents.

TBA (0.67%): It contains 0.67 g of TBA dissolved in ethanol or other suitable solvents.

TBA (8%): It contains 2 g of TBA dissolved in ethanol or other suitable solvents.

Testosterone (1%) solution: It contains 1 g of testosterone in 100 mL of arachis oil.

Tetracaine hydrochloride (0.5%): It contains 0.5 parts of this acid in 99.5 parts of a vehicle.

Trichloro acetic acid (10%): Add 10 mL of this acid to 90 mL of distilled water.

Trichloroacetic acid (20%): Add 20 mL of this acid to 80 mL of distilled water.

Tris-HCl buffer: The Tris-HCl buffer contains required amount of Tris Base, Sodium Azide, and HCl or NaOH. To prepare your required Tris-HCl buffer dissolve Tris Base and Sodium Azide in approx. 90% of final volume with cold distilled water. Add cold distilled water again to obtain the final volume. Adjust to pH 8.0 ± 0.1 with HCl or NaOH as needed and filter the solution.

Triton X-100 (0.01%): It contains 0.01 mL of Triton X-100 in a 100-mixture (with distilled water or suitable vehicle).

Triton X-100 (1%): It contains 1 mL of Triton X-100 in a 100-mixture (with distilled water or suitable vehicle).

Tween 80 (1%): It contains 1 mL of tween 80 in a 100 mixture (with distilled water or 0.9% NaCl solution).

Tyrode's solution: It contains KCl 50 mM + NaCl 91.04 mM + $MgCl_2$ 1.05 mM + $NaHCO_3$ 11.9 mM + NaH_2PO_4 0.42 mM + Glucose 5.5 mM + EDTA 0.1 mM.

Urethrane (25%) solution: It contains 25 mL of urethrane in a 100 mixture.

Verapamil (0.01 to 3 mM): Its MW is 454.602 g/mole. Dissolve MW × 0.01 to 3 μg of it in 1000 mL of ethanol or other suitable solvents.

Verapamil (1 μM): Dissolve MW × 1 μg of it in 1000 mL ethanol or other suitable solvents.

Wagner's reagent: Dissolve 2 g of I_2 and 6 g of KI in 100 mL of distilled water.

Xanthine substrate (0.15 M) solution: Its MW is 152.11 g/mole. Dissolve MW × 0.15 g of it in a minimal volume of NaOH. Add deionized water to a final volume of 1000 mL.

Yeast extract (0.5%): It contains 0.5% yeast powder in a 100 g culture medium.

Yeast extract (1%): It contains 1% yeast powder in a 100 g culture medium.

α-ketoglutarate (228.5 mM): Its MW is 146.11 g/mole. Dissolve MW × 228.5 mg of it in 1000 mL of ethanol or other suitable solvents.

References

Ames, B. N., Profet, M., & Gold, L. S. (1990). Nature's chemicals and synthetic chemicals: comparative toxicology. *Proceedings of the National Academy of Sciences*, *87*(19), 7782-7786.

Boström, J., Falk, N., & Tyrchan, C. (2011). Exploiting personalized information for reagent selection in drug design. *Drug Discovery Today*, *16*(5-6), 181-187.

Cheng, K. L., Ueno, K., & Imamura, T. (1992). *CRC Handbook of organic analytical reagents*. CRC press.

Index

S

T

U

V